How Hormones Affect Behavioral and Neural Development: Introduction to the Special Issue on "Gonadal Hormones and Sex Differences in Behavior"

Sheri A. Berenbaum
Department of Behavioral and Social Sciences
School of Medicine and
Department of Psychology
Southern Illinois University, Carbondale

As the articles in this special issue demonstrate, gonadal hormones have powerful effects on the development of the brain and behavior in human beings, as in other species. Both androgens and estrogens affect behavior throughout development, from early prenatal life through adulthood, as demonstrated in studies with a variety of methods in several species. High levels of testosterone and other androgens that are present early in development are shown to facilitate the development of male-typical characteristics, and to inhibit the development of female-typical characteristics. Some of these effects are suggested to be mediated by the conversion of androgen to estradiol in the brain. Ovarian hormones are also shown to play an important role in the development and maintenance of female-typical characteristics, and their effects on the brain appear to extend beyond the prenatal and early postnatal periods. Nevertheless, there are not simple relations between the amount of hormone present and behavior. Behavioral effects of hormones are not uniform across behaviors or across individuals. Variations have been shown to relate to the timing of exposure, the organism's sensitivity to the hormones, the specific hormone involved, and modification by the physical and social environment, although not all factors have been studied in all species, and many have not been studied directly in people. The articles in this special issue also describe attempts to identify the mechanisms—neural and basic behavioral—that mediate hormonal effects on complex human behaviors.

Requests for reprints should be sent to Sheri Berenbaum, Department of Behavioral and Social Sciences, School of Medicine, Southern Illinois University, Carbondale, IL 62901–6517. E-mail: sberenbaum@som.siu.edu

The articles in this special issue testify to the breadth and vitality of research into the ways that hormones affect the development of sex-typical behavior and illustrate several important themes that have emerged in human psychoneuroendocrinology. First, it is now clear that hormones do affect human behavior, and the important questions relate to the mechanisms and details of hormone action. Second, there are many ways to study hormone effects on human behavior, and the articles in this issue describe these methods and their products. Third, traditional conceptions of hormone–behavior relations have generally stood the test of time, but recent developments have begun to reveal the complexity of these relations.

Renewed interest in hormonal influences on human behavior among neuropsychologists was stimulated by Geschwind and Galaburda's (1985) proposals regarding the role of testosterone on brain development and the immune system. There has been an extraordinary amount of work testing their hypotheses regarding associations among left-handedness, learning disabilities, and immune dysfunction. Most studies have failed to support those hypotheses (see Bryden, McManus, & Bulman-Fleming, 1994, and McManus & Bryden, 1991, for a review and thoughtful discussion of the topic).

On the other hand, major progress continues to be made in understanding hormonal influences on behavior through studies of behavioral sexual differentiation, a field propelled by the work of Young, Goy, and their colleagues (American Psychological Association, 1997; Goy, 1996; Goy & McEwen, 1980; Phoenix, Goy, Gerall, & Young, 1959). It is this perspective that guides most of the work reported in this special issue.

This introduction is intended to provide both an overview of the articles that appear in the special issue and a discussion of themes and issues involved in studying the effects of gonadal hormones on behavioral and neural sex differences. The first section of the article provides background for readers unfamiliar with this area. The second section outlines broad themes, and includes brief descriptions of the articles that appear in the issue in the context of those themes. The next two sections address factors that may help to explain the complexity of hormonal influences on human behavior and to reconcile apparently divergent findings. One section addresses behavioral issues and the other deals with specific details of hormone effects. The fifth section is concerned with the behavioral and neural mechanisms mediating the behavioral effects of gonadal hormones. In these middle sections, articles in the special issue are discussed again as they relate to a particular topic or illustrate a specific point. The final section provides specific ties between the articles in the special issue and the concerns of developmental neuropsychologists.

SOME BACKGROUND

Many studies in a variety of nonhuman mammalian species, including rodents and primates, have shown that gonadal hormones play a major role in the development of sex differences in behavior and in the brain (for reviews, see Arnold & Gorski, 1984; Beatty, 1992; Becker, Breedlove, & Crews, 1992; Breedlove, 1994; Goy & McEwen, 1980; MacLusky & Naftolin, 1981). In both genetic males and females, high levels of androgen present during critical periods of development are associated with male-typical behavior. For example, female rodents and primates exposed to high levels of androgen prenatally and neonatally are more likely than unexposed females to mount other females as sex partners and less likely to be sexually receptive to males, whereas male rodents deprived of androgen during these sensitive periods show the opposite pattern of sexual behavior. Further, regions of the brain involved in sexual behavior, particularly the hypothalamus, show sex differences and changes with excess or reduced levels of masculinizing hormones (Gorski, Gordon, Shryne, & Southam, 1978; Raisman & Field, 1973; for reviews, see Breedlove, 1992, 1994; Goy & McEwen, 1980; MacLusky & Naftolin, 1981).

Gonadal hormones also affect nonsexual behaviors. In rats and primates, exposure to high levels of androgen during sensitive periods of brain development is associated with increased rough play and aggression (Beatty, 1992; Meaney, 1988). Some aspects of learning are also affected by the levels of gonadal hormones present early in development. Female rats given masculinizing hormones during critical periods of development learn the radial-arm maze as well as normal males, and better than normal females and male rats castrated neonatally; the superior performance of males and exposed females may be related to the use of geometric cues (Williams, Barnett, & Meck, 1990; Williams & Meck, 1991). Regions of the rat brain thought to subserve aspects of spatial learning, including the hippocampus, have also been shown to be affected by gonadal hormones (Juraska, 1991; Roof & Havens, 1992; Williams & Meck, 1991). In rhesus monkeys, androgens present in the prenatal or postnatal periods affect learning abilities that show sex differences as well as the maturation of the cortical regions subserving these abilities (Bachevalier & Hagger, 1991; Clark & Goldman-Rakic, 1989).

Studies of hormone effects on human behavior are largely consistent with studies in other species (for reviews, see Berenbaum, Korman, & Leveroni, 1995; Collaer & Hines, 1995; Hampson & Kimura, 1992). Most of these studies involve girls and women who were exposed to high levels of masculinizing hormones early in development because of a genetic disease such as congenital adrenal hyperplasia (CAH), or because their mothers took drugs with masculinizing actions during pregnancy, such as androgenizing progestins or diethylstilbestrol (DES). Girls and women with CAH have been found to be masculinized on a variety of behaviors, including toy play, aggression, spatial ability, handedness, and sexual orientation (Berenbaum & Hines, 1992; Berenbaum & Resnick, 1997; Berenbaum & Snyder, 1995; Dittmann, Kappes, & Kappes, 1992; Dittmann et al., 1990; Ehrhardt & Baker, 1974; Hampson, Rovet, & Altmann, this issue; Nass et al., 1987; Resnick, Berenbaum, Gottesman, & Bouchard, 1986; Zucker et al., 1996). Girls exposed to androgenizing progestins are more likely than unexposed sisters to report using aggression in conflict situations (Reinisch, 1981). Women exposed to DES are more likely than control women to report lesbian or bisexual fantasies and arousal (Meyer-Bahlburg et al., 1995).

Increasingly, studies of early hormone effects on human behavior have involved normal participants with typical variations in prenatal hormones, providing important converging evidence for studies of clinical samples. Females thought to be exposed to high average levels of testosterone by virtue of sharing a uterine environment with a male cotwin appear to show some behavioral masculinization: Compared to females with a female cotwin, they have higher spatial ability (Cole-Harding, Morstad, & Wilson, 1988), higher sensation seeking (Resnick, Gottesman, & McGue, 1993), and a male-typical pattern of auditory function (McFadden, 1993, this issue). Seven-year-old girls who had high levels of testosterone in utero (assessed in amniotic fluid at 14–16 weeks of gestation) had faster mental rotation than girls who had low levels of prenatal testosterone (Grimshaw, Sitarenios, & Finegan, 1995).

Behavioral—and brain—changes that occur as a result of high or low levels of gonadal hormones present early in development are considered to be *organizational*, because hormones make permanent changes in the wiring and sensitivity of the brain (Phoenix et al., 1959). But, hormonal effects on behavior are not confined to early development. Hormones may continue to affect behavior through permanent changes in the brain at later periods (Arnold & Breedlove, 1985). Typically, however, later hormones do not produce long-lasting permanent changes, but instead have *activational* effects; that is, they activate neural systems that were organized early in life. Studies in a variety of species, including human beings, have increasingly revealed the behavioral importance of these activational hormones for nonsexual behaviors (for reviews, see Becker, 1992; Kimura & Hampson, 1994). Circulating testosterone has been associated with aggression (Olweus, Mattsson, Schalling, & Low, 1980) and spatial ability (Gouchie & Kimura, 1991; Janowsky, Oviatt, & Orwoll, 1994). Estrogen appears to facilitate memory, so that postmenopausal women taking estrogen supplements have better memory than women not taking estrogen (Phillips & Sherwin, 1992; Resnick, Metter, & Zonderman, 1997). Estrogen is also important for other aspects of cognitive function, particularly articulatory and motor skills (Hampson, 1990; Hampson & Kimura, 1992; Kimura & Hampson, 1994; Saucier & Kimura, this issue; Szekely, Hampson, Carey, & Goodale, this issue).

THEMES IN HORMONE–BEHAVIOR RELATIONS

Consistency of findings across methods and species continues to provide support for two fundamental principles in psychoneuroendocrinology. First, sexual differentiation of the mammalian brain and behavior parallel sexual differentiation of the body: High levels of androgens (and metabolites) present during critical periods cause development to proceed in a masculine direction, whereas low levels produce feminine development. Second, hormones exert behavioral effects at various times in development through permanent changes in the wiring and sensitivity of the brain (organizational effects) and through ongoing changes to neural circuitry (activational effects). Although these two principles remain correct in broad form, recent work in both human and nonhuman species—much of it presented in articles in this special issue—reveals complexities and provides questions and answers about the ways in which hormones affect behavior.

Several articles in this special issue expand our knowledge about the effects of early (organizational) hormones on a variety of behaviors and aspects of brain structure and function in a variety of species. These studies reflect the range of methodology available to study the behavioral effects of early hormones. Clark and Galef (this issue) show that, in rodents, a variety of behavioral, morphological, and reproductive characteristics are affected by intrauterine position, which reflects exposure to variable levels of testosterone. Their results encourage studies of human opposite-sex twins (as illustrated in the work of McFadden, this issue), and remind us of the value of examining both physical and behavioral traits, and the complexity of hormonal effects on behavior, including the importance of hormone sensitivity and environmental responses to the organism. Fitch, Cowell, and Denenberg (this issue) clearly demonstrate that sexual differentiation is not determined simply by the amount of androgens present in early development, but depends on an active feminizing process induced by ovarian hormones. Michael and Zumpe (this issue) describe how steroid hormones are taken up in the primate brain, and suggest that masculinization occurs at least in part through the conversion of testosterone to estradiol. McFadden (this issue) provides a comprehensive review of sex differences in the human auditory system and indicates how hormones present at several times in development are likely to be responsible for these sex differences. He also demonstrates the value of examining hormonal influences on basic sensory and perceptual processes.

The effects of early hormones on human behavior are considered in four articles. Two studies address the behavioral effects of early androgens in children with CAH. Hampson, Rovet, and Altmann (this issue) provide the first evidence that preadolescent girls with CAH have higher spatial ability than their sisters, supporting the notion that early androgens facilitate the development of spatial ability. Leveroni and Berenbaum (this issue) suggest that early androgens can also inhibit the development of female-typical behavior by showing that girls with CAH have less interest in infants than their sisters. Buchanan, Pavlovic, and Rovet (this issue) report on a study of women with Turner syndrome, illustrating both estrogen effects on human spatial ability and a model for understanding how hormones affect cognition. Tenhula and Bailey (this issue) take a novel approach to studying hormonal influences on behavior, in this case sexual orientation, by examining the relation between sexual orientation and pubertal indicators likely to be influenced by early hormones; they echo Clark and Galef (this issue) in illustrating the value of examining basic reproductive characteristics in studies of hormonal influences on behavior.

Other articles in this special issue address the exciting work being done on the behavioral effects of adult, circulating hormones (activational effects); again, this work demonstrates the use of various methodological approaches. Two articles concern the effects of estrogen on motor skills and spatial abilities, and, with different methods, reach similar conclusions. Saucier and Kimura (this issue) studied women at different points in the menstrual cycle, whereas Szekely et al. (this issue) studied women taking oral contraceptives during high and low estrogen conditions. Both studies are noteworthy for repeated testing of the same group of women at different levels of estrogen, allowing important within-subject comparisons. Both studies showed that ovarian hormones differentially affect motor performance, with estrogen enhancing performance on a manual sequencing and praxis task (Saucier & Kimura, this issue; Szekely et al., this issue), but having no effect on a targeting task (Saucier & Kimura, this issue) or on visually guided movements (Szekely et al., this issue). Janowsky, Chavez, Zamboni, and Orwoll (this issue) use their findings on relations between normal variations in circulating testosterone and estrogen and normal variations in cognitive abilities to argue that such relations are more complex than previously believed. Their study is noteworthy for the assessment of both male-typical and female-typical hormones and an extensive battery of cognitive tests.

The articles in this special issue are significant in a variety of ways. The methods reflect state-of-the-art techniques, and, in fact, several articles report the first studies with a particular method. There is clear convergence of evidence from studies with different methods. The results reported in the special issue contribute substantially to our knowledge of hormonal effects on behavior, and several articles provide the first reports of hormonal effects on a given behavior, or provide a solution to a difficult question. All of the articles address theoretical and conceptual issues in understanding not only whether hormones affect behavior, but how they do so. All of the articles illustrate the complexity of hormonal effects on behavior and all of them point to common themes in understanding hormone–behavior relations and suggest directions for future work in psychoneuroendocrinology. Some of these are highlighted in the following sections.

BEHAVIORAL CONSIDERATIONS

Masculinity Versus Femininity

Feminine and masculine development do not merely reflect opposite ends of a single continuum, and they rarely exist in two distinct forms. Further, sex-typed behaviors are multidimensional. Although these points are often made (Constantinople, 1973; Huston, 1983), studies are rarely designed to examine separately the continua of male-typical and female-typical behavior and to consider several components of each. Although it is more common to see two discrete forms of behavior in nonhuman species, even there it is clear that both male-typical and female-typical behaviors can coexist. For example, a female rat may try to mount other females, but also be sexually receptive to males. Hormones can differentially affect not just masculine and feminine behaviors (Davis, Chaptal, & McEwen, 1979; Debold & Whalen, 1975), but the different components of these behaviors (e.g., lordosis and proprioception; see Fitch & Denenberg, in press).

When behaviors are assessed on continua, it can be very difficult to differentiate masculinization from defeminization and feminization from demasculinization. It is usual to label as male-typical those behaviors that are more common or higher in males than in females, such as aggression, spatial ability, and play with boys' toys, and to label as female-typical those behaviors that are more common or higher in females than in males, such as emotional expressiveness and perception, verbal memory, perceptual speed and accuracy, and maternal behavior. Although most studies of hormone effects on behavior have focused on changes in male-typical behavior associated with varying levels of androgens, articles in this special issue illustrate that things are changing. Studies in girls with CAH show that high levels of androgen can inhibit the development of some aspects of female-typical behavior, including maternal behavior (Leveroni & Berenbaum, this issue) and perhaps perceptual speed (Hampson et al., this issue). Buchanan et al. (this issue) suggest that some of the cognitive deficits in women with Turner syndrome result from low levels of female-typical estrogen. Fitch et al. (this issue) demonstrate the important role of ovarian hormones in the development of female-typical traits, and indicate how such findings require new conceptualizations of feminine and masculine behavior. They also present interesting proposals for examining the development of both male-typical and female-typical behaviors.

Explaining Sex Differences in Performance Versus Process

It has been generally believed that gonadal hormones only affect behaviors that show sex differences. In fact, it has been argued that evaluations of behavioral effects of gonadal hormones are valid only when the measures used differentiate typical males and females (e.g., Berenbaum et al., 1995; Hampson et al., this issue; Resnick et al., 1986). It is also generally believed that the same factors that produce differences between the sexes produce variations within sex. For example, sex differences in early androgens may contribute to sex differences in spatial ability, and natural variations in levels or availability of androgens among normal males and females might contribute to within-sex variability in spatial ability. This perspective is reflected in several articles in this special issue, in comparisons of girls with known differences in early hormones (Hampson et al., this issue; Leveroni & Berenbaum, this issue), and in comparisons of adults with measured differences in circulating hormones (Janowsky et al., this issue; Saucier & Kimura, this issue). A modification of this approach, illustrated by Tenhula and Bailey (this issue), involves studies of covariation in sex-typed traits. If differences in androgen exposure contribute to within-sex variation, then traits that are masculinized during similar developmental periods should be correlated within sex (Bailey, Gaulin, Agyei, & Gladue, 1994; Gladue & Bailey, 1995).

There has been increasing consideration of the fact that hormones can produce sex differences in brain organization and behavioral processes without necessarily producing average differences in performance. This topic is discussed in several articles in this special issue. Fitch et al. (this issue) provide examples of cases in which sex differences are not manifested in average behavioral differences, but in different patterns of brain–behavior correlations. Buchanan et al. (this issue) suggest that estrogen affects visual working memory, which does not appear to show sex differences. Janowsky et al. (this issue) suggest that activational hormones act on neural systems besides those that cause sex differences. This topic deserves further study with measures specifically designed to test hypotheses about the nature of sex differences (performance vs. process).

Developmental Change

There are two issues of particular importance to developmentalists. First, because behavior may change in form as well as in level, it is important that the behaviors examined be age appropriate and that attention be paid to equivalence of constructs across ages (similar tests may not always measure similar constructs at different ages). This issue is apparent in studies of hormonal influences on spatial ability, given the difficulties in assessing sex-differentiated spatial abilities in young children. Hampson et al.'s (this issue) study reveals the value of using age-appropriate cognitive measures. Second, hormonal effects may vary across age, in part because of neural development, and it is important to study the developmental course of hormone effects. Such studies will also provide basic information about brain development. Michael and Zumpe (this issue) provide direct data about age changes in steroid uptake in several regions of the primate brain, and Fitch et al. (this issue) discuss developmental changes in the effects of gonadal hormones.

DELINEATING DETAILS OF HORMONE EFFECTS

It has become increasingly important to specify the details of hormone action that indicate why some behaviors are more strongly influenced by early hormones than others. Hormonal effects on behavior probably depend on a variety of factors, and delineation of these factors is more likely to occur when they are studied from several perspectives, as illustrated by the articles in this special issue.

Organizational Versus Activational Hormones

The distinction between organizational and activational hormones is no longer as clear as it once was (Arnold & Breedlove, 1985; Fitch & Denenberg, in press). This is illustrated in several articles in this special issue. Fitch et al. (this issue) suggest that ovarian hormone effects on behavior differ from androgen effects in dimensions related to the organization–activation distinction. McFadden's (this issue) review of sex differences in auditory characteristics clearly demonstrates the value of considering the effects of both early and circulating hormones. Clark and Galef (this issue) show that male gerbils with high prenatal levels of testosterone also have high adult circulating levels of testosterone, and are more responsive to exogenous hormones than are males with low prenatal testosterone. This suggests that organizational and activational hormones are correlated and that they work jointly to affect behavior. It will be interesting to examine this further, for example, by studying whether females with a male cotwin have higher levels of circulating testosterone than do females with a female cotwin, and whether behavioral masculinization is greatest in females with a male cotwin who also have high circulating levels.

Androgens Versus Ovarian Hormones

Androgens have generally been considered to be the only hormones necessary for sexual differentiation, with masculine development resulting from high levels of androgens and feminine development proceeding when androgen levels are low. It is now clear, however, that ovarian hormones play an active role in sexual differentiation (Fitch & Denenberg, in press; Fitch et al., this issue; Stewart & Cygan, 1980; Toran-Allerand, 1984). Fitch et al. (this issue) discuss the evidence for the importance of ovarian hormones and indicate how this evidence affects our theories and studies of human behavioral and neural sex differences. Studies in females with Turner syndrome, such as the one described by Buchanan et al. (this issue), can contribute to our understanding of the effects of ovarian hormones on human behavior.

Sensitive Periods

In considering permanent effects of gonadal hormones on the brain and behavior (the traditional organizational effects), it is widely accepted that these effects are maximal during circumscribed sensitive periods. The sensitive periods for hormonal effects on human behavior have been considered to be those times during which androgens (especially testosterone) are substantially higher in males than in females. This includes prenatal weeks 8 to 24, postnatal months 1 to 5, and a prolonged period beginning in adolescence and continuing throughout adulthood (Smail, Reyes, Winter, & Faiman, 1981). The early prenatal period has been generally thought to be the main critical period for organizational effects of hormones on brain development and later behavior, but there has been increased awareness that the other periods may be important, too.

Studies in nonhuman animals are very important for detailing sensitive periods, because experimental manipulations can be carefully controlled to increase or decrease hormone levels only during specific periods. In primates, there appear to be several distinct sensitive periods for androgen effects on behavior, with different behaviors masculinized by exposure early versus late in gestation (Goy, Bercovitch, & McBrair, 1988). For example, female rhesus macaques exposed to androgen early in gestation (and thus with virilized genitalia) show increased mounting behavior, whereas those exposed late in gestation (with no genital virilization) show increased rough play.

The fact that behavioral effects of hormones may vary according to the time of hormone exposure is discussed in several articles in this special issue. Fitch et al. (this issue) suggest that the behavioral effects of ovarian hormones and androgen differ in time course, specifically that ovarian hormones exert effects well beyond the prenatal and neonatal periods. Hampson et al. (this issue) speculate that androgens present in the early postnatal period are important for the development of aspects of spatial ability. Tenhula and Bailey (this issue) suggest that hormones might affect sexual orientation and pubertal timing at different developmental points.

Apparent inconsistencies in studies of hormonal influences on human behavior might be resolved with additional attention to the fact that behaviors might be differentially affected at different points in development. In particular, it will be interesting to compare groups with exposure to unusual levels of androgens and ovarian hormones during different developmental periods. For example, findings that females with a male cotwin are masculinized on auditory characteristics (McFadden, 1993, this issue) and spatial ability (Cole-Harding et al., 1988), but not on toy play (Henderson & Berenbaum, 1997) suggest that the critical period for the masculinization of toy play is later than the critical period for the development of the other traits, because the amnion is permeable (permitting the transfer of testosterone from the male to the female fetus) only early in prenatal development. The deficits in visual working memory in girls with Turner syndrome observed by Buchanan et al. (this issue) might be studied in relation to estrogen in early or middle childhood, as a test of Fitch et al.'s (this issue) hypothesis that ovarian estrogen continues to produce permanent changes to the brain in the postnatal period.

It will be very interesting to study, in a sample of normal children, later behavior in relation to both androgen and ovarian hormones determined at several points considered to be sensitive periods for the effects of these hormones. For example, given the speculations that androgen acts primarily during prenatal and early postnatal development, and that ovarian hormones act primarily during postnatal development, it might be hypothesized that some aspects of childhood and adolescent sex-typed behavior would be related to prenatal androgens (determined from amniotic fluid), other aspects to androgens in the early postnatal period (determined from serum collected directly from the child), and yet other aspects of behavior to ovarian hormones in the prepubertal period (determined from serum from the child).

Information on timing of behavioral effects of hormones also helps to constrain hypotheses about the neural substrates of behavior, a particular concern to developmental neuropsychologists. For example, if androgen effects on spatial ability extend into the early postnatal period, this means that the neural substrates for spatial ability continue to develop postnatally. This also has implications for environmental interventions.

Dose

The absolute level of the hormone necessary to change behavior is likely not the same for all behaviors. Some behaviors may be affected only by extreme variations in hormones, whereas others may be affected by relatively minor variations. Studies in populations with well-characterized hormone excess, such as CAH, should ultimately provide information on this issue, as illustrated in the following two examples. First, sex-typical play may be changed only with high levels of androgen characteristic of girls with CAH (and typical boys), but not likely to be found in typical girls, even those with a boy cotwin. Second, a behavior that strongly differentiates females with CAH from their unaffected sisters may reflect the fact that the behavior is masculinized or defeminized with a lower dose of androgen than a behavior that only weakly differentiates the groups (assuming, of course, that the behaviors are equally well measured); such differences would be expected to parallel the sex differences in the general population. This might explain why it has been possible to detect and replicate differences between girls with CAH and their sisters in sex-typed play and spatial ability, but not as easy to detect differences in perceptual speed (see Hampson et al., this issue).

Dose effects do not have to be linear. In fact, associations between circulating testosterone and spatial ability may be curvilinear (Kimura & Hampson, 1994). Similarly, very high levels of early androgens may sometimes produce demasculinization, although they often have no effect (Baum & Schretlen, 1975; Diamond, Llacuna, & Wong, 1973), and this is discussed in this special issue. As shown by Clark and Galef (this issue), high levels of exogenous testosterone appear to reduce the expression of male-typical asymmetries in male gerbils, and large doses of testosterone appear to be less effective than small doses at masculinizing asymmetries in female gerbils. This effect can also occur in human beings, although it does not always: Hampson et al. (this issue) show that boys with CAH have lower spatial ability than their brothers, but Leveroni and Berenbaum (this issue) show that boys with CAH do not have enhanced interest in infants. Further studies may help to pinpoint the reasons why excess androgen results in demasculinization of some behaviors but not others.

There may also be threshold effects, such that the amount of hormone is linearly related to behavior only at some levels of the hormone. For example, if spatial ability is facilitated by a moderate amount of testosterone, then there will be a linear relation between testosterone and spatial ability only in females, because all males exceed the threshold.

Fitch et al. (this issue) provide another perspective on dose effects. They suggest that the direction of estrogen effects depends on the amount present, with estrogen producing masculinized behavior at high levels and feminized behavior at low levels (Stewart & Cygan, 1980).

Specific Hormones and Their Interactions

Masculinizing hormones come in many forms, and each affects different aspects of physical and behavioral sexual differentiation. For example, dihydrotestosterone is the metabolite responsible for differentiation of the external genitalia (Siiteri & Wilson, 1974); dihydrotestosterone and another form of testosterone, testosterone propionate, have different effects on learning abilities in monkeys (Bachevalier & Hagger, 1991). Some metabolites are more potent masculinizing agents than others (e.g., dihydrotestosterone is more potent than testosterone in masculinizing the external genitalia, and both are more potent that dihydroepiandrostenedione). In some species, it is estradiol metabolized from androgen in the brain that is responsible for the masculine-typical development of some behaviors. For example, in rodents, estradiol masculinizes sexual behavior and learning (Breedlove, 1992; Goy & McEwen, 1980; Williams & Meck, 1991), but testosterone itself or dihydrotestosterone masculinizes rough play (Meaney, 1988). Masculinized sexual orientation in women women exposed to DES in utero is thought to reflect a similar mechanism in people, that is, the masculinizing effects of estradiol. Michael and Zumpe (this issue) discuss the important role of estradiol in sexual differentiation of the macaque brain, suggesting that masculinization of behavior and the brain in all species occurs (at least in part) through aromatization of testosterone to estradiol.

Further, the effects of specific hormones depend on other hormones present, so that the presence of one hormone may promote or prevent the effect of another hormone (Goy & McEwen, 1980). For example, progesterone has been shown to act as an antiandrogen in female rodents, providing protection against the masculinizing effects of androgen (Hull, 1981; Hull, Franz, Snyder, & Nishita, 1980; Shapiro, Goldman, Bongiovanni, & Marino, 1976), and may serve a similar protective role in human females (Ehrhardt & Meyer-Bahlburg, 1979; Ehrhardt, Meyer-Bahlburg, Feldman, & Ince, 1984). Thus, androgens may affect behavior only when they are high enough to counteract progesterone (as in girls with CAH) or when progesterone levels are low. This might explain why it may be more difficult to see changes in sex-typed behavior in typical females (those with a male cotwin or with only slightly elevated levels of androgens in amniotic fluid) than in females with exposure to high levels of androgens (such as CAH or androgenizing progestins). Janowsky et al. (this issue) also suggest that circulating progesterone may modify the behavioral effects of estrogen.

Sensitivity to Hormones

It is likely that individuals vary not only in the levels of hormones to which they are exposed, but in their sensitivity to those hormones. Clark and Galef (this issue) note that response to exogenous testosterone in gerbils depends on their early exposure. Mutations in the human androgen receptor gene cause androgen resistance to varying degrees, with phenotypic abnormalities in men ranging from complete insensitivity to androgen and thus female differentiation to men with infertility and minor undervirilization (McPhaul, Marcelli, Zoppi, Griffin, & Wilson, 1993). It will be interesting to see if these receptor variations are related to behavioral variations. The likelihood of such effects is revealed by studies showing that early exposure to testosterone produces increased aggression in one mouse strain but not another, and that this strain difference in behavioral reactivity to neonatal testosterone is genotype dependent (Michard-Vanhee, 1988). Michael and Zumpe's (this issue) findings that the brains of male and female macaques are similar with respect to estrogen receptors suggest that sensitivity may not cause behavioral differences between the sexes, but they do not rule out a role for hormone receptor sensitivity in producing within-sex variation.

Variations in hormone sensitivity might account for observations that not all females with CAH have high spatial ability (Hampson et al., this issue) or reduced interest in infants (Leveroni & Berenbaum, this issue). Neurohormonal theories of sexual orientation have generally been concerned only with levels of prenatal hormones, but future work might profitably consider individual differences in sensitivity to hormones. Female homosexuality might arise not from very high levels of masculinizing hormones during early development, but from increased sensitivity to typical levels (Tenhula & Bailey, this issue).

Effects of Circulating Hormones: Between- and Within-Individual Variations

Studies of behavioral effects of circulating hormones have considered these hormones to be sources of behavioral differences both between individuals, as illustrated in the study of Janowsky et al. (this issue), and within individuals, as illustrated in the studies of Saucier and Kimura (this issue) and Szekely et al. (this issue). The usual expectation is that the same factors (e.g., level of estrogen) will account for variation between and within individuals, and studies that fail to support these expectations are usually considered to have methodological limitations. However, this is not always the case, and, in fact, Saucier and Kimura (this issue) have a nice demonstration of significant relations between estrogen and manual praxis within subjects (across the menstrual cycle), but not between subjects (no significant correlations between estrogen and motor performance on the first testing occasion). Janowsky et al. (this issue) also failed to detect relations between estrogen and cognition (although other issues are also involved in interpreting their results). Thus, it is interesting to consider the possibility that some hormonal variations may be important only for behavioral variation within an individual, whereas other hormonal variations may be more strongly related to variations across individuals. This seems to be a topic worth studying.

HOW DO HORMONES AFFECT BEHAVIOR?

Some of the most exciting questions in human psychoneuroendocrinology relate to the mechanisms—neural and behavioral—whereby hormones affect behavior, as several articles in this special issue indicate. (There is also a lot of exciting work focused on the cellular and molecular mechanisms mediating hormonal effects on the brain and behavior—e.g., McCarthy, 1994—but that work is beyond the scope of this special issue.)

Direct Effects

Hormones may affect behavior directly through changes to brain regions immediately involved in the behavior. Studies in other species show that gonadal hormones affect hypothalamic areas involved in aspects of sexual behavior (for reviews, see Breedlove, 1992, 1994; Goy & McEwen, 1980; MacLusky & Naftolin, 1981) and hippocampal areas involved in aspects of spatial learning (Juraska, 1991; Roof & Havens, 1992; Williams & Meck, 1991). Gonadal hormones affect neuronal size, survival, and outgrowth; synapse number and organization; dendritic branching patterns; gross nuclear volume; cortical thickness; and neurotransmitter systems.

Fitch et al. (this issue) show how ovarian hormones affect the development of the corpus callosum in the rat. The corpus callosum and other commissures are important brain structures in human beings, aspects of which appear to be related to sex (e.g., Allen & Gorski, 1991; Cowell, Allen, Zalatimo, & Denenberg, 1992; de Lacoste-Utamsing & Holloway, 1982; Witelson, 1989; see Driesen & Raz, 1995, for a review), sexual orientation (Allen & Gorski, 1992), and components of human cognition (Hines, Chiu, McAdams, Bentler, & Lipcamon, 1992). Michael and Zumpe (this issue) describe their work delineating hormone uptake in primate brain regions involved in sex-typical behavior; it is likely that some of the same regions act as sites of hormone action in people. There has been an explosion of investigations into sex differences in the human brain (Gur et al., 1995; Harasty, Double, Halliday, Kril, & McRitchie, 1997; Shaywitz et al., 1995; Witelson, Glezer, & Kigar, 1995; for reviews, see Farace & Turkheimer, 1997; Resnick & Maki, in press), and it is only a matter of time before reports appear on these sexually differentiated regions in relation to both early and adult hormones, for example, in individuals with CAH and in women at different phases of the menstrual cycle. It is worth noting, however, that hormonal effects on behavior may not always be revealed by brain sex differences. This is discussed by Michael and Zumpe (this issue), who did not find sex differences in steroid receptor distribution and number in the macaque brain, suggesting that sex differences in steroid uptake mechanisms do not account for sex differences in primate behavior.

Indirect Effects Through Other Traits

From psychological perspectives, it is interesting to consider some of the indirect mediating mechanisms from hormones to behaviors. For example, how and why do high levels of early androgen result in high scores on modern tests of spatial ability, or interest in playing with toy trucks, or reduced attention to babies? In this issue, several authors discuss these mechanisms; some also briefly mention possible evolutionary mechanisms. Some behavioral effects of hormones are mediated by effects on physical structures. Clark and Galef (this issue) show that hormones affect sexual behavior in part through effects on genital musculature. It is worthwhile to consider whether any of the behavioral changes seen in people in association with variations in hormones (either early in development or in adulthood) can be attributed to hormonal effects on peripheral musculature.

Other effects may be mediated by basic perceptual or sensory processes. McFadden (this issue) suggests that sex differences in higher cognitive function may result not simply from prenatal hormones operating at specific cortical sites, but also from hormones acting at peripheral sites that contribute to the activation of the cortical sites. His comments should encourage researchers to consider fundamental sensory and perceptual processes that might account for sex differences in cognition or perceptual asymmetries.

Still other effects are likely to be mediated by basic cognitive processes and the neural substrates that subserve them. Buchanan et al. (this issue) take the much-needed step of applying cognitive approaches to understanding the spatial deficit in Turner syndrome, and they attempt to delineate neural and cognitive mechanisms from genes to performance. In examining behavioral effects of estrogen, Saucier and Kimura (this issue) and Szekely et al. (this issue) go beyond general examination of hormone effects to questions regarding specificity of hormone action, and suggest that estrogen facilitates left-hemisphere regions subserving praxis. Szekely et al.'s (this issue) analysis of the fundamental components of motor tasks provides a model for studying components of higher order behaviors.

Effects Through the Environment

It is also interesting to consider the ways in which the effects of hormones are mediated or moderated by aspects of the environment, either social (e.g., parent childrearing practices) or physical (e.g., prenatal exposure to alcohol). Wallen (1996) showed how the social environment modifies the expression of hormonally influenced sex-typed behavior in juvenile rhesus monkeys, such that the behaviors that are the least variable across social contexts are the most affected by prenatal hormones. This suggests that, in people, hormonal effects are most likely to be seen on behaviors that show large sex differences across contexts. Perhaps it is not surprising, then, that toy and activity preferences consistently differentiate girls with CAH from controls, because sex differences in these preferences are observed across cultures and situations, but that it is more difficult to find differences in aggression, because there are many forms and meanings to aggression (Berenbaum & Resnick, 1997; Berenbaum & Snyder, 1995; Dittmann et al., 1990; Ehrhardt & Baker, 1974).

In considering the ways in which the environment might modify hormonal effects on human behavior, it is worth distinguishing hormone–environment correlations from hormone–environment interactions (similar to the genotype–environment correlations and interactions discussed by Scarr & McCartney, 1983). Individuals with differing levels of hormones may be exposed to different environments, either because they select different environments or because others provide them with different environments (hormone–environment correlations), as noted in several articles in this special issue. Clark and Galef (this issue) report that hormones affect not only the behavior of the organism but others' responses to the individual (such as mother's grooming and peers' attraction to the individual). Leveroni and Berenbaum (this issue) discuss how hormone–environment correlations might affect the development of maternal behavior. Hampson et al. (this issue) consider whether the boy-typical toy preferences of CAH girls result in experiences that facilitate the development of spatial ability. Michael and Zumpe (this issue) also suggest that early androgen effects on sexual behavior decrease with age and experience.

Individuals with different levels of hormones may also respond differently to the same environment (hormone–environment interactions). In rodents, for example, sex differences and testosterone effects on the size of the corpus callosum are moderated by an environmental intervention, handling (Fitch & Denenberg, in press). Hormone–environment interactions have not been well studied in people, but would include, for example, girls with CAH imitating aggressive behavior more readily than girls without CAH. Such moderating effects of the environment might make it difficult to see behavioral differences between individuals with exposure to high versus low levels of hormones, but could help to reveal mechanisms whereby hormones affect behavior.

WHAT DO THESE STUDIES MEAN FOR DEVELOPMENTAL NEUROPSYCHOLOGY?

Developmental neuropsychologists have reason to celebrate and benefit from the advances that have been made in understanding hormonal influences on behavior. These studies directly help to explain the neural substrates of most of the behaviors neuropsychologists study, including emotion, cognition, motor behavior, asymmetry, and developmental disabilities. These studies directly pinpoint how brain structures and functions are involved in specific behaviors, specify the developmental course of specific behaviors and their neural substrates, and highlight the components of behavior, thereby suggesting distinctions that are honored by the nervous system. Saucier and Kimura (this issue) and Szekely et al. (this issue) present independent convincing evidence that left-hemisphere regions involved in praxis are modulated by estrogen, and that fine motor skills are neurally distinct from visually guided movements and extrapersonal motor skills. Janowsky et al. (this issue) suggest that circulating hormones affect neural systems in addition to those that cause sex differences, so we might look more widely in the brain for effects of circulating hormones. Hampson et al.'s (this issue) finding of enhanced spatial ability in girls with CAH extends similar findings in adults (Resnick et al., 1986), and encourages the search for specific neural systems that mediate this effect. Buchanan et al.'s (this issue) studies identify visual working memory as one of the core cognitive causes of the visuospatial deficit in girls with Turner syndrome, and, as such, indicate that it would be profitable to examine neural regions subserving visual working memory to understand genetic and brain mechanisms involved in sex-differentiated spatial ability. McFadden (this issue) suggests that sex and lateral differences in cortical function may result from sex and ear differences in auditory characteristics and simple abilities. Fitch et al. (this issue) show how estrogen may account for the sex differences in plasticity reported in the neuropsychological literature. Tenhula and Bailey (this issue) remind us to consider brain regions subserving basic reproductive and sexual functions.

The articles in this special issue are interesting and worthwhile reading in their own right, but they may also act to stimulate developmental neuropsychologists to consider hormones in their own studies. Perhaps we can look forward to the day when studies describing hormonal influences on sex-typed behavior appear regularly in the pages of this journal.

ACKNOWLEDGMENTS

Preparation of this article was supported in part by National Institutes of Health Grant HD19644. I thank Barbara Bulman-Fleming, Gina Grimshaw, Lisabeth DiLalla, and Catherine Leveroni for thoughtful and helpful comments on an earlier version of this article.

REFERENCES

Allen, L. S., & Gorski, R. A. (1991). Sexual dimorphism of the anterior commissure and the massa intermedia of the human brain. *Journal of Comparative Neurology, 312,* 97–104.

Allen, L. S., & Gorski, R. A. (1992). Sexual orientation and the size of the anterior commissure in the human brain. *Proceedings of the National Academy of Sciences, 89,* 7199–7202.

American Psychological Association. (1997). Awards for distinguished scientific contributions: Robert W. Goy. *American Psychologist, 52,* 310–312.

Arnold, A. P., & Breedlove, S. M. (1985). Organizational and activational effects of sex steroids on brain and behavior: A reanalysis. *Hormones and Behavior, 19,* 469–498.

Arnold, A. P., & Gorski, R. A. (1984). Gonadal steroid induction of structural sex differences in the central nervous system. *Annual Review of Neuroscience, 7,* 413–442.

Bachevalier, J., & Hagger, C. (1991). Sex differences in the development of learning abilities in primates. *Psychoneuroendocrinology, 16,* 177–188.

Bailey, J. M., Gaulin, S., Agyei, Y., & Gladue, B. A. (1994). Effects of gender and sexual orientation on evolutionarily relevant aspects of human mating psychology. *Journal of Personality and Social Psychology, 66,* 1081–1093.

Baum, M. J., & Schretlen, P. (1975). Neuroendocrine effects of perinatal androgenization in the male ferret. *Progress in Brain Research, 42,* 343–355.

Beatty, W. W. (1992). Gonadal hormones and sex differences in nonreproductive behaviors. In A. A. Gerall, H. Moltz, & I. L. Ward (Eds.), *Handbook of behavioral neurobiology: Vol. 11. Sexual differentiation* (pp. 85–128). New York: Plenum.

Becker, J. B. (1992). Hormonal influences on extrapyramid sensorimotor function and hippocampal plasticity. In J. B. Becker, S. M. Breedlove, & D. Crews (Eds.), *Behavioral endocrinology* (pp. 325–356). Cambridge, MA: MIT Press.

Becker, J. B., Breedlove, S. M., & Crews, D. (Eds.). (1992). *Behavioral endocrinology.* Cambridge, MA: MIT Press.

Berenbaum, S. A., & Hines, M. (1992). Early androgens are related to childhood sex-typed toy preferences. *Psychological Science, 3,* 203–206.

Berenbaum, S. A., Korman, K., & Leveroni, C. (1995). Early hormones and sex differences in cognitive abilities. *Learning and Individual Differences, 7,* 303–321.

Berenbaum, S. A., & Resnick, S. M. (1997). Early androgen effects on aggression in children and adults with congenital adrenal hyperplasia. *Psychoneuroendocrinology, 22,* 505–515.

Berenbaum, S. A., & Snyder, E. (1995). Early hormonal influences on childhood sex-typed activity and playmate preferences: Implications for the development of sexual orientation. *Developmental Psychology, 31,* 31–42.

Breedlove, S. M. (1992). Sexual differentiation of the brain and behavior. In J. B. Becker, S. M. Breedlove, & D. Crews (Eds.), *Behavioral endocrinology* (pp. 39–68). Cambridge, MA: MIT Press.

Breedlove, S. M. (1994). Sexual differentiation of the human nervous system. *Annual Review of Psychology, 45,* 389–418.

Bryden, M. P., McManus, I. C., & Bulman-Fleming, M. B. (1994). Evaluating the empirical support for the Geschwind–Behan–Galaburda model of cerebral lateralization. *Brain and Cognition, 26,* 103–167.

Buchanan, L., Pavlovic, J., & Rovet, J. (1998/this issue). A reexamination of the visuospatial deficit in Turner syndrome: Contributions of working memory. *Developmental Neuropsychology, 14,* 341–367.

Clark, M. M., & Galef, B. G., Jr. (1998/this issue). Effects of intrauterine position on the behavior and genital morphology of litter-bearing rodents. *Developmental Neuropsychology, 14,* 197–211.

Clark, A. S., & Goldman-Rakic, P. S. (1989). Gonadal hormones influence the emergence of cortical function in nonhuman primates. *Behavioral Neuroscience, 103,* 1287–1295.

Cole-Harding, S., Morstad, A. L., & Wilson, J. R. (1988). Spatial ability in members of opposite-sex twin pairs [Abstract]. *Behavior Genetics, 18,* 710.

Collaer, M. L., & Hines, M. (1995). Human behavioral sex differences: A role for gonadal hormones during early development? *Psychological Bulletin, 118,* 55–107.

Constantinople, A. (1973). Masculinity-femininity: An exception to a famous dictum? *Psychological Bulletin, 80,* 389–407.

Cowell, P. E., Allen, L. S., Zalatimo, N. S., & Denenberg, V. H. (1992). A developmental study of sex and age interactions in the human corpus callosum. *Developmental Brain Research, 66,* 187–192.

Davis, P. G., Chaptal, C. V., & McEwen, B. S. (1979). Independence of the differentiation of masculine and feminine behavior in rats. *Hormones and Behavior, 12,* 12–19.

Debold, J. F., & Whalen, R. E. (1975). Differential sensitivity of mounting and lordosis control systems to early androgen treatment in male and female hamsters. *Hormones and Behavior, 6,* 196–209.

de Lacoste-Utamsing, C., & Holloway, R. L. (1982). Sexual dimorphism in the corpus callosum. *Science, 216,* 1431–1432.

Diamond, M., Llacuna, A., & Wong, C. L. (1973). Sex behavior after neonatal progesterone, testosterone, estrogen, or antiandrogens. *Hormones and Behavior, 4,* 73–88.

Dittmann, R. W., Kappes, M. E., & Kappes, M. H. (1992). Sexual behavior in adolescent and adult females with congenital adrenal hyperplasia. *Psychoneuroendocrinology, 17,* 153–170.

Dittmann, R. W., Kappes, M. H., Kappes, M. E., Borger, D., Stegner, H., Willig, R. H., & Wallis, H. (1990). Congenital adrenal hyperplasia I: Gender-related behaviors and attitudes in female patients and their sisters. *Psychoneuroendocrinology, 15,* 401–420.

Driesen, N. R., & Raz, N. (1995). The influence of sex, age, and handedness on corpus callosum morphology: A meta-analysis. *Psychobiology, 23,* 240–247.

Ehrhardt, A. A., & Baker, S. W. (1974). Fetal androgens, human central nervous system differentiation, and behavior sex differences. In R. C. Friedman, R. R. Richart, & R. L. Vande Weile (Eds.), *Sex differences in behavior* (pp. 33–51). New York: Wiley.

Ehrhardt, A. A., & Meyer-Bahlburg, H. F. L. (1979). Prenatal sex hormones and the developing brain: Effects on psychosexual differentiation and cognitive functioning. *Annual Review of Medicine, 30,* 417–430.

Ehrhardt, A. A., Meyer-Bahlburg, H. F. L., Feldman, J. F., & Ince, S. E. (1984). Sex-dimorphic behavior in childhood subsequent to prenatal exposure to exogenous progestogens and estrogens. *Archives of Sexual Behavior, 13,* 457–477.

Farace, E., & Turkheimer, E. (1997). Gender differences in brain morphometry and function. In E. D. Bigler (Ed.), *Neuroimaging II: Clinical applications. Human brain function: Assessment and rehabilitation* (pp. 127–151). New York: Plenum.

Fitch, R. H., Cowell, P. E., & Denenberg, V. H. (1998/this issue). The female phenotype: Nature's default? *Developmental Neuropsychology, 14*, 213–231.

Fitch, R. H., & Denenberg, V. H. (in press). A role for ovarian hormones in sexual differentiation of the brain. *Behavioral and Brain Sciences.*

Geschwind, N., & Galaburda, A. M. (1985). Cerebral lateralization: Biological mechanisms, associations, and pathology. *Archives of Neurology, 42,* 428–459, 521–552, 634–654.

Gladue, B. A., & Bailey, J. M. (1995). Aggressiveness, competitiveness, and human sexual orientation. *Psychoneuroendocrinology, 20,* 475–485.

Gorski, R. A., Gordon, J. H., Shryne, J. E., & Southam, A. M. (1978). Evidence for a morphological sex difference within the medial preoptic area of the rat brain. *Brain Research, 143,* 333–346.

Gouchie, C., & Kimura, D. (1991). The relationship between testosterone levels and cognitive ability patterns. *Psychoneuroendocrinology, 16,* 323–334.

Goy, R. W. (1996). Editor's note. Special issue: Sexual differences in behavior. *Hormones and Behavior, 30,* 299.

Goy, R. W., Bercovitch, F. B., & McBrair, M. C. (1988). Behavioral masculinization is independent of genital masculinization in prenatally androgenized female rhesus macaques. *Hormones and Behavior, 22,* 552–571.

Goy, R. W., & McEwen, B. S. (1980). *Sexual differentiation of the brain.* London: Oxford University Press.

Grimshaw, G. M., Sitarenios, G., & Finegan, J. K. (1995). Mental rotation at 7 years: Relations with prenatal testosterone levels and spatial play experience. *Brain and Cognition, 29,* 85–100.

Gur, R. C., Mozley, L. H., Mozley, P. D., Resnick, S. M., Karp, J. S., Alavi, A., Arnold, S. E., & Gur, R. E. (1995). Sex differences in regional cerebral glucose metabolism during a resting state. *Science, 267,* 528–531.

Hampson, E. (1990). Estrogen-related variations in human spatial and articulatory-motor skills. *Psychoneuroendocrinology, 15,* 97–111.

Hampson, E., & Kimura, D. (1992). Sex differences and hormonal influences on cognitive function in humans. In J. B. Becker, S. M. Breedlove, & D. Crews (Eds.), *Behavioral endocrinology* (pp. 357–398). Cambridge, MA: MIT Press.

Hampson, E., Rovet, J., & Altmann, D. (1998/this issue). Spatial reasoning in children with congenital adrenal hyperplasia due to 21-hydroxylase deficiency. *Developmental Neuropsychology, 14,* 299–320.

Harasty, J., Double, K. L., Halliday, G. M., Kril, J., & McRitchie, D. A. (1997). Language-associated cortical regions are proportionally larger in the female brain. *Archives of Neurology, 54,* 171–176.

Henderson, B. A., & Berenbaum, S. A. (1997). Sex-typed play in opposite-sex twins. *Developmental Psychobiology, 31,* 115–123.

Hines, M., Chiu, L., McAdams, L. A, Bentler, P. M., & Lipcamon, J. (1992). Cognition and the corpus callosum: Verbal fluency, visuospatial ability, and language lateralization related to midsagittal surface areas of callosal subregions. *Behavioral Neuroscience, 106,* 3–14.

Hull, E. M. (1981). Effects of neonatal exposure to progesterone on sexual behavior of male and female rats. *Physiology and Behavior, 26,* 401–405.

Hull, E. M., Franz, J. R., Snyder, A. M., & Nishita, J. K. (1980). Perinatal progesterone and learning, social and reproductive behavior in rats. *Physiology and Behavior, 24,* 251–256.

Huston, A. C. (1983). Sex-typing. In P. H. Mussen (Ed.), *Handbook of child psychology: Vol. 4. Socialization, personality, and social development* (pp. 387–467). New York: Wiley.

Janowsky, J. S., Chavez, B., Zamboni, B. D., & Orwoll, E. (1998/this issue). The cognitive neuropsychology of sex hormones in men and women. *Developmental Neuropsychology, 14,* 421–440.

Janowsky, J. S., Oviatt, S. K., & Orwoll, E. S. (1994). Testosterone influences spatial cognition in older men. *Behavioral Neuroscience, 108,* 325–332.

Juraska, J. M. (1991). Sex differences in cognitive regions of the rat brain. *Psychoneuroendocrinology, 16,* 105–119.
Kimura, D., & Hampson, E. (1994). Cognitive pattern in men and women is influenced by fluctuations in sex hormones. *Current Directions in Psychological Science, 3,* 57–61.
Leveroni, C. L., & Berenbaum, S. A. (1998/this issue). Early androgen effects on interest in infants: Evidence from children with congenital adrenal hyperplasia. *Developmental Neuropsychology, 14,* 321–340.
MacLusky, N. J., & Naftolin, F. (1981). Sexual differentiation of the central nervous system. *Science, 211,* 1294–1303.
McCarthy, M. M. (1994). Molecular aspects of sexual differentiation of the rodent brain. *Psychoneuroendocrinology, 19,* 415–427.
McFadden, D. M. (1993). A masculinizing effect on the auditory systems of human females having male co-twins. *Proceedings of the National Academy of Science, 90,* 11900–11904.
McFadden, D. M. (1998/this issue). Sex differences in the auditory system. *Developmental Neuropsychology, 14,* 261–298.
McManus, I. C., & Bryden, M. P. (1991). Geschwind's theory of cerebral lateralization: Developing a formal, causal model. *Psychological Bulletin, 110,* 237–253.
McPhaul, M. J., Marcelli, M., Zoppi, S., Griffin, J. E., & Wilson, J. D. (1993). Genetic basis of endocrine disease 4. The spectrum of mutations in the androgen receptor gene that causes androgen resistance. *Journal of Clinical Endocrinology and Metabolism, 76,* 17–23.
Meaney, M. J. (1988). The sexual differentiation of social play. *Trends in Neuroscience, 11,* 54–58.
Meyer-Bahlburg, H. F. L., Ehrhardt, A. A., Rosen, L. R., Gruen, R. S., Veridiano, N. P., Vann, F. H., & Neuwalder, H. F. (1995). Prenatal estrogens and the development of homosexual orientation. *Developmental Psychology, 31,* 12–21.
Michael, R. P., & Zumpe, D. (1998/this issue). Developmental changes in behavior and in steroid uptake by the male and female macaque brain. *Developmental Neuropsychology, 14,* 233–260.
Michard-Vanhee, C. (1988). Aggressive behavior induced in female mice by an early single injection of testosterone is genotype dependent. *Behavior Genetics, 18,* 1–12.
Nass, R., Baker, S., Speiser, P., Virdis, R., Balsamo, A., Cacciari, E., Loche, A., Dumic, M., & New, M. (1987). Hormones and handedness: Left-hand bias in female congenital adrenal hyperplasia patients. *Neurology, 37,* 711–715.
Olweus, D., Mattsson, A., Schalling, D., & Low, H. (1980). Testosterone, aggression, physical, and personality dimensions in normal adolescent males. *Psychosomatic Medicine, 42,* 253–269.
Phillips, S. M., & Sherwin, B. B. (1992). Effects of estrogen on memory function in surgically menopausal women. *Psychoneuroendocrinology, 17,* 485–495.
Phoenix, C. H., Goy, R. W., Gerall, A. A., & Young, W. C. (1959). Organizing action of prenatally administered testosterone propionate on the tissues mediating mating behavior in the female guinea pig. *Endocrinology, 65,* 369–382.
Raisman, G., & Field, P. M. (1973). Sexual dimorphism in the neuropil of the preoptic area of the rat and its dependence on neonatal androgen. *Brain Research, 54,* 1–20.
Reinisch, J. M. (1981). Prenatal exposure to synthetic progestins increases potential for aggression in humans. *Science, 211,* 1171–1173.
Resnick, S. M., Berenbaum, S. A., Gottesman, I. I., & Bouchard, T. J. (1986). Early hormonal influences on cognitive functioning in congenital adrenal hyperplasia. *Developmental Psychology, 22,* 191–198.
Resnick, S., M., Gottesman, I. I., & McGue, M. (1993). Sensation seeking in opposite-sex twins: An effect of prenatal hormones? *Behavior Genetics, 23,* 323–329.
Resnick, S. M., & Maki, P. M. (in press). Sex differences in regional brain structure and function. In P. W. Kaplan (Ed.), *The neurology of women.* New York: Demos Vermande.

Resnick, S. M., Metter, E. J., & Zonderman, A. B. (1997). Estrogen replacement therapy and longitudinal decline in visual memory: A possible protective effect? *Neurology, 49,* 1491–1497.
Roof, R. L., & Havens, M. D. (1992). Testosterone improves maze performance and induces development of a male hippocampus in females. *Brain Research, 572,* 310–313.
Saucier, D. M., & Kimura, D. (1998/this issue). Intrapersonal motor but not extrapersonal targeting skill is enhanced during the midluteal phase of the menstrual cycle. *Developmental Neuropsychology, 14,* 385–398.
Scarr, S., & McCartney, K. (1983). How people make their own environments: A theory of genotype → environment effects. *Child Development, 54,* 424–435.
Shapiro, B. H., Goldman, A. S., Bongiovanni, A. M., & Marino, J. M. (1976). Neonatal progesterone and feminine sexual development. *Nature, 264,* 795–796.
Shaywitz, B. A., Shaywitz, S. E., Pugh, K. R., Constable, R. T., Skudlarski, P., Fulbright, R. K., Bronen, R. A., Fletcher, J. M., Shankweiler, D. P., Katz, L., & Gore, J. C. (1995). Sex differences in the functional organization of the brain for language. *Nature, 373,* 607–609.
Siiteri, P. K., & Wilson, J. D. (1974). Testosterone formation and metabolism during male sexual differentiation in the human embryo. *Journal of Clinical Endocrinology and Metabolism, 38,* 113–125.
Smail, P. J., Reyes, F. I., Winter, J. S. D., & Faiman, C. (1981). The fetal hormone environment and its effect on the morphogenesis of the genital system. In S. J. Kogan & E. S. E. Hafez (Eds.), *Pediatric andrology* (pp. 9–19). The Hague, Netherlands: Martinus Nijhoff.
Stewart, J., & Cygan, D. (1980). Ovarian hormones act early in development to feminize adult open-field behavior in the rat. *Hormones and Behavior, 14,* 20–32.
Szekely, C., Hampson, E., Carey, D. P., & Goodale, M. A. (1998/this issue). Oral contraceptive use affects manual praxis but not simple visually guided movements. *Developmental Neuropsychology, 14,* 399–420.
Tenhula, W. N., & Bailey, J. M. (1998/this issue). Female sexual orientation and pubertal onset. *Developmental Neuropsychology, 14,* 369–383.
Toran-Allerand, C. D. (1984). Gonadal hormones and brain development: Implications for the genesis of sexual differentiation. *Annals of the New York Academy of Sciences, 435,* 101–110.
Wallen, K. (1996). Nature needs nurture: The interaction of hormonal and social influences on the development of behavioral sex differences in rhesus monkeys. *Hormones and Behavior, 30,* 364–378.
Williams, C. L., Barnett, A. M., & Meck, W. H. (1990). Organizational effects of early gonadal secretions on sexual differentiation in spatial memory. *Behavioral Neuroscience, 104,* 84–97.
Williams, C. L., & Meck, W. H. (1991). The organizational affects of gonadal steroids on sexually dimorphic spatial ability. *Psychoneuroendocrinology, 16,* 155–176.
Witelson, S. F. (1989). Hand and sex differences in the isthmus and genu of the human corpus callosum: A postmortem morphological study. *Brain, 112,* 799–835.
Witelson, S. F., Glezer, I. I., & Kigar, D. L. (1995). Women have greater density of neurons in posterior temporal cortex. *Journal of Neuroscience, 15,* 3418–3428.
Zucker, K. J., Bradley, S. J., Oliver, G., Blake, J., Fleming, S., & Hood, J. (1996). Psychosexual development of women with congenital adrenal hyperplasia. *Hormones and Behavior, 30,* 300–318.

Effects of Intrauterine Position on the Behavior and Genital Morphology of Litter-Bearing Rodents

Mertice M. Clark and Bennett G. Galef, Jr.
Department of Psychology
McMaster University
Hamilton, Canada

We review the literature describing hormonally mediated effects of intrauterine position on the genital morphology and reproductive behaviors of litter-bearing rodents. We emphasize work carried out in our own laboratory in which male and female Mongolian gerbils served as subjects. The results of the studies we consider indicate that biologically significant aspects of the variance in morphology and reproductive strategy seen in all populations of adult rodents reflect variance in perinatal levels of exposure to gonadal hormones induced by intrauterine position. We conclude that studies of correlations between intrauterine position and adult characteristics provide opportunities to examine the impact of normal variation in perinatal exposure to hormones on adult mammalian phenotypes.

Variation in perinatal exposure to gonadal hormones produces variation in the characteristics of adult mammals (Becker, Breedlove, & Crews, 1992). Consequently, identifying features of the perinatal environment that alter exposure to gonadal hormones received by animals early in life can help to explain the phenotypic variability found in natural mammalian populations. Such explanation is potentially important because whenever we can identify a cause of apparently random variations in phenotype, we increase not only our basic understanding of the biological world, but also our ability to control events that may affect the lives of both humans and other animals.

Laboratory studies of domesticated rodents have identified several charac-

---

Requests for reprints should be sent to Mertice M. Clark, Department of Psychology, McMaster University, Hamilton, Ontario L8S 4K1, Canada. E-mail: mclark@mcmaster.ca

teristics of the normal uterine environment that can cause fetal mammals to receive differing levels of exposure to gonadal hormones. We focus here on effects of one of these features of intrauterine life, intrauterine position (IUP), on both perinatal exposure to hormones and the adult phenotypes of male and female rodents.

IUP EFFECTS ON THE GENITAL MORPHOLOGY AND BEHAVIOR OF RODENTS

House Mouse and Norway Rat

In many litter-bearing rodent species such as the house mouse (*Mus domesticus*) or Norway rat (*Rattus norvegicus*), the IUP that a male or female fetus occupies relative to fetuses of the same or opposite sex influences the hormonal milieu in which that fetus matures (Clemens, Gladue, & Coniglio, 1978; Gandelman, vom Saal, & Reinisch, 1977; Meisel & Ward, 1981). For example, male mouse fetuses that occupy IUPs between two male fetuses (2M males) have greater blood concentrations of testosterone (T) than do brothers maturing in IUPs between two female fetuses (2F males).[1] Similarly, female fetuses located between males (2M females) have higher T titers than do their sisters gestated between females (2F females).

The opposite relation is observed for blood concentrations of estradiol (E); mouse fetuses of both sexes from 2F IUPs have significantly greater blood concentrations of E than do fetuses of the same sex from 2M IUPs (vom Saal, Grant, McMullen, & Laves, 1983), and levels of both T and E found in fetal rodents that develop in IUPs between one male and one female fetus are intermediate between those of fetuses that develop in 2M and 2F IUPs (vom Saal, 1984, 1989).

Although there has been some controversy as to how steroid hormones travel from one fetus to the next and, consequently, as to whether the sex of immediate intrauterine neighbors is the most important determinant of levels of fetal exposure to T (Houtsmuller, Juranek, Gebauer, Slob, & Rowland, 1994; Houtsmuller & Slob, 1990; Meisel & Ward, 1981; Richmond & Sachs, 1984), recent studies both of dye transport within the uterus of pregnant mice and of movement of radioactively labeled T between fetuses indicate that androgens secreted by the gonads of male fetuses late in gestation diffuse through the amniotic fluid and cross fetal membranes to adjacent fetuses (Even, Dhar, & vom Saal, 1992; vom Saal & Dhar, 1992). This diffusion causes fetuses located between male fetuses to receive relatively high levels of exposure to exogenous T during prenatal development.

---

[1] At different times during the exploration of IUP effects, different classification schemes have been used to assign fetuses to IUPs. To simplify the exposition, we discuss all experiments as though fetuses had been classified in terms of the number of both adjacent male and adjacent female fetuses, although that was not always the case in the original research.

Genital morphology. In house mice, several hormonally sensitive, morphological features have been reported to be correlated with IUP, including anogenital distance (AGD), body weight (Kinsley, Miele, et al., 1986), seminal vesicle weight, and prostate gland and preputial gland weights (Even & vom Saal, 1991; Nonneman, Ganjam, Welshons, & vom Saal, 1992). AGD has received the greatest attention.

At birth, the amount of tissue that separates the anus and genital papilla of 2M females is greater than the corresponding amount of tissue in 2F females (Clemens et al., 1978; vom Saal & Bronson, 1978, 1980). By using a weight-corrected index of the AGD in female house mice, it may also be possible for researchers to discriminate female mice from 2M and 2F IUPs as adolescents (Vandenbergh & Huggett, 1995).

As would be expected if observed differences in AGD at birth found in female rodents are mediated by their prenatal levels of exposure to T, administration of antiandrogens to either pregnant rats (Clemens et al., 1978) or pregnant mice (vom Saal, 1989) increases the AGD of their female offspring.

Behavior. Effects of IUP on the reproductive behavior of mice are numerous. Male mice from 2M IUPs are more aggressive and (perhaps unexpectedly) less sexually active, less infanticidal, and more paternal than are their male littermates from 2F IUPs (vom Saal, 1984, 1989).

Female mice from 2M IUPs have their first estrus at a later age than do their sisters from 2F IUPs. The former animals have longer estrus cycles and a shorter reproductive life than do the latter. They give birth to fewer litters during their lifetimes and to a greater percentage of males per litter. They are also both less attractive to males and more aggressive toward other females than are females from 2F IUPs (Kinsley, Konen, Miele, Ghiraldi, & Svare, 1986; Vandenbergh & Huggett, 1995; vom Saal, 1984, 1989; vom Saal & Bronson, 1978).

Some investigators have failed to observe some effects of IUP on behavior or morphology of female house mice (Jubilan & Nyby, 1992; Simon & Cologer-Clifford, 1991). However, the reality of IUP effects on the phenotypes of female house mice are suggested by two observations: First, many of these effects have been reported repeatedly both within and across laboratories. Second, parallel and very robust effects of IUP on morphology and reproductive behavior have been found in females of another litter-bearing rodent species, the Mongolian gerbil (*Meriones unguiculatus*).

Mongolian Gerbils

Females. Our interest in the impact of IUP on adult reproduction was the result of a serendipitous discovery made while routinely recording the age at vaginal opening of female Mongolian gerbils as one of a number of measures of their rate of maturation (Clark & Galef, 1985). We found that age at vaginal introitus was bimodally distributed in our colony; some females exhibited vaginal perforation before their eyes opened on Day 16 postpartum, others only after they were weaned on Day 25, and there was a period from Day 22 to 27 when essentially no vaginal opening occurred (Clark, Spencer, & Galef, 1986).

When we examined the entire reproductive lives of samples of these early- and late-maturing gerbils, we found marked differences in their reproductive profiles. Early-maturing females (a) were less likely to behave aggressively toward others; (b) were more likely to be impregnated by strange males with whom they were paired than were late-maturing females (Clark et al., 1986); (c) reproduced for the first time at an earlier age; (d) had more litters during their lifetimes; (e) produced more young in each litter and, consequently, over a lifetime; and (f) produced more than twice as many offspring as did late-maturing females.

Further, at both delivery and weaning, litters of early-maturing females contained a greater proportion of daughters than did litters of late-maturing females, and a greater proportion of the females in the litters of early-maturing than of late-maturing females were themselves early-maturing.

Early-maturing females spent less time and effort caring for their offspring than did late-maturing females: Late-maturing females spent more time nursing their young and were more likely to retrieve pups displaced from the nest than were early-maturing females (Clark & Galef, 1986).

Some differences in the reproductive behavior of early- and late-maturing females reflected reliable differences in their ages at parturition or in the sizes and sex ratios of the litters they delivered. However, even when we controlled experimentally for such factors, differences in the sex ratios of litters produced by early- and late-maturing females persisted, as did differences in the age at sexual maturation of their daughters (Clark & Galef, 1986).

As mentioned previously, early-maturing female gerbils tend to be born as members of relatively large, female-biased litters, whereas late-maturing females are more often members of relatively small, male-biased litters. A necessary consequence of changes in the size or sex composition of litters is change in the probability that any fetus in those litters will occupy an IUP between either two males or two females: As the proportion of males in a litter increases, the probability that a fetus in that litter will occupy a 2M IUP increases; and as the size of a litter decreases, the probability of a fetus being located at the end of a line of pups in a uterine horn increases, so the probability of its being between two fetuses of either sex decreases. Consequently, it seemed reasonable to ask whether, for example, the correlation we had observed between age at sexual maturation of a dam and age at sexual maturation of her daughters was mediated by differences in the IUPs occupied by daughters born to mothers that had matured early or late.

In fact, we found that both the sex ratios of the litters a gerbil dam produced and the rates of maturation of her daughters were affected by her IUP: (a) Females from 2M IUPs delivered litters with a reliably greater proportion of males than did females from 2F IUPs (Clark & Galef, 1994, 1995a, 1995b; Clark, Karpiuk, & Galef, 1993; Vandenbergh & Huggett, 1994, reported a similar effect in house mice); and (b) daughters born to both early- and late-maturing gerbil dams that occupied 2F IUPs were almost sure to be early-maturing themselves, whereas daughters from 2M IUPs born to both early- and late-maturing dams produced roughly equal numbers of early- and late-maturing daughters (Clark & Galef, 1988).

We also found that, within each sex, gerbil fetuses from 2M IUPs had higher circulating levels of T than did gerbil fetuses from 2F IUPs (Clark, Crews, & Galef, 1991), a result suggesting that differences in prenatal exposure to T, consequent on IUP, might mediate the differences we had observed in the reproductive profiles of female gerbils from different IUPs.

However, additional findings indicated that differences in the age at vaginal introitus of daughters born to early- and late-maturing dams could not be totally explained in terms of the IUPs that the dams had occupied: 2M daughters of early-maturing dams that gestated in 2M IUPs were twice as likely to mature early as were similarly located daughters of late-maturing dams, and fetuses located in IUPs between one male and one female fetus and gestated by late-maturing dams had higher blood titers of T than did fetuses in similar IUPs that were gestated by early-maturing dams (Clark et al., 1991).

Thus, although IUP accounted for much variance both in age at vaginal opening and circulating levels of T in female gerbil fetuses, there were clearly additional effects of a dam herself on both levels of gonadal hormones to which her young were exposed and rates of maturation of her daughters. Indeed, we found that, on the last day of gestation, late-maturing dams had higher circulating levels of T and lower circulating levels of E than did early-maturing dams (Clark et al., 1991). Probably, effects of gerbil dams on the reproductive life histories of their daughters, like the effects of IUP on reproductive life histories of female Mongolian gerbils, are mediated by variance in prenatal exposure to gonadal hormones.

Caution in interpreting the correlations between circulating levels of T and E in dams late in gestation and the reproductive profiles of the daughters they bear is appropriate, because it is always possible that the sex ratio of the litter that a dam is gestating is affecting her circulating levels of hormones rather than that a dam's endogenous hormone levels are affecting her fetuses. For example, Clark, Crews, and Galef (1993) examined the frequency of T-dependent behaviors exhibited by individual Mongolian gerbils during successive pregnancies and found that, on the last days of gestation, both the number and proportion of males in the litters females were gestating affected the frequency with which those females scent marked (scent marking in female gerbils is an androgen-sensitive behavior). And, as one might expect, on the last day of gestation, the number and percentage of males in the litters females were gestating were positively correlated with their circulating levels of T and negatively correlated with their circulating levels of E (Clark, Crews, & Galef, 1993).

Males. IUP has biologically significant effects on the reproductive profiles of male, as well as female, Mongolian gerbils. Indeed, male gerbils gestated in 2F IUPs appear to be at considerable reproductive disadvantage in comparison with their brothers gestated in 2M IUPs.

To compare the potency of male gerbils from different IUPs, we paired individual adult males that had been gestated in 2M and 2F IUPs with a succession of randomly selected virgin females and examined the size of the litter produced by each female with which a male had been paired. We found that males gestated in 2M IUPs sired significantly more offspring than did males gestated in 2F IUPs (Clark, Tucker, & Galef, 1992; Clark, Vonk, & Galef, 1997).

Although litters sired by 2M males were slightly smaller than those sired by 2F males, the primary cause of the reduced fecundity of males from 2F IUPs was their failure to impregnate their consorts. Males from 2F IUPs were five times more likely than were males from 2M IUPs to fail to impregnate a female during a 3-week period of cohabitation with her (Clark, Tucker, & Galef, 1992).

Observation of the reproductive behavior of males from different IUPs revealed apparent inadequacies in the copulatory performance of 2F males that may help to explain at least some of their lack of success in impregnating females. When paired with an unfamiliar virgin female, 2F males exhibited longer latencies to intromit, longer latencies to ejaculate, and were significantly less likely than were 2M males to achieve ejaculation (Clark, Malenfant, Winter, & Galef, 1990; Clark, Vonk, & Galef, 1997). The observed greater sexual success of 2M than of 2F male Mongolian gerbils is not consistent with vom Saal's (1984, 1989) reports of greater sexual activity in 2F than 2M male house mice. However, the apparent inconsistency probably reflects differences in indices of sexual behavior rather than a true interspecies difference in response to IUP. Reported differences in effects of IUP on parental behavior of male house mice and male Mongolian gerbils (discussed later) may also reflect differences in measurement.

Examination of the genital musculature of 2M male gerbils revealed that their bulbocavernosus and levator ani muscles (which wrap around the base of the penis and rectum and mediate penile reflexes involved in copulation; Hart & Melese-d'Hospital, 1983) were roughly 50% larger than were those of 2F males (Forger, Galef, & Clark, 1996). Such deficits in the genital musculature of males from 2F IUPs may have contributed to their relatively limited reproductive success (Sachs, 1982).

In rats, prenatal exposure to T permanently increases the size of the genital musculature by increasing both the number and size of muscle fibers (Breedlove, Jacobson, Gorski, & Arnold, 1982; Cihak, Gutman, & Hanzlikova, 1970; Tobin &

Joubert, 1991), so it is not unreasonable to propose that differences observed in the genital musculature of Mongolian gerbils from different IUPs reflected, at least in part, differences in levels of prenatal exposure to T.

Male gerbils from 2F IUPs suffer from yet another potential reproductive disadvantage. Female gerbils can discriminate 2M from 2F males on the basis of their scents and, when in estrus, prefer to associate with 2M males. Female gerbils not only scent mark more frequently when they encounter the scent marks of 2M males than when they encounter those of 2F males (Clark & Galef, 1994), they also, when in estrus, choose to spend more time near 2M males than 2F males, when given a choice between them (Clark, Tucker, & Galef, 1992).

The differences in the copulatory behavior of adult males from different IUPs and the differing response of females to 2M and 2F males described here may be a result of differences both in the circulating levels of T in adult males from different IUPs and in the responsiveness of males from different IUPs to whatever T is in their plasma. Adult male gerbils that, as fetuses, occupied 2M IUPs, have higher circulating levels of T than do adult male gerbils that, as fetuses, matured in 2F IUPs (Clark, vom Saal, & Galef, 1992). Castrated 2M males are also more responsive to exogenous T than castrated 2F males (Clark, Bishop, vom Saal, & Galef, 1993). Consequently, 2M males should be more likely to express T-sensitive behavioral and morphological characteristics than are their 2F fellows.

The reduced attractiveness to females and lower sexual competence of 2F male gerbils described earlier are also characteristics one might expect natural selection to have acted vigorously to suppress, and there is some evidence that such selection may be at work. By segregating her male and female fetuses in different uterine horns, a gerbil dam could protect her sons from prenatal contact with females and the reduced attractiveness and potency that such contact entails. In fact, female Mongolian gerbils do tend to gestate their male fetuses in their right and their female fetuses in their left uterine horns, thus producing fewer 2F male offspring and 2M female offspring than one would otherwise expect (Clark & Galef, 1990).

The right ovaries of female gerbils produce a greater proportion of male-destined eggs than do their left ovaries. Consequently, when we surgically exchanged right and left ovaries within female gerbils, they produced more male fetuses in their left than in their right uterine horns, whereas females whose left and right ovaries we removed and reimplanted in their original locations, continued to produce more males in their right than in their left uterine horns (Clark, Ham, & Galef, 1994).

There is also evidence of a second way in which gerbil dams may be able to increase the future potency of sons. It has been known for some time that the amount of anogenital licking that a male Norway rat pup receives from its dam before it is weaned can influence the pattern of its copulatory behavior as an adult (Moore,

1983). When adult, those male rats that, as pups, were the recipients of relatively large amounts of anogenital licking by their dams exhibited shorter ejaculatory latencies and shorter interintromission intervals than did brothers that received less anogenital grooming. It is, however, not known whether these variations in copulatory behavior affect the ability to impregnate females (Moore, 1983).

We have found that the greater the number of male intrauterine neighbors a male gerbil pup had while a fetus, the more time its dam spends grooming its anogenital area. In 13 of 16 litters containing pups from more than one IUP, males adjacent to greater numbers of males in utero received a greater amount of anogenital grooming from their dam than did male pups adjacent to fewer males in utero (Clark, Bone, & Galef, 1989). And, as mentioned earlier, there is a correlation between the IUP that a male gerbil fetus occupies and its reproductive success when adult; male gerbils from 2F IUPs that receive relatively little maternal anogenital grooming (like male rats that received little maternal anogenital grooming) have longer ejaculation latencies and longer postejaculatory intervals than do male gerbils from 2M IUPs. Consequently, observed effects of IUP on copulatory performance in male gerbils may be mediated by differences in the amount of anogenital grooming that mothers direct toward pups from different IUPs. Experiments needed to directly test that hypothesis have yet to be conducted.

Whatever the underlying mechanism, the relative lack of reproductive success of 2F male gerbils is difficult to understand from an evolutionary perspective. The fitness costs of reduced potency are obvious; its fitness benefits are more difficult to imagine.

In a thoughtful review of the literature on effects of T on the reproductive behavior of birds, Ketterson and Nolan (1994) described several species in which exposure to high levels of T both increases sexual behavior and decreases parental behavior. They discussed such negative correlations among T-sensitive behavioral traits both as design constraints limiting adaptation and as trade-offs persisting because they permit organisms to adjust their reproductive tactics in response to variations in environmental conditions.

We have recently begun to explore the possibility that adult 2F male gerbils (with low circulating levels of T), although clearly less potent than their 2M brothers (with high circulating levels of T), might exhibit compensatory increases in their parental behavior, increasing their reproductive success by increasing the investment they make in the relatively few young that they do produce. To date, the data are promising. At least in the laboratory, 2F male Mongolian gerbils (unlike 2F male mice; vom Saal, 1984, 1989) are consistently more attentive to young of their species than are 2M males (Clark, Desousa, Vonk, & Galef, 1997). Possibly, under adverse environmental conditions, the relatively great investment that 2F male gerbils are willing to make in their offspring compensates for their reduced potency. Experiments needed to directly test that hypothesis have not been conducted.

Effects of IUP on Sexually Dimorphic Asymmetries in Mongolian Gerbils

Informal observation of young gerbils revealed a phenomenon that we rarely saw in young Norway rats, the other rodent species bred in substantial numbers in our vivarium. Because it was not unusual for one of the eyes of a gerbil pup to open 1 or even 2 days before the other, we frequently found gerbil pups with only one of their eyes open.

We became interested in this asynchronous eye opening because our informal observations suggested that there was a correlation between the sex of a pup and the order in which its eyes opened. A formal study revealed that, indeed, the right eyes of female gerbil pups opened first almost twice as often as did the right eyes of male gerbil pups (Clark, Robertson, & Galef, 1993).

Observation of the order of eye opening in cesarean-delivered male and female gerbils from 2M and 2F IUPs revealed further that, regardless of sex, 2F gerbil pups exhibited primacy of right-eye opening (the female pattern) with significantly higher frequency than did 2M gerbil pups. The influence of IUP on lateralization of eye opening is consistent with the hypothesis that prenatal exposure to gonadal hormones causes the sex-correlated asymmetry in eye-opening we had originally observed (Clark, Robertson, & Galef, 1993), and led us to search for other sexually dimorphic asymmetries in these animals.

In a series of studies, we failed to find, in Mongolian gerbils: (a) the sex difference in neonatal postural asymmetry observed in 1-day-old rat pups by both Ross, Glick, and Meilbach (1981) and Rosen, Berrebi, Yutzey, and Denenberg (1983); (b) the sex difference in rotational direction selected by adult rats described by Glick and Ross (1981); or (c) the sex difference in paw preference in a reaching task reported by Collins (1975) in house mice. However, in the course of these unsuccessful studies, we did notice an apparent difference between male and female gerbils in their use of right and left forepaws when standing immobile in the species-typical tripodal stance (see Figure 1).

In a tripodal stance, male gerbils were more likely than were females to rest on their right forepaws and to hold their left forepaws in the air. Regardless of sex, gerbils from 2M IUPs were more likely than were gerbils from 2F IUPs to rest on their right forepaws (Clark, Robertson, & Galef, 1993).

The results of further experiments were consistent with the hypothesis that perinatal exposure to gonadal hormones played a role in development of asymmetry in the tripodal stance of Mongolian gerbils. We found that, as adults, female gerbils that we had injected with low levels of T in the days immediately following their birth were more likely to use their right forelimbs for support when in the tripodal stance (the male pattern) than were control females that we had injected with vehicle. On the other hand, and unexpectedly, male gerbils we injected shortly after birth with low levels of T, as adults, rested on their left forepaws (the female pattern)

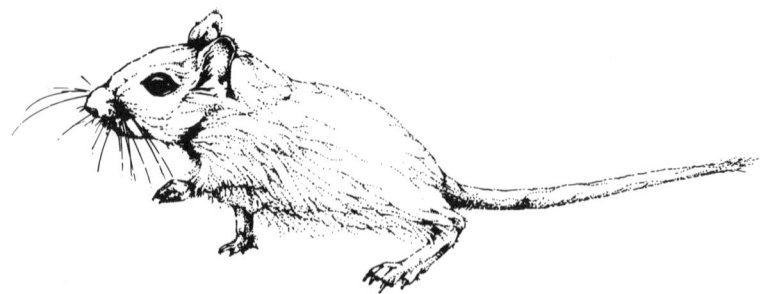

FIGURE 1   Drawing from a photograph of a young adult male gerbil resting on its right forepaw, the male pattern of the tripodal stance.

more frequently than did control subjects injected with oil (Clark, Robertson, & Galef, 1996).

The experimental findings, like those of an earlier report of effects of hormonal manipulations on tail posture in female (but not in male) rats (Rosen et al., 1983), demonstrated effects of perinatal administration of T on behavioral lateralization. Such results are consistent with a larger body of correlational evidence (see Bradshaw & Rogers, 1993; James, 1988; Rogers, 1989, for reviews) that, as Geschwind and Galaburda (1987) hypothesized, implicates T in the development of lateral asymmetries. On the other hand, the direction of the effects we and Rosen et al. (1983) observed were not always consistent with expectations based on the Geschwind and Galaburda (1987) hypothesis. For example, we found that exposing neonatal gerbils to exogenous T increased expression of the female pattern of forepaw use by males and either masculinized or left unaffected the pattern of forepaw use by females, with large doses of T having less effect than small ones (Clark et al., 1996).

EFFECTS OF PERINATAL STRESS ON ADULT REPRODUCTION

The experiments described here demonstrate that experiences of rodents during the perinatal period, especially their prenatal exposure to steroid hormones originating in their uterine neighbors, can have important effects on adult morphology and behavior. Of course, it has been known for some time that variables other than IUP can affect levels of fetal exposure to exogenous gonadal hormones and, consequently, can influence the probability of expression of hormone-sensitive characteristics in adult mammals. In particular, stress applied to pregnant rodents has been shown to affect many of the same anatomical, physiological, and behavioral traits affected by IUP. Age at vaginal opening, length of estrus cycle, and litter sex ratios are all greater in daughters of stressed than unstressed females, and daughters of stressed dams are both less fertile and less fecund than are daughters of unstressed dams (Herrenkohl, 1979; Herrenkohl & Politch, 1978; Kinsley & Svare, 1988; Politch & Herrenkohl, 1984; Ward & Weisz, 1980). Similarly, daughters born to pregnant mice housed at high densities (a potential social stressor) have greater anogenital distances and reduced copulatory receptivity relative to uncrowded control mice (Allen & Haggett, 1977; Zielinski, Vandenbergh, & Montano, 1991).

Sons of stressed rat dams, like their sisters, show effects of the stressors applied to their mothers. Sons of stressed dams are less willing to copulate with females in estrus than are sons of unstressed dams (Ward, 1971). This impairment in the sexual behavior of sons of stressed dams is believed to reflect a shift away from a sensitive period for central nervous system development in the age at which sons of stressed dams experience a species-typical surge in circulating levels of T (Ward & Weisz, 1980).

Given the apparent hormonal basis of effects of both IUP and stress on adult phenotypes, it is not surprising to find also that effects of stressors and IUP interact. For example, vom Saal et al. (1990) reported that stress applied to mice during the last week of their pregnancies results in (a) higher circulating levels of T in both male and female mouse fetuses, and (b) increases in anogenital distance and estrus cycle lengths in 2F, but not in 2M, female mice.

CONCLUSIONS

More than a century ago, Darwin focused attention on the quantitative variation in both morphological and behavioral characteristics to be observed in members of any natural population. Elucidating the mechanisms responsible for such individual differences in phenotype is one of the basic tasks of developmental neuropsychology and psychobiology.

Although we know today that naturally occurring phenotypic variability has both genetic and environmental causes, recent advances in molecular biology have led to an ever-increasing focus on genotype as a source of this variability. Results such as those described here make clear that naturally occurring variation in perinatal experience has effects on adult morphology and behavior that can be as important as those produced by the expression of alternative alleles found in natural populations.

Although there is, as yet, relatively little relevant data, it seems reasonable to suppose that normally occurring variation in perinatal exposure to gonadal hormones can affect temperament and life-history strategy in members of our species as well as others (Udry, Morris, & Kovenock, 1995). Consequently, studies of the effects of normal variation in hormonal exposure caused by gestation in different IUPs in the uteri of litter-bearing rodents may provide more than basic information about sources of phenotypic variability in litter-bearing mammals. Such studies may also provide a useful model system in which to explore the role of normal variation in perinatal exposure to gonadal hormones in producing variation in the morphology and behavior of adult *Homo sapiens*.

ACKNOWLEDGMENTS

Some portions of this review appear in Clark and Galef (in press).

REFERENCES

Allen, T., & Haggett, B. (1977). Group housing of pregnant female mice reduces copulatory receptivity of female progeny. *Physiology & Behavior, 19,* 61–68.

Becker, J. B., Breedlove, S. M., & Crews, D. (1992). *Behavioral endocrinology.* Cambridge, MA: MIT Press.

Bradshaw, J., & Rogers, L. (1993). *The evolution of lateral asymmetries, language, tool use and intellect.* San Diego, CA: Academic.

Breedlove, S. M., Jacobson, C. D., Gorski, R. A., & Arnold, A. P. (1982). Masculinization of the female spinal cord following a single neonatal injection of testosterone propionate but not estradiol benzoate. *Brain Research, 237,* 173–181.

Cihac, R., Gutman, E., & Hanzlikova, V. (1970). Involution and hormone-persistence of the *M. Sphincter (levitor) ani* in female rats. *Journal of Anatomy, 106,* 93–110.

Clark, M. M., Bishop, A. M., vom Saal, F. S., & Galef, B. G., Jr. (1993). Responsiveness to testosterone of male gerbils from known intrauterine positions. *Physiology & Behavior, 53,* 1183–1187.

Clark, M. M., Bone, S., & Galef, B. G., Jr. (1989). Intrauterine positions and schedules of urination: Correlates of differential maternal anogenital stimulation. *Developmental Psychobiology, 22,* 389–400.

Clark, M. M., Crews, D., & Galef, B. G., Jr. (1991). Concentrations of sex steroid hormones in pregnant and fetal Mongolian gerbils. *Physiology & Behavior, 49,* 239–243.

Clark, M. M., Crews, D., & Galef, B. G., Jr. (1993). Androgen mediated effects of male fetuses on the behavior of dams late in pregnancy. *Developmental Psychobiology, 26,* 25–35.

Clark, M. M., Desousa, D., Vonk, J., & Galef, B. G., Jr. (1997). Parenting and potency: Alternate routes to reproductive success in male Mongolian gerbils. *Animal Behaviour, 54,* 635–642.

Clark, M. M., & Galef, B. G., Jr. (1985). Measures of growth, development and sexual maturation in Mongolian gerbils (*Meriones unguiculatus*): Effects of photic period during ontogeny. *Developmental Psychobiology, 18,* 191–202.

Clark, M. M., & Galef, B. G., Jr. (1986). Postnatal effects on reproduction and maternal care in early- and late-maturing gerbils. *Physiology & Behavior, 36,* 997–1003.

Clark, M. M., & Galef, B. G., Jr. (1988). Effects of uterine position on rate of sexual development in female Mongolian gerbils. *Physiology & Behavior, 42,* 15–18.

Clark, M. M., & Galef, B. G., Jr. (1990). Sexual segregation in the left and right horns of gerbil uterus: "The male embryo is usually on the right and the female on the left" (Hippocrates). *Developmental Psychobiology, 23,* 29–38.

Clark, M. M., & Galef, B. G., Jr. (1994). Sex-ratio and inheritance. *Nature, 367,* 327–328.

Clark, M. M., & Galef, B. G., Jr. (1995a). A gerbil dam's fetal intrauterine position affects the sex ratios of the litters she gestates. *Physiology & Behavior, 57,* 297–299.

Clark, M. M., & Galef, B. G., Jr. (1995b). Prenatal influences on reproductive life-history strategies. *Trends in Ecology & Evolution, 10,* 151–153.

Clark, M. M., & Galef, B. G., Jr. (in press). Perinatal influences on the reproductive behavior of adult rodents. In T. Mousseau & C. Fox (Eds.), *Maternal effects as adaptations.* New York: Oxford University Press.

Clark, M. M., Ham, M., & Galef, B. G., Jr. (1994). Differences in the sex ratios of offspring originating in the left and right ovaries of Mongolian gerbils *(Meriones unguiculatus). Journal of Reproduction and Fertility, 101,* 393–396.

Clark, M. M., Karpiuk, P., & Galef, B. G., Jr. (1993). Hormonally mediated inheritance of acquired characteristics in Mongolian gerbils. *Nature, 364,* 712.

Clark, M. M., Malenfant, S. A., Winter, D. A., & Galef, B. G., Jr. (1990). Fetal uterine position affects copulation and scent marking by adult male gerbils. *Physiology & Behavior, 47,* 301–305.

Clark, M. M., Robertson, R. K., & Galef, B. G., Jr. (1993). Intrauterine position effects on sexually dimorphic asymmetries of Mongolian gerbils: Testosterone, eye opening, and paw preference. *Developmental Psychobiology, 26,* 185–194.

Clark, M. M., Robertson, R. K., & Galef, B. G., Jr. (1996). Effects of perinatal testosterone on handedness of gerbils: Support for part of the Geschwind–Galaburda hypothesis. *Behavioral Neuroscience, 110,* 1–5.

Clark, M. M., Spencer, C. A., & Galef, B. G., Jr. (1986). Reproductive life history correlates of early and late sexual maturation in Mongolian gerbils *(Meriones unguiculatus). Animal Behaviour, 34,* 551–560.

Clark, M. M., Tucker, L., & Galef, B. G., Jr. (1992). Stud males and dud males: Intrauterine position effects on the reproductive success of male gerbils. *Animal Behaviour, 43,* 215–221.

Clark, M. M., vom Saal, F. S., & Galef, B. G., Jr. (1992). Foetal intrauterine position correlates with endogenous testosterone levels of adult male Mongolian gerbils. *Physiology & Behavior, 51,* 957–960.

Clark, M. M., Vonk, J. M., & Galef, B. G., Jr. (1997). Reproductive profiles of adult Mongolian gerbils gestated as the sole fetuses in a uterine horn. *Physiology & Behavior, 61,* 77–81.

Clemens, L. G., Gladue, B. A., & Coniglio, L. P. (1978). Prenatal endogenous androgenic influences on masculine sexual behavior and genital morphology in male and female rats. *Hormones and Behavior, 10,* 40–53.

Collins, R. L. (1975). When left-handed mice live in right-handed worlds. *Science, 187,* 181–184.

Even, M. D., Dhar, M. G., & vom Saal, F. S. (1992). Transport of steroids between fetuses via amniotic fluid in relation to the intrauterine position phenomenon in rats. *Journal of Reproduction and Fertility, 96,* 709–716.

Even, M. D., & vom Saal, F. S. (1991). Seminal vesicle and preputial gland response to steroids in male mice is influenced by prior intrauterine position. *Physiology & Behavior, 51,* 11–16.

Forger, N., Galef, B. G., Jr., & Clark, M. M. (1996). Intrauterine position affects motoneuron number and muscle size in a sexually dimorphic neuromuscular system. *Brain Research, 735,* 119–124.

Gandelman, R., vom Saal, F. S., & Reinisch, J. M. (1977). Contiguity to male foetuses affects morphology and behavior of female mice. *Nature, 266,* 722–724.

Geschwind, N., & Galaburda, A. M. (1987). *Cerebral lateralization.* Cambridge, MA: MIT Press.

Glick, S. D., & Ross, D. A. (1981). Right-sided population bias and lateralization of activity in normal rats. *Brain Research, 205,* 222–225.

Hart, B. L., & Melese-d'Hospital, P. Y. (1983). Penile mechanisms and the role of the striated penile muscles in penile reflexes. *Physiology & Behavior, 31,* 807–813.

Herrenkohl, L. (1979). Prenatal stress reduces fertility and fecundity in female offspring. *Science, 206,* 1097–1099.

Herrenkohl, L., & Politch, J. (1978). Effects of prenatal stress on the estrus cycle of female offspring as adults. *Experientia, 34,* 1240–1241.

Houtsmuller, E. J., Juranek, J., Gebauer, C. E., Slob, A. K., & Rowland, D. L. (1994). Males located caudally in the uterus affect sexual behavior of male rats in adulthood. *Behavioural Brain Research, 62,* 119–125.

Houtsmuller, E. J., & Slob, A. K. (1990). Masculinization and defeminization of female rats by males located caudally in the uterus. *Physiology & Behavior, 48,* 555–560.

James, W. H. (1988). Testosterone levels, handedness and sex ratio at birth. *Journal of Theoretical Biology, 133,* 261–266.

Jubilan, B. M., & Nyby, J. G. (1992). The intrauterine position phenomenon and precopulatory behaviors of house mice. *Physiology & Behavior, 51,* 857–872.

Ketterson, E. D., & Nolan, V. (1994). Hormones and life histories: An integrative approach. In L. A. Real (Ed.), *Behavioral mechanisms in evolutionary ecology* (pp. 327–353). Chicago: University of Chicago Press.

Kinsley, C. H., Konen, C. M., Miele, J. L., Ghiraldi, L. A., & Svare, B. (1986). Intrauterine position modulates maternal behaviors in female mice. *Physiology & Behavior, 36,* 793–799.

Kinsley, C., Miele, J., Wagner, C. K., Ghiraldi, L., Broida, J., & Svare, B. (1986). Prior intrauterine position influences body weight in male and female mice. *Hormones and Behavior, 20,* 201–211.

Kinsley, C., & Svare, B. (1988). Prenatal stress alters maternal aggression in mice. *Physiology & Behavior, 42,* 7–13.

Meisel, R. L., & Ward, I. (1981). Fetal female rats are masculinized by male littermates located caudally in the uterus. *Science, 213,* 239–241.

Moore, C. L. (1983). Maternal contributions to the development of masculine sexual behavior in laboratory rats. *Developmental Psychobiology, 17,* 347–356.

Nonneman, D. J., Ganjam, V. K., Welshons, W. V., & vom Saal, F. S. (1992). Intrauterine position effects on steroid metabolism and steriod receptors of reproductive organs in male mice. *Biology of Reproduction, 47,* 723–729.

Politch, J., & Herrenkohl, L. (1984). Effects of prenatal stress on reproduction in male and female mice. *Physiology & Behavior, 32,* 95–99.

Richmond, G., & Sachs, B. D. (1984). Further evidence for masculinization of female rats by males located caudally *in utero. Hormones and Behavior, 18,* 484–490.

Rogers, L. J. (1989). Laterality in animals. *International Journal of Comparative Psychology, 3,* 5–25.

Rosen, G. D., Berrebi, A. S., Yutzey, D. A., & Denenberg, V. H. (1983). Prenatal testosterone causes shift of asymmetry in neonatal tail posture of the rat. *Developmental Brain Research, 9,* 99–101.

Ross, D. A., Glick, S. D., & Meilbach, R. C. (1981). Sexually dimorphic brain and behavioral asymmetries in the neonatal rat. *Proceedings of the National Academy of Sciences, 78,* 1958–1961.

Sachs, B. D. (1982). Role of the rat's striated penile muscles in penile reflexes, copulation and the induction of pregnancy. *Journal of Reproduction and Fertility, 66,* 433–443.

Simon, N. G., & Cologer-Clifford, A. (1991). In utero contiguity to males does not influence morphology, behavioral sensitivity to testosterone of hypothalamic androgen binding in CF-1 female mice. *Hormones and Behavior, 25,* 518–530.

Tobin, C., & Joubert, Y. (1991). Testosterone-induced development of the rat levator ani muscle. *Developmental Biology, 146,* 131–138.

Udry, J. R., Morris, N. M., & Kovenock, J. (1995). Androgen effects on women's gendered behavior. *Journal of Biosocial Science, 27,* 359–368.

Vandenbergh, J. G., & Huggett, C. L. (1994). Mother's prior intrauterine position affects the sex ratio of her offspring in house mice. *Proceedings of the National Academy of Sciences, USA, 91,* 11055–11059.

Vandenbergh, J. G., & Huggett, C. L. (1995). The anogenital distance index, a predictor of the intrauterine position effects on reproduction in female house mice. *Laboratory Animal Science, 45,* 567–573.

Vom Saal, F. S. (1984). The intrauterine position phenomenon: Effects on physiology, aggressive behavior and population dynamics in house mice. In K. Flannelly, R. Blanchard, & D. Blanchard (Eds.), *Biological perspectives on aggression* (pp. 135–179). New York: Liss.

Vom Saal, F. S. (1989). Sexual differentiation in litter-bearing mammals: Influence of sex of adjacent fetuses in utero. *Journal of Animal Science, 67,* 1824–1840.

Vom Saal, F. S., & Bronson, F. (1978). In utero proximity of female mouse fetuses to males: Effect on reproductive performance during later life. *Biology of Reproduction, 19,* 842–853.

Vom Saal, F. S., & Bronson, F. H. (1980). Sexual characteristics of adult female mice are correlated with their blood testosterone levels during prenatal development. *Science, 208,* 597–599.

Vom Saal, F. S., & Dhar, M. G. (1992). Blood flow in the uterine loop artery and loop vein is bidirectional in the mouse: Implications for transport of steroids between fetuses. *Physiology & Behavior, 52,* 163–171.

Vom Saal, F. S., Grant, W., McMullen, C., & Laves, K. (1983). High fetal estrogen titers correlate with enhanced sexual performance and decreased aggression in male mice. *Science, 220,* 1306–1308.

Vom Saal, F. S., Quadagno, D. M., Even, M. D., Keisler, L. W., Keisler, D. H., & Kahn, S. (1990). Paradoxical effects of maternal stress on fetal steroids and postnatal reproductive traits in female mice from different intrauterine positions. *Biology of Reproduction, 43,* 751–761.

Ward, I. L. (1971). Prenatal stress feminizes and demasculinizes the behavior of males. *Science, 175,* 82–84.

Ward, I. L., & Weisz, J. (1980). Maternal stress alters plasma testosterone in fetal males. *Science, 207,* 328–329.

Zielinski, W. J., Vandenbergh, J. G., & Montano, M. M. (1991). Effects of social stress and intrauterine position on sexual phenotypes in wild-type house mice (*Mus musculus*). *Physiology & Behavior, 49,* 117–123.

The Female Phenotype: Nature's Default?

Roslyn Holly Fitch
Biobehavioral Sciences Graduate Degree Program
University of Connecticut, Storrs

Patricia E. Cowell
Department of Human Communication Sciences
University of Sheffield
Sheffield, England

Victor H. Denenberg
Biobehavioral Sciences Graduate Degree Program
University of Connecticut, Storrs

Traditional mammalian developmental models focus on the presence or absence of testosterone as the critical factor differentiating males from females. In this view, a female phenotype occurs by default in the absence of masculinizing hormones. Accumulating evidence, however, suggests that ovarian hormones also play an important role in development of the female brain. The existence of an active ovarian influence on female development (which supplements passive feminization via the absence of testosterone) changes our assumptions and ideas about sexual differentiation and has important theoretical and scientific implications for the study of behavioral similarities and differences between the sexes, and their neural substrates.

"Accuse not nature: She hath done her part."

—John Milton

Requests for reprints should be sent to Roslyn Holly Fitch, Biobehavioral Sciences Graduate Degree Program, University of Connecticut, Box U-154, Horsebarn Hill Road, Storrs, CT 06269. E-mail: hfitch@psych.psy.uconn.edu

The traditional model of mammalian sexual differentiation asserts that each critical stage relies on the production of a substance by the male—Testis Determination Factor, Mullerian Inhibiting Substance, and ultimately, testosterone. In contrast, the female is assumed to develop via a passive or default mechanism in the absence of proactive factors including gonadal steroids. Despite the wide acceptance of this model, researchers have previously suggested that estrogen (presumably of ovarian origin) plays an active role in feminization of the brain (e.g., Dohler, 1991; Dohler, Hancke, et al., 1984; Fitch & Denenberg, 1995, in press; Gerall, Dunlap, & Hendricks, 1973; Hendricks, 1992; Toran-Allerand, 1976, 1992), and evidence to support this view has accumulated in the animal literature over the past 20 years.

ANIMAL STUDIES

In studies of rodents, prepubertal ovariectomy (OVX) has been found to significantly alter a variety of sexually dimorphic behaviors in a male-typical direction, including decreased receptive sexual behavior (lordosis; Blizard & Denef, 1973; Sodersten, 1976), decreased proceptive sexual behavior (darting, hopping, ear wiggling; Gerall et al., 1973), decreased open field behavior (Blizard & Denef, 1973; Denti & Negroni, 1975; Stewart & Cygan, 1980), decreased activity in a plus maze (Leret, Molina-Holgado, & Gonzalez, 1994; Zimmerberg & Farley, 1993), depressed active avoidance performance (Denti & Negroni, 1975), and decreased behavioral response to amphetamine (AMPH; Forgie & Stewart, 1994). At the anatomical level, neonatal treatment with an estrogen antagonist or estrogen mRNA antisense has been shown to reduce the volume of the sexually dimorphic nucleus of the preoptic area (SDN–POA) in female rats (Dohler, Hancke, et al., 1984; Dohler, Srivastava, et al., 1984; McCarthy, Schlenker, & Pfaff, 1993). Prepubertal OVX has been found to increase cortical thickness (Diamond, Johnson, & Ehlert, 1979; Stewart & Kolb, 1988) and cross-sectional size of the corpus callosum (CC; Fitch, Cowell, Schrott, & Denenberg, 1991; Mack, Cowell, & Denenberg, 1992; Mack, Fitch, et al., 1996) in female rats, whereas OVX followed by estrogen treatment was found to decrease cortical thickness (Pappas, Diamond, & Johnson, 1979) and callosal size (Mack, Fitch, Cowell, Schrott, & Denenberg, 1993) relative to OVX only. One study found prepubertal OVX to alter patterns of asymmetry in cortical thickness (Diamond, Dowling, & Johnson, 1981), although another group failed to replicate this finding (Stewart & Kolb, 1988). Prepubertal OVX was also found to prevent a female-typical loss of dendritic spines in the visual cortex of rats (Munoz-Cueto, Garcia-Segura, & Ruiz-Marcos, 1990).

Some feminizing effects of ovarian steroids have also been observed when male rats are gonadectomized. Specifically, neonatal gonadectomy followed by low-dose estrogen was found to lower spatial behavior in male rats to female-typical levels (Dawson, Cheung, & Lau, 1975), and postpubertal gonadectomy followed by low-dose estrogen and progesterone treatment was found to enlarge a hypothalamic nucleus normally larger in female as compared to male rats (the anteroventral preoptic nucleus or AVPv; Bloch & Gorski, 1988), as well as decreasing the size of other hypothalamic nuclei to female-typical size.

Other effects of ovarian steroids on neurophysiology and neurochemistry have been seen in the adult female brain, although these effects are largely nonpermanent (i.e., are transient, or activational). OVX and estrogen replacement have been shown to alter dendritic spine density of ventromedial hypothalamic neurons, and this measure varies endogenously across the estrous cycle (Frankfurt, Gould, Woolley, & McEwen, 1990). Similarly, exposure to pulsatile estrogen was shown to potentiate dopaminergic and behavioral response to AMPH in female but not male rats, and this responsiveness also varies across the estrous cycle in females (Becker, 1990; Becker & Cha, 1989; Castner & Becker, 1990; Forgie & Stewart, 1994). Adult OVX has been shown to lead to an increase in dendritic arbor of pyramidal neurons in parietal cortex (Stewart & Kolb, 1994), as well as a decrease in hippocampal dendritic spine density (Gould, Woolley, Frankfurt, & McEwen, 1990). The latter effect is blocked by concurrent treatment with estrogen and progesterone. Moreover, hippocampal dendritic spine density was shown to vary across the estrous cycle (Woolley, Gould, Frankfurt, & McEwen, 1990; Woolley & McEwen, 1992).

These findings are all consistent with an active role for ovarian steroids in development and phenotypic characterization (i.e., differentiation) of the female brain, including evidence that specific neurophysiologic and neurochemical parameters of the female brain vary with fluctuating levels of ovarian hormones. These latter findings suggest that chronic cyclicity is not merely a feature of the hypothalamic–pituitary–gonadal axis in females, but that it also has critical neurophysiologic consequences for the intact female brain. The relevance of this issue to sexual differentiation is discussed further later.

Given the long-standing observation that masculinization of many systems is dependent on the biosynthesis of estrogen from testosterone (intracellular aromatization; see Toran-Allerand, 1984, 1986, for reviews), one might question how estrogen could exert masculinizing effects in males and concomitant feminizing effects in females. We suggest three interrelated mechanisms that could account for these sexually dimorphic estrogenic effects: (a) marked sex differences in estrogen levels (high for aromatized estrogen in males, relatively low for estrogen of ovarian origin in females); (b) documented variation in topographic distribution and density of target estrogen receptor populations as a function of sex (Brown, MacLusky, Shanabrough, & Naftolin, 1990; DonCarlos & Handa, 1994; Kuhnemann, Brown, Hochberg, & MacLusky, 1994) and age (MacLusky, Chaptal, & McEwen, 1979; MacLusky, Lieberburg, & McEwen, 1979; Miranda & Toran-Allerand, 1992; O'Keefe & Handa, 1990; Shugrue, Stumpf, MacLusky, Zielinsky, & Hochberg, 1990), and (c) evidence of sex differences in critical periods for estrogen action. Although the first two points are relatively straightforward, evidence to support a temporal distinction in sensitive periods for testicular and ovarian effects is discussed in further detail later.

The concept of critical, or sensitive, periods in development has played a central role in theories of sexual differentiation. Accumulated evidence has led to the view that testosterone exerts masculinizing effects on the central nervous system of male rats during the period between about gestational Day 17 and postnatal Days 8 to 10, depending on the system being studied (e.g., Rhees, Shryne, & Gorski, 1990a, 1990b; but see Bloch & Mills, 1995). This perinatal period of sensitivity to the masculinizing effects of testosterone appears to be similar in mice (e.g., see Wagner & Clemens, 1989). In the case of the rat CC, masculinization of gross anatomy appears to result purely from the prenatal action of testicular androgens (Mack, McGivern, Hyde, & Denenberg, 1996).

A different set of temporal parameters appears to apply to female brain development. The sensitive period for permanent structural and behavioral ovarian effects does not end by Day 10 in female rodents, as generally appears to be true in males, but, depending on the system under study, appears to extend much later in life. Support for a later sensitive period in females includes evidence that: (a) prepubertal OVX decreases female sexual behavior (Gerall et al., 1973), (b) exposure to low doses of estrogen as late as Day 30 to 40 increases the open field behavior of OVX rats to female-typical levels (Stewart & Cygan, 1980), (c) OVX on Days 25 to 26 decreases the locomotor response to AMPH in female rats (Forgie & Stewart, 1994), (d) ethinylestradiol exposure from Days 40 to 90 leads to a thinner cortex in ovariectomized female rats (Pappas et al., 1979), (e) OVX of female rats on Day 30 prevents the female-typical decrease in cortical pyramidal dendritic spines (Munoz-Cueto et al., 1990), and (f) Day 12 OVX significantly increases callosal size in female rats to that of males, whereas estrogen replacement to OVX females commencing on Day 25 decreases callosal size below intact female values (Fitch et al., 1991, Mack et al., 1992; Mack et al., 1993). In addition, postpubertal castration of male rats followed by low-dose estrogen and progesterone treatment increases the size of the AVPv hypothalamic nucleus and decreases the size of other sexually dimorphic nuclei (Bloch & Gorski, 1988). These findings all suggest a sensitive period for ovarian effects on neurophysiology that extends up to or around puberty in rodents.

Thus, it may be that an early and high level of intracellular estrogen in males (derived from aromatization of testosterone) interacts with sex- and age-specific estrogen receptor populations to induce male-typical characteristics, whereas a later and lower level of estrogen (of ovarian origin) in females interacts with sex- and age-specific estrogen receptor populations to induce female-typical characteristics. Work by Stewart and Cygan (1980; see also Stewart, Vallentyne, & Meaney, 1979) highlights this distinction by demonstrating masculinizing effects of early high-dose estrogen treatment (25 ug estradiol benzoate on P2 and 3) and feminizing effects of later low-dose estrogen replacement (silastic implants of estradiol 17B on P30–40, delivering physiological levels of about 108 pg/ml serum) on ovariectomized female rats, for the same measure of open field behavior.

HUMAN STUDIES

Clearly, evidence from animal studies supports the role of ovarian hormones in normative development of the female brain. In the human literature there also exists growing evidence pointing to an active role for ovarian hormones in neurobehavioral function across the life span (e.g., Hampson, 1990; Hampson & Kimura, 1988; Kimura & Hampson, 1993; Sherwin, 1994). For example, one study found that sex differences in size of the fiber tract interconnecting the cerebral hemispheres, the corpus callosum, were highly dependent on age. Specifically, anterior regions in the callosa of women continued to increase in size even through the 5th decade, whereas male anterior callosal measures appeared to peak in the 2nd to 3rd decades and decline in size thereafter (Cowell, Allen, Zalatimo, & Denenberg, 1992). Another recent study suggested that these differences in gross anatomy may be related to particular cytoarchitectural components of the anterior CC that continue to develop well into adulthood in women but not men (Aboitiz, 1996).

There are multiple factors that may contribute to these divergent paths of callosal development across the human life span. It is possible that high levels of estrogen in the early childbearing years have an inhibitory effect on CC growth, and that this inhibition declines with gradual reductions in estrogen levels through midadulthood. It is also possible that differences in interhemispheric function influence sex-specific trends in anterior CC size. For example, it has been shown in women that certain lexical and rhyming tasks involve activation of right and left language centers in the frontal lobe, which sends fibers through the anterior CC (Shaywitz et al., 1995; Wood, Flowers, & Naylor, 1991). In men, these same tasks are associated primarily with activation of the left hemisphere, which would suggest the need for a different pattern of interhemispheric connections as compared to women.

In addition to these differing CC developmental trends in early to middle adulthood, evidence suggests that the anterior CC in women declines in width to the size seen in men by the 7th decade of life (Cowell et al., 1994). These combined results suggest that estrogen may play a complex, multidimensional role in the neurophysiology of the CC across the female life span, including specific inhibition of the attainment of maximum adult size, maintenance of fiber tracts needed for female-typical patterns of cerebral asymmetry, and possibly general neuroprotectivity against the effects of age (Cowell et al., 1994). However, the effects of advanced age on the female brain appear to vary from region to region. Thus, as seen in animals, the effects of estrogen in humans may vary depending on which aspect of the female brain or behavior is examined. For example, age-related decreases in volume in the human brain are greater in men than in women in the frontal and temporal cortices (Cowell et al., 1994; Murphy et al., 1996), whereas in the parietal cortex and hippocampus, decrements are greater in women than in men (Murphy et al., 1996). Further research will be required to resolve (a) which human neurobehavioral systems showing sex differences in aging are under the direct influence of endocrine changes, and (b) whether such sex differences arise as a function of hormonal fluctuations in women, men, or both.

Neurocognitive studies on the role of ovarian hormones have also revealed significant effects of estrogen decline in middle adulthood and estrogen replacement therapy after menopause. Preliminary evidence suggests that estrogen depletion and replacement modulate a wide array of cognitive, emotional, and neurophysiological factors (e.g., Kampen & Sherwin, 1994; Paganini-Hill & Henderson, 1994; Schneider, Farlow, Henderson, & Pogoda, 1996). The clinical relevance of conceptual modifications to the study of sexual dimorphism in humans is clear. The next step in this area of research is to systematically examine the effects of hormone treatment on the brain structure and function of menopausal women with and without estrogen, healthy women with variations in estrogen exposure (e.g., birth control pills, pregnancy; see Szekely, Hampson, Carey, & Goodale, this issue), and individuals with clinical syndromes involving endocrine dysfunction.

Preliminary evidence from patients with endocrine dysfunction, in fact, suggests an active role for ovarian hormones in normative female development. For example, it has long been known that women with Turner's syndrome (a genetic disorder characterized by one X chromosome and ovarian dysgenesis) show a wide array of phenotypic alterations and cognitive deficits (e.g., Collaer & Hines, 1995; Ross, Stefanatos, Roeltgen, Kushner, & Cutler, 1995; see also Buchanan, Pavlovic, & Rovet, this issue). More recently, it has also been shown that the brains of girls with Turner's syndrome are characterized by a variety of anomalies in parietal cortex (Murphy et al., 1993; Reiss, Mazzacocco, Greenlaw, Freund, & Ross, 1995) and hippocampus (Murphy, 1993). Taken together with the findings on the aging female brain (Murphy et al., 1996), these findings indicate maintenance of the parietal lobe and hippocampus may require estrogen levels higher than those in both Turner's syndrome girls and healthy women above the age of 60. Because spatial ability is adversely affected in women with Turner's syndrome (Reiss et al., 1995), in healthy aging women (see Halpern, 1992), and in aging women with memory loss (Small, LaRue, Komo, Kaplan, & Mandelkern, 1995), one may speculate that the early development and continued maintenance of the parietal cortex, hippocampus, and related cognitive functions involve both an early and an extended sensitivity of the female brain to estrogen.

Clearly, the animal and human literatures reviewed here provide a strong basis for the assertion that ovarian hormones influence development, organization, and function of the female brain across the life span. These findings should not cause

THE FEMALE PHENOTYPE 219

us to abandon the traditional model of androgen-mediated sexual differentiation, but rather to call for the supplementation of this model via recognition of active ovarian effects on female development (which are distinct from the passive component of female development that occurs in the absence of testosterone). Moreover, although the findings just discussed strongly support the importance of normal ovarian function for neurodevelopment in females, some of the theoretical implications of revising our model of sexual differentiation are more subtle and pertain to our philosophical understanding of and approach to sex difference research in general. Several such issues are discussed in the following section.

IMPLICATIONS OF OVARIAN EFFECTS ON NEUROPHYSIOLOGY FOR SEX DIFFERENCE RESEARCH

Implications for Evolutionary Perspectives on Sexual Differentiation

Neuroendocrinologists interested in evolutionary pressures on sex-specific patterns of development (i.e., the selective advantage underlying sex-specific patterns of differentiation) suggest that the female phenotype emerges via passive mechanisms because the mammalian fetus already develops within an intense milieu of female (maternal ovarian) hormones. Thus, the production of hormones by the fetal ovaries would be inconsequential relative to the overwhelming presence of maternal ovarian hormones. In contradistinction to the lack of gonadal activation on the part of the female fetus, to prompt the development of a fetus with features distinct from those of the mother (i.e., a male) something different (testosterone) must be added to the in utero maternal–fetal mix. From this perspective, testicular activity can have an early (prenatal) onset, whereas ovarian activity would be delayed until after birth and the dissipation of maternal ovarian hormones.

Moreover, in many species the fetus appears to avoid developmental consequences of exposure to maternal ovarian hormones altogether, via the presence of steroid-binding blood-borne proteins (e.g., alpha-fetoprotein, which binds and inactivates plasma estrogen). In rodents, circulating alpha-fetoprotein levels are high prenatally and in the immediate postnatal period, but decline by around Day 7 (Ali, Kaul, & Sahib, 1981; Ali & Sahib, 1983; Raynaud, Mercier-Bodard, & Baulieu, 1971). The presence of alpha-fetoprotein could thus cancel any developmental consequences of ovarian hormones—of either maternal or fetal origin—during the prenatal and early postnatal period.

This evidence strongly suggests little advantage for ovarian activity during the prenatal and early postnatal period. Accordingly, evidence shows that the female ovaries become active much later in development than the testes. In rodents, the testes secrete significant amounts of testosterone as early as embryonic Day 17, whereas the ovaries do not appear to secrete active substances until around the 2nd postnatal week (Funkenstein, Nimrod, & Lindner, 1980; Levina, Gyevai, & Horvath, 1975; Mannan & O'Shaughnessy, 1991; Sokka & Huhtaniemi, 1995; Weniger, Zeis, & Chouraqui, 1993). This series of developmental events would logically necessitate that if fetal ovarian hormones are to have effect, they must do so after the exposure to and clearance of the maternal ones; hence, the need for a later sensitive period for female differentiation. The need for an extended sensitive period in females remains less clear from an early developmental perspective. One possible advantage conferred by an extended sensitivity of neurobehavioral systems to ovarian hormones is a greater degree of ongoing plasticity in certain aspects of the adult female brain, a topic discussed further later.

Implications for Defining the Parameters of Sexual Differentiation

Accumulating evidence suggests that even when subjected to equivalent hormonal priming conditions, the transient changes seen in female neurochemistry, neurophysiology, and behavior in response to fluctuating estrogen cannot always be reproduced in males (e.g., Becker, 1990; Becker & Ramirez, 1981; Forgie & Stewart, 1994; Stewart & Kolb, 1994). These research findings indicate that the initial organization of female brains for cyclicity also has secondary consequences that are expressed as ongoing plasticity of specific neurobehavioral systems. Thus, in addition to changing our views about the factors that play a role in sexual differentiation (i.e., to include reference to ovarian hormones as active participants in the early differentiation process), we must also address and incorporate accumulating evidence for patterns of ongoing neurophysiologic plasticity in the adult female brain. Such phenomena call into question the traditional boundaries defining sexually differentiating factors, that have until now been confined to early organizational (permanent) male–female differences.

The work of Becker and colleagues reveals that postpubertal female brains continue to show neurophysiologic changes throughout adulthood that also act to distinguish them from male brains. Does this indicate that some activational hormonal effects, previously thought to be unrelated to sexual differentiation, may actually reflect another type of critical sex difference? In the past, such effects would probably have been considered irrelevant to sexual differentiation, as they reflect activational (nonpermanent) changes. However, we suggest that if these changes are actually chronic and ongoing across the female life span, then they may also have serious implications for how we define the female brain per se. Although these factors appear to represent critical aspects of female brain organization, they have not, to our knowledge, been adequately addressed within the framework of the sexual differentiation model.

Important examples of ongoing plasticity in the neurophysiology and behavior of the adult human female brain also come from the field of schizophrenia research. The data suggest a clinical course in women that points to a relation between ovarian hormones and symptomatology. Women experience more frequent and severe symptoms and require more medication as they grow older (Seeman, 1983). This pattern contrasts with that seen in men who require less medication with advancing age, and supports the view that declining estrogen levels are a risk factor for female patients with schizophrenia (Seeman, 1983). Women may also experience relative freedom from the acute symptoms of schizophrenia during pregnancy, followed by increased risk of postpartum relapse (Riecher-Rossler, Hafner, Stumbaum, Maurer, & Schmidt, 1994). These trends have led some authors to propose that in some cases, estrogen treatment may be used in conjunction with more conventional medications to aid in the treatment of this disorder (Riecher-Rossler et al., 1994). Indeed, another psychiatric condition, clinical depression associated with menopause, has been shown to respond to estrogen therapy (Sherwin, 1994). Research on the neurobehavioral correlates to estrogen-based treatments for psychiatric disorders provides a unique opportunity to explore further the clinical ramifications and theoretical implications for the notion that the female brain is not simply a male brain minus testosterone, but a uniquely estrogen-dependent system in terms of differentiation, development, and function in later life.

Implications for Traditional Definitions of Feminization and Defeminization

A revised model of sexual differentiation will have repercussions for how we define feminization and defeminization as developmental processes. Defeminization of behavior has been considered to reflect suppression of female attributes, which can occur with early testosterone exposure (e.g., reduction of lordosis behavior in female rats given neonatal testosterone). It is not yet clear how this definition can be reconciled with situations in which evidence shows different behavioral consequences following early androgen exposure versus removal of ovarian hormones. As one example, different effects on the female rat SDN–POA are seen following early androgen exposure that enlarges the SDN–POA to male-like size (Gorski, 1984) versus the estrogen-receptor blocker tamoxifen, which decreases size of the SDN–POA below that seen in normal females (Dohler, Hancke, et al., 1984). Which process is defeminizing? Both treatments affect SDN–POA size in a direction "away from" intact female values.

With respect to behavior, early androgen exposure (e.g., through adrenal hyperplasia) increases visuospatial scores in females (an effect that might be considered defeminizing; Masica, Money, Ehrhardt, & Lewis, 1969; Resnick, Berenbaum, Gottesman, & Bouchard, 1986; see also Hampson et al., this issue). At the same time, evidence suggests that females with Turner's syndrome exhibit ovarian dysgenesis and concomitant deficits in visuospatial skills (although it is not yet clear whether these cognitive effects are genetic, hormonal, or both; e.g., Collaer & Hines, 1995; Ross et al., 1995; see also Buchanan et al., this issue). Based on traditional definitions, it is difficult to ascertain which of these processes would more aptly represent the defeminization of visuospatial behavior.

Previously, use of the behavioral or neuroanatomical end product to define an underlying developmental process as feminizing or defeminizing was possible because of an assumption of movement along a single underlying hormonal axis characterized by more or less exposure to testosterone. However, because the process of sexual differentiation can be shown to reflect dual—perhaps orthogonal—underlying axes of hormonal exposure, it appears that even our basic descriptive terminology must be redefined.

Are Androgenic Masculinization and Estrogenic Feminization Independent or Interactive Processes?

Do both early androgenic induction of male-typical characteristics, and later estrogenic (and perhaps, progesterone-mediated) induction of female-typical characteristics, occur to some extent in both males and females, as both males and females produce all hormones in varying amounts and at different times? Or does early androgen exposure eliminate any later window for feminization? Some data suggest that the ovaries cannot override early androgen exposure in producing female-typical patterns of sexually dimorphic behaviors (e.g., Forgie & Stewart, 1994), whereas others suggest that the presence of the ovaries has a modifying influence on the effects of early androgen exposure (e.g., Blizard & Denef, 1973; Sodersten, 1976). The fact that this issue remains theoretically unresolved and largely ignored in research practice is evident in animal studies in which intact females are used to assess the effects of exogenous androgenic manipulations. In such a paradigm, researchers make the tacit assumption that the presence of the ovaries does not interfere in any way with developmental androgen-based effects. Indeed, gonadectomized females are rarely used as a baseline in hormonal studies, even though control males are routinely gonadectomized to eliminate endogenous hormonal interference. In the human literature, this issue also remains largely unresolved, although it is particularly relevant to individuals with endocrine dysfunction. For example, it is unclear to what degree excess androgen production in females with adrenal hyperplasia interacts with normal ovarian secretions to influence neural development. This issue remains a topic for future research.

Implications for the Study of Sex Differences in Cognition

Group differences in performance. Many of the cognitive behaviors that have been consistently shown to differ in males and females have been attributed to the early effects of androgens (e.g., Benbow, 1988). Animal research supports this assertion by showing neonatal androgen effects on virtually every sexually dimorphic cognitive task that has been studied in animals (see Beatty, 1992, or Van Haaren, Van Hest, & Heinsbroek, 1990, for review). However, evidence suggests that ovarian hormones also affect cognitive performance in animals (e.g., Denti & Negroni, 1975).

As an example of the complex and multidimensional form of some sex differences, we refer to the work of researchers who have looked beyond mean cognitive performance. When we measure spatial navigation behavior in male and female rats, it is tacitly assumed that we are measuring the same underlying process. However, evidence suggests that male and female rats utilize fundamentally different strategies in some forms of maze-learning, and that reliance on a particular strategic approach is influenced by early hormonal exposure (see Williams & Meck, 1991). What implications do these findings have for evidence of sex differences in human cognition?

There are a wide variety of types of sex differences that arise in the human literature and a comprehensive theory should accommodate them all. Effects range from straightforward differences in mean cognitive or behavioral performance to more complex neurobehavioral sex differences such as those documented by Williams and Meck (1991). In some cases, a behavioral measure may not show a mean sex difference at all, and yet reveal a completely different pattern of brain–behavior correlations. For example, Witelson showed that men and women in the same hand preference category (nonconsistent right-handers) had disparate neuroanatomical profiles as measured by regional callosum size and various other cortical measures (Witelson, 1991; Witelson & Kigar, 1992a, 1992b). This research in both rodents and humans outlines a scenario whereby the presence of two distinct hormonal processes in development could account for qualitative, in addition to quantitative, differences in male and female brain organization and cognitive function (see also Halpern, 1992). It is also possible, as with the example of Witelson's work with hand preference, that the presence of masculinizing and feminizing influences in development contribute to different—even orthogonal—patterns of brain organization in men and women with respect to the same cognitive task. Thus, masculinization and feminization processes may produce not merely group differences in mean performance or preferred cognitive strategies, but fundamental sex differences in neurocognitive processing that are not even necessarily observable at the behavioral level. The fact that many sex differences present themselves as differences in cognitive strategies and differences in brain–behavior relations has profound implications for the interpretation of sex differences on standardized tests of cognitive performance.

Mathematical models of group difference and variance. Accumulating evidence also suggests that male and female scores on cognitive tests are not always characterized by equivalent distributions and variances, as assumed within most statistical models (Feingold, 1995). For example, one study determined that female scores on a mental rotation test were bimodal; 80% of the women scored approximately the same as the male group, whereas a second group of women (20%) scored much lower than the men and remaining women (Kail, Carter, & Pelligrino, 1979; see also Favreau & Everett, 1996). Such an observation, although rarely addressed by traditional statistical tests, could reflect the fact that female performance on visuospatial tasks appears to fluctuate on the basis of estrogen exposure (Hampson, 1990), with the implication that a constantly changing subset of normally cycling women tested at any given time might show depressed performance on such a task. Such an interpretation contrasts with the views that (a) there is a fixed subpopulation of women whose visuospatial ability is always lower than the male average; or (b) women, as a population, have lower mean performance than men. The preceding is concerned with variation in female performance across the menstrual cycle. A different phenomenon is that a much higher overall variance in measures of performance on cognitive tasks has been observed for males as compared to females (e.g., Lubinski & Benbow, 1992). This is consistent with evidence of a much higher proportion of males at the high end of the cognitive spectrum (e.g., genius categories; Benbow, 1988), as well as at the low end (e.g., having neurodevelopmental disorders including retardation, autism, dyslexia, and language disorders; Finucci, Isaacs, Whitehouse, & Childs, 1983; Gualtieri & Hicks, 1985; Liederman & Flannery, 1993; Msall, Buck, Rogers, & Catanzaro, 1992; Msall et al., 1993; Neils & Aram, 1986; Spinillo et al., 1995). Commenting on this phenomenon, Geschwind and Galaburda (1985) suggested that males may be at risk for both cognitive disability and genius, due to early exposure to a "male factor," which was most likely testosterone.

Another possibility is that ovarian hormones are actively involved in promoting effective reorganization following neurodevelopmental trauma, and hence may also act to reduce cognitive variance in the female population. Findings that support this view include evidence that estrogen has protective effects against the onset, recurrence, and severity of certain mental disorders such as schizophrenia (Goldstein, Seidman, Santangelo, Knapp, & Tsuang, 1994; Oades & Schepker, 1994; Riecher-Rossler et al., 1994; Seeman, 1983, 1986; Seeman & Lang, 1990), as well as memory loss and Alzheimer's disease after menopause (Kampen & Sherman, 1994; Paganini-Hill & Henderson, 1994; Sherwin, 1994). Within the animal literature, progesterone has been shown to act as a neuroprotectant against cerebral trauma in female rats (Roof, Duvdevani, & Stein, 1993). These findings may be related to observations that female premature infants show better recovery than male premature infants following intracranial hemorrhage, as measured by IQ (Raz et al., 1995), as well as observations that female rats show better cognitive recovery from both neonatal and adult lesions as compared to males (Fitch, Brown, Tallal, & Rosen, 1997; Roof, Zhang, & Glasier, 1993).

The concept that estrogen may play a protective role in females could account for the smaller number of females in the lower tails of cognitive distributions, although it does not account for observations of lower incidence of cognitive genius in females. Perhaps the plasticity resulting from ovarian effects and chronic cyclicity carries (statistically) a cognitive price. Restriction of range at one end of the distribution may cause a restriction at the other end as well. Moreover, endogenous estrogen does not appear to protect against all neurofunctional disorder, as women suffer more frequently than men from certain syndromes such as depressive disorder. The basis for these differing effects is not well understood and clearly requires further empirical study.

We must also acknowledge that models that attribute sex differences in cognition to biologic factors are highly contentious. Controversy surrounds both the assertion of increased developmental disability among boys (which has been attributed to teacher and clinician bias in identifying and referring more boys than girls; e.g., Shaywitz, Escobar, Shaywitz, Fletcher, & Makuch, 1992), and the failure of girls to score at genius levels on standardized tests in equal numbers to boys (an effect that has been attributed to social, parental, and educational bias; see Halpern, 1992). Nevertheless, we must recognize that developmental hormonal factors influence group cognitive performance and variability as a function of sex and, moreover, that the developmental role of ovarian hormones influences patterns and variability of female cognitive performance (both individual variability across time, as well as the population variance) in ways that have not, to date, been addressed theoretically or studied empirically.

SUMMARY

Traditional models of sexual differentiation have emerged from the data showing a powerful influence of testosterone on differentiation of the male phenotype in mammals. Therefore, the work of researchers in this area has rested on the assumption that testosterone exposure represents the single overriding hormonal factor that distinguishes the male from the female neurobehavioral phenotype. The conceptual and empirical repercussions of this assumption to other fields of research (particularly those pertaining to sex differences in brain and behavior) have been profound. In this article, we have reviewed evidence demonstrating that ovarian hormones also play a key role in sexual differentiation of the brain. This evidence prompts a modification of the traditional model of sexual differentiation, specifically the addition of an active developmental role for the ovaries. This conceptual change opens up many new avenues of study in terms of developmental sex differences in both neurophysiology and behavior, and may ultimately affect the way in which we approach this field of research.

REFERENCES

Aboitiz, F. (1996). *Corpus callosum morphology in relation to cerebral asymmetries in the post-mortem human.* Paper presented at The NATO Advanced Study Institute for the Role of the Corpus Callosum in Sensory Motor Integration: Anatomy, Physiology and Behavior; Individual Differences and Clinical Applications, Castelvecchio, Lucca, Italy.

Ali, M., Kaul, H. K., & Sahib, M. K. (1981). Ontogeny and distribution of alpha-fetoprotein in feto-neonatal rat brain. *Brain Research, 227,* 618–621.

Ali, M., & Sahib, M. K. (1983). Changes in alpha-fetoprotein and albumin synthesis rates and their levels during fetal and neonatal development of the rat brain. *Brain Research, 282,* 314–317.

Beatty, W. W. (1992). Gonadal hormones and sex differences in nonreproductive behaviors. In A. A. Gerall, H. Moltz, & I. L. Ward (Eds.), *Handbook of behavioral neurobiology* (Vol. 11, pp. 85–128). New York: Plenum.

Becker, J. B. (1990). Direct effect of 17B-estradiol on striatum: Sex differences in dopamine release. *Synapse, 5,* 157–164.

Becker, J. B., & Cha, J. (1989). Estrous-cycle variation in amphetamine induced behaviors and striatal dopamine release assessed with microdialysis. *Behavioral Brain Research, 35,* 117–125.

Becker, J. B., & Ramirez, V. D. (1981). Experimental studies on the development of sex differences in the release of dopamine from striatal tissue fragments in vitro. *Neuroendocrinology, 32,* 168–173.

Benbow, C. P. (1988). Sex differences in mathematical reasoning ability in intellectually talented pre-adolescents: Their nature, effects and possible causes. *Behavioral and Brain Sciences, 11,* 169–183.

Blizard, D., & Denef, C. (1973). Neonatal androgen effects on open-field activity and sexual behavior in the female rat: The modifying influence of ovarian secretions during development. *Physiology and Behavior, 11,* 65–69.

Bloch, G. J., & Gorski, R. A. (1988). Estrogen/progesterone treatment in adulthood affects the size of several components of the medial preoptic area in the male rat. *Journal of Comparative Neurology, 275,* 613–622.

Bloch, G. J., & Mills, R. (1995). Prepubertal testosterone treatment of neonatally gonadectomized male rats: Defeminization and masculinization of behavioral and endocrine function in adulthood. *Neuroscience and Biobehavioral Reviews, 19,* 187–200.

Brown, T. J., MacLusky, N. J., Shanabrough, M., & Naftolin, F. (1990). Comparison of age- and sex-related changes in cell nuclear estrogen-binding capacity and progestin receptor induction in the rat brain. *Endocrinology, 126,* 2965–2972.

Buchanan, L., Pavlovic, J., & Rovet, J. (1998/this issue). A reexamination of the visuospatial deficit in Turner syndrome: Contributions of working memory. *Developmental Neuropsychology, 14,* 341–367.

Castner, S. A., & Becker, J. B. (1990). Estrogen and striatal dopamine release: A microanalysis study. *Society for Neuroscience Abstracts, 16,* 130.

Collaer, M. L., & Hines, M. (1995). Human behavioral sex differences: A role for gonadal hormones during early development? *Psychological Bulletin, 118,* 55–107.

Cowell, P. E., Allen, L. S., Zalatimo, N. S., & Denenberg, V. H. (1992). A developmental study of sex and age interactions in the human corpus callosum. *Developmental Brain Research, 66,* 187–192.

Cowell, P. E., Turetsky, B. I., Gur, R. C., Shtasel, D. L., Grossman, R. I., & Gur, R. E. (1994). Sex differences in aging of the human frontal and temporal lobes. *Journal of Neuroscience, 14,* 4748–4755.

Dawson, J., Cheung, Y. M., & Lau, R. T. S. (1975). Developmental effects of neonatal sex hormones on spatial and activity skills in the white rat. *Biological Psychology, 3,* 213–229.

Denti, A., & Negroni, J. (1975). Activity and learning in neonatally hormone treated rats. *Acta Physiologica Latinoamerica, 25,* 99–106.

Diamond, M., Dowling, G., & Johnson, R. (1981). Morphologic cerebral cortical asymmetry in male and female rats. *Experimental Neurology, 71,* 261–268.

Diamond, M., Johnson, R. E., & Ehlert, J. (1979). A comparison of cortical thickness in male and female rats—normal and gonadectomized, young and adult. *Behavioral Neurology, 26,* 485–491.

Dohler, K. D. (1991). The pre- and postnatal influence of hormones and neurotransmitters on sexual differentiation of the mammalian hypothalamus. *International Reviews in Cytology, 131,* 1–57.

Dohler, K. D., Hancke, J. L., Srivastava, S. S., Hofmann, C., Shryne, J. E., & Gorski, R. A. (1984). Participation of estrogens in female sexual differentiation of the brain: Neuroanatomical, neuroendocrine and behavioral evidence. In G. J. De Vries, J. P. C. De Bruin, H. B. M. Uylings, & M. A. Corner (Eds.), *Progress in brain research* (Vol. 61, pp. 99–117). New York: Elsevier.

Dohler, K. D., Srivastava, S., Shryne, J., Jarzab, B., Sipos, A., & Gorski, R. A. (1984). Differentiation of the sexually dimorphic nucleus in the preoptic area of the rat brain is inhibited by postnatal treatment with an estrogen antagonist. *Neuroendocrinology, 38,* 297–301.

DonCarlos, L. L., & Handa, R. J. (1994). Developmental profile of estrogen receptor mRNA in the preoptic area of male and female neonatal rats. *Developmental Brain Research, 79,* 283–289.

Favreau, O. E., & Everett, J. C. (1996). A tale of two tails. *American Psychologist, 51,* 268–269.

Feingold, A. (1995). The additive effects of differences in central tendency and variability are important in comparisons between groups. *American Psychologist, 50,* 5–13.

Finucci, J. M., Isaacs, S. D., Whitehouse, C. C., & Childs, B. (1983). Classification of spelling errors and their relationship to reading ability, sex, grade placement, and intelligence. *Brain and Language, 20,* 340–345.

Fitch, R. H., Brown, C. B., Tallal, P. T., & Rosen, G. D. (1997). The effects of sex and MK–801 on auditory processing deficits associated with developmental microgyric lesions in rats. *Behavioral Neuroscience, 111,* 404–412.

Fitch, R. H., Cowell, P. E., Schrott, L. M., & Denenberg, V. H. (1991). Corpus callosum: Ovarian hormones and feminization. *Brain Research, 542,* 313–317.

Fitch, R. H., & Denenberg, V. H. (1995). A role for ovarian hormones in sexual differentiation of the brain. *Psycoloquy* [On-line]. Available: 95.6.05.sex-brain.1.fitch

Fitch, R. H., & Denenberg, V. H. (in press). A role for ovarian hormones in sexual differentiation of the brain. *Behavioral Brain Sciences.*

Forgie, M. L., & Stewart, J. (1994). Effect of prepubertal ovariectomy on amphetamine-induced locomotion in adult female rats. *Hormones and Behavior, 28,* 241–260.

Frankfurt, M., Gould, E., Woolley, C. S., & McEwen, B. S. (1990). Gonadal steroids modify dendritic spine density in ventromedial hypothalamic neurons: A golgi study in the adult rat. *Neuroendocrinology, 51,* 530–535.

Funkenstein, B., Nimrod, A., & Lindner, H. R. (1980). The development of steroidogenic capability and responsiveness to gonadotropins in cultured neonatal rat ovaries. *Endocrinology, 106,* 98–106.

Gerall, A., Dunlap, J., & Hendricks, S. (1973). Effects of ovarian secretions on female behavioral potentiality in the rat. *Journal of Comparative and Physiological Psychology, 82,* 449–465.

Geschwind, N., & Galaburda, A. M. (1985). Cerebral lateralization: Biological mechanisms, associations, and pathology. *Archives of Neurology, 42,* 428–654.

Goldstein, J. M., Seidman, L. J., Santangelo, S., Knapp, P. H., & Tsuang, M. T. (1994). Are schizophrenic men at higher risk for developmental deficits than schizophrenic women? Implications for adult neuropsychological functions. *Journal of Psychiatric Research, 28,* 483–498.

Gorski, R. (1984). Critical role for the medial preoptic area in the sexual differentiation of the brain. In G. J. De Vries, J. P. C. De Bruin, H. B. M. Uylings, & M. A. Corner (Eds.), *Progress in Brain Research* (Vol. 61, pp. 129–145). New York: Elsevier.

Gould, E., Woolley, C. S., Frankfurt, M., & McEwen, B. S. (1990). Gonadal steroids regulate dendritic spine density in hippocampal pyramidal cells in adulthood. *Journal of Neuroscience, 10,* 86–1291.

Gualtieri, T., & Hicks, R. (1985). An immunoreactive theory of selective male affliction. *The Behavioral and Brain Sciences, 8,* 427–441.

Halpern, D. F. (1992). *Sex differences in cognitive abilities.* Hillsdale, NJ: Lawrence Erlbaum Associates, Inc.

Hampson, E. (1990). Variations in sex-related cognitive abilities across the menstrual cycle. *Brain and Cognition, 14,* 26–43.

Hampson, E., & Kimura, D. (1988). Reciprocal effects of hormonal fluctuations on human motor and perceptual-spatial skills. *Behavioral Neuroscience, 102,* 456–459.

Hampson, E., Rovet, J., & Altmann, D. (1998/this issue). Spatial reasoning in children with congenital adrenal hyperplasia due to 21-hydroxylase deficiency. *Developmental Neuropsychology, 14,* 299–320.

Hendricks, S. E. (1992). Role of estrogens and progestins in the development of female sexual behavior potential. In A. A. Gerall, H. Moltz, & I. L. Ward (Eds.), *Handbook of behavioral neurobiology: Vol. 11. Sexual differentiation* (pp. 129–155). New York: Plenum.

Kail, R., Carter, P., & Pelligrino, J. (1979). The locus of sex differences in spatial ability. *Perception & Psychophysics, 26,* 182–186.

Kampen, D. L., & Sherwin, B. B. (1994). Estrogen use and verbal memory in healthy postmenopausal women. *Obstetrics and Gynecology, 83,* 979–983.

Kimura, D., & Hampson, E. (1993). Neural and hormonal mechanisms mediating sex differences in cognition. In P. A. Vernon (Ed.), *Biological approaches to the study of human intelligence* (pp. 375–397). Norwood, NJ: Ablex.

Kuhnemann, S., Brown, T. J., Hochberg, R. B., & MacLusky, N. J. (1994). Sex differences in the development of estrogen receptors in the rat brain. *Hormones & Behavior, 28,* 483–491.

Leret, M. L., Molina-Holgado, F., & Gonzalez, M. I. (1994). The effect of perinatal exposure to estrogens on the sexually dimorphic response to novelty. *Physiology and Behavior, 55,* 371–373.

Levina, S. E., Gyevai, A., & Horvath, E. (1975). Responsiveness of the ovary to gonadotropins in pre- and perinatal life: Oestrogen secretion in tissue and organ cultures. *Journal of Endocrinology, 65,* 219–223.

Liederman, J., & Flannery, K. (1993). Male prevalence for reading disability is found in a large sample free from ascertainment bias. *Society for Neuroscience Abstracts, 19,* 1462.

Lubinski, D., & Benbow, C. P. (1992). Gender differences in abilities and preferences among the gifted: Implications for the math-science pipeline. *Current Directions in Psychological Science, 1,* 61–66.

Mack, C. M., Cowell, P. E., & Denenberg, V. H. (1992). Corpus callosum: Interactive effects of handling and ovariectomy in the rat. *Society for Neuroscience Abstracts, 18,* 213.

Mack, C. M., Fitch, R. H., Cowell, P. E., Schrott, L. M., & Denenberg, V. H. (1993). Ovarian estrogen acts to feminize the rat's corpus callosum. *Developmental Brain Research, 71,* 115–119.

Mack, C. M., Fitch, R. H., Hyde, L. A., Seaman, A. J., Bimonte, H. E., Wei, W., & Denenberg, V. (1996). Lack of activational influence of ovarian hormones on the size of the female rat's corpus callosum. *Physiology and Behavior, 60,* 431–434.

Mack, C. M., McGivern, R. F., Hyde, L. A., & Denenberg, V. (1996). Absence of postnatal testosterone fails to demasculinize the male rat's corpus callosum. *Developmental Brain Research, 95,* 252–254.

MacLusky, N. J., Chaptal, C., & McEwen, B. S. (1979). The development of estrogen receptor systems in the rat brain and pituitary: Postnatal development. *Brain Research, 178,* 143–160.

MacLusky, N. J., Lieberburg, I., & McEwen, B. S. (1979). The development of estrogen receptors in the rat brain and pituitary: Perinatal development. *Brain Research, 178,* 129–142.

Mannan, M. A., & O'Shaughnessy, P. J. (1991). Steroidogenesis during postnatal development in the mouse ovary. *Journal of Endocrinology, 130,* 101–106.

Masica, D. N., Money, J., Ehrhardt, A. A., & Lewis, V. G. (1969). IQ, fetal sex hormones, and cognitive patterns: Studies of the testicular feminizing syndrome of androgen insensitivity. *Johns Hopkins Medical Journal, 124,* 34–43.
McCarthy, N. M., Schlenker, E. H., & Pfaff, D. W. (1993). Enduring consequences of neonatal treatment with antisense oligodeoxynucleotides to estrogen receptor messenger ribonucleic acid on sexual differentiation of rat brain. *Endocrinology, 133,* 433–439.
Miranda, R. C., & Toran-Allerand, C. D. (1992). Developmental expression of estrogen receptor mRNA in the rat cerebral cortex: A nonisotopic *in situ* hybridization histochemistry study. *Cerebral Cortex, 2,* 1–15.
Msall, M. E., Buck, G. M., Rogers, B. T., & Catanzaro, N. L. (1992). Kindergarten readiness after extreme prematurity. *American Journal of Diseases of Children, 146,* 1371–1375.
Msall, M. E., Buck, G. M., Rogers, B. T., Duffy, L. C., Mallen, S. R., & Catanzaro, N. L. (1993). Predictors of mortality, morbidity, and disability in a cohort of infants < or = 28 weeks' gestation. *Clinical Pediatrics, 32,* 521–527.
Munoz-Cueto, J. A., Garcia-Segura, L. M., & Ruiz-Marcos, A. (1990). Developmental sex differences and effect of ovariectomy on the number of cortical pyramidal cell dendrite spines. *Brain Research, 515,* 64–68.
Murphy, D. M., DeCarli, C., Daly, E., Haxby, J. V., Allen, G., White, B. J., McIntosh, A. R., Powell, C. M., Horwitz, B., Rapoport, S. I., & Schapiro, M. B. (1993). X-chromosome effects on female brain: A magnetic resonance imaging study of Turner's syndrome. *Lancet, 342,* 1197–1200.
Murphy, D. M., DeCarli, C., McIntosh, A. R., Daly, E., Mentis, M. J., Pietrini, P., Szczepanik, J., Schapiro, M. B., Grady, C. L., Horwitz, B., & Rapoport, S. I. (1996). Sex differences in human brain morphometry and metabolism: An *in vivo* quantitative magnetic resonance imaging and positron emission tomography study on the effect of aging. *Archives of General Psychiatry, 53,* 585–594.
Neils, J. R., & Aram, D. M. (1986). Handedness and sex of children with developmental language disorders. *Brain and Language, 28,* 53–65.
Oades, R. D., & Schepker, R. (1994). Serum gonadal steroid hormones in young schizophrenic patients. *Psychoneuroendocrinology, 19,* 373–385.
O'Keefe, J. A., & Handa, R. J. (1990). Transient elevation of estrogen receptors in the neonatal rat hippocampus. *Developmental Brain Research, 57,* 119–127.
Paganini-Hill, A., & Henderson, V. W. (1994). Estrogen deficiency and risk of Alzheimer's disease in women. *American Journal of Epidemiology, 140,* 256–261.
Pappas, C. T. E., Diamond, M. C., & Johnson, R. E. (1979). Morphological changes in the cerebral cortex of rats with altered levels of ovarian hormones. *Behavioral and Neural Biology, 26,* 298–310.
Raynaud, J. P., Mercier-Bodard, C., & Baulieu, E. E. (1971). Rat estradiol binding plasma protein. *Steroids, 18,* 767–788.
Raz, S., Lauterbach, M. D., Hopkins, T. L., Glogowski, B. K., Porter, C. L., Riggs, W. W., & Sander, C. G. (1995). A female advantage in recovery from early cerebral insult. *Developmental Psychology, 31,* 958–966.
Reiss, A. L., Mazzacocco, M. M., Greenlaw, R., Freund, L. S., & Ross, J. L. (1995). Neurodevelopmental effects of X monosomy: A volumetric imaging study. *Annals of Neurology, 38,* 731–738.
Resnick, S., Berenbaum, S. A., Gottesman, I. I., Bouchard, T. J., Jr. (1986). Early hormonal influences on cognitive functioning in congenital adrenal hyperplasia. *Developmental Psychology, 22,* 191–198.
Rhees, R. W., Shryne, J. E., & Gorski, R. A. (1990a). Onset of the hormone-sensitive perinatal period for sexual differentiation of the sexually dimorphic nucleus of the preoptic area. *Journal of Neurobiology, 21,* 781–786.
Rhees, R. W., Shryne, J. E., & Gorski, R. A. (1990b). Termination of the hormone-sensitive period for differentiation of the sexually dimorphic nucleus of the preoptic area in male and female rats. *Developmental Brain Research, 52,* 17–23.

Riecher-Rossler, A., Hafner, H., Stumbaum, M., Maurer, K., & Schmidt, R. (1994). Can estradiol modulate schizophrenic symptomatology? *Schizophrenia Bulletin, 20,* 203–214.
Roof, R. L., Duvdevani, R., & Stein, D. G. (1993). Gender influences outcome of brain injury: Progesterone plays a protective role. *Brain Research, 607,* 333–336.
Roof, R. L., Zhang, Q., Glasier, M. M., & Stein, D. G. (1993). Gender-specific impairment on Morris water maze task after entorhinal cortex lesion. *Behavioral Brain Research, 57,* 47–51.
Ross, J. L., Stefanatos, G., Roeltgen, D., Kushner, H., & Cutler, G. B., Jr. (1995). Ullrich–Turner syndrome: Neurodevelopmental changes from childhood through adolescence. *American Journal of Medical Genetics, 58,* 74–82.
Schneider, L. S., Farlow, M. R., Henderson, V. W., & Pogoda, J. M. (1996). Effects of estrogen replacement therapy on response to tacrine in patients with Alzheimer's disease. *Neurology, 46,* 1580–1584.
Seeman, M. V. (1983). Interaction of sex, age, and neuroleptic dose. *Comprehensive Psychiatry, 24,* 125–128.
Seeman, M. V. (1986). Current outcome in schizophrenia: Women vs. men. *Acta Psychiatrica Scandinavica, 73,* 609–617.
Seeman, M. V., & Lang, M. (1990). The role of estrogens in schizophrenic gender differences. *Schizophrenia Bulletin, 16,* 185–194.
Shaywitz, B. A., Shaywitz, S. E., Pugh, K. R., Constable, R. T., Skudlarski, P., Fulbright, R. K., Bronen, R. A., Fletcher, J. M., Shankweiler, D. P., Katz, L., & Gore, J. C. (1995). Sex differences in the functional organization of the brain for language. *Nature, 373,* 607–609.
Shaywitz, S. E., Escobar, M. D., Shaywitz, B. A., Fletcher, J. M., & Makuch, R. (1992). Evidence that dyslexia may represent the lower tail of a normal distribution of reading ability. *New England Journal of Medicine, 326,* 145–150.
Sherwin, B. B. (1994). Estrogenic effects on memory in women. *Annals of the New York Academy of Sciences, 743,* 213–230.
Shugrue, P. J., Stumpf, W. E., MacLusky, N. J., Zielinski, J. E., & Hochberg, R. B. (1990). Developmental changes in estrogen receptors in mouse cerebral cortex between birth and postweaning: Studied by autoradiography with 11b–Methoxy–16a–[125I] Iodoestradiol. *Endocrinology, 126,* 1112–1124.
Small, G. W., La Rue, A., Komo, S., Kaplan, A. & Mandelkern, M. A. (1995). Predictors of cognitive change in middle-aged and older adults with memory loss. *American Journal of Psychiatry, 152,* 1757–1764.
Sodersten, P. (1976). Lordosis behavior in male, female, and androgenized female rats. *Journal of Endocrinology, 70,* 409–420.
Sokka, T. A., & Huhtaniemi, I. T. (1995). Functional maturation of the pituitary–gonadal axis in the neonatal female rat. *Biology of Reproduction, 52,* 1404–1409.
Spinillo, A., Fazzi, E., Orcesi, S., Accorsi, P., Beccaria, F., & Capuzzo, E. (1995). Perinatal factors and 2-year minor neurodevelopmental impairment in low birth weight infants. *Biology of the Neonate, 67,* 39–46.
Stewart, J., & Cygan, D. (1980). Ovarian hormones act early in development to feminize open field behavior in the rat. *Hormones and Behavior, 14,* 20–32.
Stewart, J., & Kolb, B. (1988). Asymmetry in the cerebral cortex of the rat: An analysis of the effects of neonatal gonadectomy on cortical thickness in three strains of rats. *Behavioral and Neural Biology, 49,* 344–360.
Stewart, J., & Kolb, B. (1994). Dendritic branching in cortical pyramidal cells in response to ovariectomy in adult female rats: Suppression by neonatal exposure to testosterone. *Brain Research, 654,* 149–154.

Stewart, J., Vallentyne, S., & Meaney, M. J. (1979). Differential effects of testosterone metabolites in the neonatal period on open-field behavior and lordosis in the rat. *Hormones and Behavior, 13,* 282–292.

Szekely, C., Hampson, E., Carey, D. P., & Goodale, M. A. (1998/this issue). Oral contraceptive use affects manual praxis but not simple visually guided movements. *Developmental Neuropsychology, 14,* 399–420.

Toran-Allerand, A. (1976). Sex steroids and the development of the newborn mouse hypothalamus and preoptic area in vitro: Implication for sexual differentiation. *Brain Research, 106,* 407–412.

Toran-Allerand, D. (1984). On the genesis of sexual differentiation of the central nervous system: Morphogenetic consequences of steroidal exposure and possible role of alpha-feto-protein. In G. J. De Vries, J. P. C. De Bruin, H. B. M. Uylings, & M. A. Corner (Eds.), *Progress in brain research* (Vol. 61, pp. 63–97). New York: Elsevier.

Toran-Allerand, D. (1986). Sexual differentiation of the brain. In W. T. Greenough & J. M. Juraska (Eds.), *Developmental neuropsychology* (pp. 175–211). London: Academic.

Toran-Allerand, D. (1992). Organotypic culture of the developing cerebral cortex and hypothalamus: Relevance to sexual differentiation. In P. Tallal & B. McEwen (Eds.), *Psychoneuroendocrinology* (Vol. 16, pp. 7–24). New York: Pergamon.

Van Haaren, F., Van Hest, A., & Heinsbroek, R. P. W. (1990). Behavioral differences between male and female rats: Effects of gonadal hormones on learning and memory. *Neuroscience and Biobehavioral Reviews, 14,* 23–33.

Wagner, C. K., & Clemens, L. G. (1989). Perinatal modification of a sexually dimorphic motor nucleus in the spinal cord of the B6D2F1 house mouse. *Physiology and Behavior, 45,* 831–835.

Weniger, J. P., Zeis, A., & Chouraqui, J. (1993). Estrogen production by fetal and infantile rat ovaries. *Reproduction, Nutrition, and Development, 33,* 129–136.

Williams, C. L., & Meck, W. H. (1991). The organizational effects of gonadal steroids on sexually dimorphic spatial ability. *Psychoneuroendocrinology, 16,* 155–176.

Witelson, S. F. (1991). Neural sexual mosaicism: Sexual differentiation of the human temporo-parietal region for functional asymmetry. *Psychoneuroendocrinology, 16,* 131–153.

Witelson, S. F., & Kigar, D. L. (1992a). Broca's region: Anatomical and functional asymmetries. *Society for Neuroscience Abstracts, 18,* 331.

Witelson, S. F., & Kigar, D. L. (1992b). Sylvian fissure morphology and asymmetry in men and women: Bilateral differences in relation to handedness in men. *The Journal of Comparative Neurology, 323,* 326–340.

Wood, F. B., Flowers, L. D., & Naylor, C. E. (1991). Cerebral laterality in functional neuroimaging. In F. L. Kitterle (Ed.), *Cerebral laterality: Theory and research, The Toledo Symposium* (pp. 103–115). Hillsdale, NJ: Lawrence Erlbaum Associates, Inc.

Woolley, C. S., Gould, E., Frankfurt, M., & & McEwen, B. S. (1990). Naturally occurring fluctuation in dendritic spine density on adult hippocampal pyramidal neurons. *Journal of Neuroscience, 10,* 4035–4039.

Woolley, C. S., & McEwen, B. S. (1992). Estradiol mediates fluctuation in hippocampal synapse density during the estrous cycle in the adult rat. *Journal of Neuroscience, 12,* 2549–2554.

Zimmerberg, B., & Farley, M. J. (1993). Sex differences in anxiety behavior in rats: Role of gonadal hormones. *Physiology and Behavior, 54,* 1119–1124.

Developmental Changes in Behavior and in Steroid Uptake by the Male and Female Macaque Brain

Richard P. Michael and Doris Zumpe
Department of Psychiatry and Behavioral Sciences
Emory University School of Medicine, Atlanta

We describe the sex differences in the development of play initiation, rough-and-tumble play, and mounting behavior in rhesus monkeys. There are also sex differences in the acquisition and maintenance of dominance rank under naturalistic conditions in this female-bonded, matrilineal society. The hormonal control of adult mating behavior, as well as the behavioral patterns expressed, are quite different in males and females, but both sexes have the capacity to show bisexual patterns of behavior in special circumstances. Using high-performance liquid chromatography and autoradiography, we found a well-marked system of neurons that can accumulate steroids in the hypothalamus and amygdala of the fetus by 120 days of gestation. In the male fetus, plasma testosterone is high at this time, so receptors are occupied. In contrast, plasma hormones in the female remain low throughout gestation. The natural masculinization of genetic male fetuses, as well as the masculinization of females whose mothers were administered androgens during pregnancy, are due at least in part to the aromatization of testosterone in the brain and the resulting occupation of estrogen receptors: This was established in fetal males castrated in utero. Many of the deleterious effects of diethylstilbestrol administered to pregnant women can also be accounted for by its uptake by the brain and the genital tract before birth. In adults, we used in vivo competition studies with unlabeled steroids to demonstrate that the major form of radioactivity in the brain after [^{3}H]testosterone administration is its aromatized metabolite [^{3}H]estradiol in the preoptic area, hypothalamus, and amygdala, and in the basal accessory amygdaloid nucleus there is strong evidence for a population of neurons containing tau receptors that accumulate only unchanged [^{3}H]testosterone. Comparison of data from fetuses, neonates, and adults revealed an

---

Requests for reprints should be sent to Richard P. Michael, Department of Psychiatry and Behavioral Sciences, Emory University School of Medicine, Georgia Mental Health Institute, 1256 Briarcliff Road, N.E., Atlanta, GA 30306–2636.

increase with age in the proportion of cells accumulating [^{3}H]estradiol in the preoptic area and hypothalamus, whereas in the amygdala a similar increase occurred between the neonatal period and adulthood. We were unable to demonstrate any significant sex differences in steroid uptake mechanisms in the brain and pituitary gland at any stage of development, but the hormonal milieu differs vastly in the 2 sexes, and this must affect brain mechanisms differently in the 2 sexes, the most plausible source of sex differences in behavior, although not necessarily a sufficient one.

Effects of hormones on behavior during development as well as in adulthood are particularly complex in anthropoid primates for the following reasons: (a) Their great neocortical development facilitates complex and variable behavioral responses, and the roles of environmental factors and social influences are consequently more pronounced; (b) puberty is much delayed in many primate species (2–3 years in macaques) and during this period the more variable adult behavioral patterns have an opportunity to develop; and (c) there follows after puberty a period of social immaturity during adolescence (1 year or more in macaques) that permits extensive learning of social roles when effective behavioral interactions with conspecifics can mature. The much-cited work of Harlow and colleagues (Harlow & Zimmerman, 1959) demonstrated in rhesus monkeys the critical role of the early postnatal environment for the subsequent development of normal adult behavior; when infants were reared in social isolation, many aspects of their adult behavioral repertoire were disrupted. Even in adult primates reared in the wild, the behavioral effects of gonadal hormones are much influenced by such variables as kinship, duration of familiarity with a conspecific, partner preferences, individual differences, dominance rank, and the amount and quality of space available. These and other factors can also modulate hormonal effects in humans, and knowledge of the role of gonadal hormones during nonhuman primate development may also be viewed in this broader perspective.

SEX DIFFERENCES IN THE BEHAVIOR OF ADULT MACAQUES

This section presents a brief review of sex differences in the social organization and behavior of adult macaques to provide a context for the ontogenetic studies involving hormonal mechanisms and behavior.

Nonhuman primate species vary widely in their social organizations, but rhesus monkeys live in social groups consisting of several adult males and females together with their young. Females born into a group remain in it for life, but males leave around puberty to join another social group, after which they emigrate again, on average every 4 years or so throughout their adult lives. Consequently, groups are female bonded and matrilineal. This is reflected in a sex difference in the acquisition of dominance rank. Daughters acquire dominance ranks just below their mothers, whereas sons typically lose dominance status as juveniles, and also after emigration into a new group, where they can eventually attain high rank again. Males, then, cycle through low and high ranks throughout their lives, whereas female rank is socially inherited and generally stable. There is evidence, reviewed elsewhere (Zumpe & Michael, 1996), that male group transfers depend on a mechanism involving decreased sexual attraction between long-familiar individuals, similar to that proposed by Westermarck (1891) for incest avoidance in humans.

Except during periods of mating activity, adult males and females do not often interact socially. Female rhesus monkeys have 28-day menstrual cycles; among mammals, only humans and anthropoid primates have menstrual cycles. The hormonal changes determining these are similar to those in humans (Hammarbäck, Damber, & Bäckström, 1989) except that there is no secondary estradiol rise during the luteal phase (Bonsall, Zumpe, & Michael, 1978). Mating is generally restricted to a few days before and after ovulation, when a male and female form temporary but exclusive consort bonds: They travel, feed, and rest together, and groom and mate repeatedly. In captivity, mating can continue throughout the cycle, but it peaks at midcycle when estrogen levels are high (Michael & Bonsall, 1977). The male typically approaches or follows a female while making lipsmacking movements at her. He frequently examines the female's perineal region by looking, sniffing, and licking, and initiates mounts by clasping the female's hips with his hands and, if the female adopts a receptive stance, he clasps both of her ankles with his feet (double foot-clasp mount), intromits, thrusts, and, after 5 to 15 such mounts, ejaculates. The female may also approach and lipsmack at the male, and may initiate a mount by adopting the receptive "presentation" posture during which she stands on all fours close to but facing away from the male, exposing her anogenital region. In addition to using the presentation posture, the female can initiate a mount with certain fast but stereotyped hand and head movements. Males and females may perform the behavior characteristic of the opposite sex in both sexual and nonsexual contexts. Both sexes use mounts and presentations in greeting and to signal dominance and submission, respectively. In addition, males may mount or present to other males in a sexual context. Likewise, females may mount both sexually unresponsive males (this can stimulate mounting by the male) and other females in a sexual context. Although there is sexual dimorphism in the frequencies with which male mounts and female presentations are made, the capacity to exhibit the behavioral patterns of both sexes is clearly apparent in adult males and females.

The effects of gonadal hormones (estrogen, androgens, and progestins) on sexual and aggressive behavior in adult macaques has been reviewed elsewhere (Michael & Zumpe, 1993) and is summarized only briefly here. In males, androgen stimulates sexual motivation and it is important for erectile potency and, consequently, for intromission and ejaculation. At plasma levels in the physiological range, testosterone (which can be aromatized to estradiol) is more effective than the nonaromatizable androgen, dihydrotestosterone (DHT), in restoring the sexual behavior of castrated males. There is evidence that male sexual motivation depends on the brain uptake of both unchanged testosterone and its locally produced metabolite estradiol (Zumpe, Clancy, Bonsall, & Michael, 1996). In females, physiological testosterone levels have no detectable behavioral effects, but administration of very high doses increases their sexual motivation, although not their attractiveness to males. Estradiol at physiological levels, however, markedly increases sexual motivation, sexual receptivity, and also sexual attractiveness. The behavioral effects of DHT in females are unknown. Progesterone, finally, has inhibitory effects on sexual motivation and behavior of both males and females, particularly at supraphysiological levels.

BEHAVIORAL EFFECTS OF PRENATAL ANDROGEN ADMINISTRATION

It is known that hormone treatments of gonadectomized adult mammals do not generally feminize the sexual behavior of males given estrogen or masculinize that of females given androgen. Nevertheless, several lines of evidence suggested that potent hormonal effects might occur during embryogenesis and early in the neonatal period, particularly at certain critical times during development. One of the most noteworthy examples from developmental biology concerns the freemartin condition in cattle (Keller & Tandler, 1916; Lillie, 1916, 1917). This is an intersex condition occurring in one of a pair of dizygotic twin calves, the other twin being a normal male, characterized by some degree of masculinization of the genetic female. There is an enlarged penislike clitoris and male duct structures are usually well preserved whereas female duct structures are rudimentary. The condition results from an anastomotic communication between the placental circulations of the twins: The more extreme the anastomosis, the more extreme is the female's masculinization. This experiment of nature could not be replicated experimentally with any facility in eutherian mammals, even after the chemical isolation of the gonadal steroids in the 1920s. But many examples of genetically determined intersex conditions may be found in the clinical literature, and much attention was given to them by Wilkins (Wilkins, Jones, Holman, & Stempfel, 1958) in the Pediatric Endocrine Clinic at Johns Hopkins and, subsequently, by Money and his associates (Money & Erhardt, 1972). One noteworthy example is congenital adrenal hyperplasia comprising some six autosomal recessive disorders that results in mild to extreme masculinization of genetic females in utero. The best experimental sex reversals in mammals were produced in the North American opossum (Burns, 1956), the neonate being accessible to manipulation at a very immature stage of development. In other mammals, pregnant females have been treated with androgens at different times during gestation, and the course of sexual differentiation in the embryo has been affected in guinea pigs (Dantchakoff, 1936), rats (Greene,

1942), rabbits (Jost, 1953), and monkeys (Wells & Van Wagenen, 1954). These studies, and many others, led the late W. C. Young to the proposition that hormones exert an organizational effect in early development and an activational effect in adulthood (Young, 1961). This seminal concept was investigated by the extensive work of Goy and associates (see the following section) on the development of behavior patterns in rhesus monkeys.

Developmental changes in the behavior of male and female rhesus monkeys were evaluated, after weaning at about 3.5 months of age, in small infant peer groups formed and observed for 30 min every weekday (Goy, 1968; Phoenix, 1974). At this age, well-marked sex differences were already apparent in threat behavior, initiation of play, rough-and-tumble play, chasing play, and in mounts, but not in sexual presentations. In every case, rates by male infants were at least twice those of female infants, and these differences were even greater at 6 months of age. The role of early androgen secretion was assessed by neonatal castration of males and by androgen treatment of pregnant females. Castration on the day of birth, when androgen levels are high, did not influence the male-typical sexual and social behavior of infant males (Goy, 1968). However, female infants whose mothers had received daily injections of testosterone propionate from about 40 to 65 days or 40 to 90 days of gestation (gestation length is 168 days) showed levels of play initiation, rough-and-tumble play, chasing play, and mounting that were intermediate between those of normal males and normal females during the 1st year of life. These behavioral differences continued throughout adolescence up to the time of puberty, normally around 3 years of age, and puberty itself was delayed in the prenatally androgenized females by an average of 7.5 months compared with normal females (Goy, 1968; Goy & Resko, 1972). After puberty, in the 5th year of life, rough play decreased to low levels in normal males and in prenatally androgenized females, and rates of typical male foot-clasp mounting were high and essentially indistinguishable in these two groups whereas they were virtually zero in normal females (Phoenix, 1974).

The external genitalia of prenatally androgenized females were masculinized, with a well-developed but empty scrotum, an enlarged, penislike clitoris, and no vagina. After puberty, these pseudohermaphroditic females menstruated via the penis. It was argued that the behavioral differences might be attributed in part to these somatic features and to the perception by the mother that the infant was a male. This interpretation caused debate, because rhesus mothers treat male and female infants differently, inspecting the genitals of males more frequently than those of females, and the development of gender identity in humans is thought to depend considerably on the differential treatment of infants by adults (Money & Erhardt, 1972). A further study was therefore aimed at comparing the behavior of female infants that were androgenized by testosterone propionate either between 40 to 64 days of gestation, which produced genital virilization and delayed puberty, or between 115 to 139 days of gestation, which did neither (Goy, Bercovitch, &

McBrair, 1988). Behavioral observations were made during 25- to 30-min tests conducted periodically between 3 and 27 months of age. Females androgenized early, like normal males, received many more genital inspections by their mothers, mounted their mothers more, and groomed them less than did normal females and females androgenized late in gestation, suggesting that behaviors directed at mothers might have been influenced by the mother's responses to genital virilization of their infant. No such influences were detected in behavioral interactions with peers. Both groups of androgenized females showed levels of mounting and play that were lower than in males and generally higher than in normal females: In females androgenized early, mounts tended to be higher, whereas in females androgenized later, rough play and play initiations (those made as well as those received from normal males) were higher. The authors interpreted this to mean that certain male-typical behaviors directed at peers (rough play and play initiation) had later critical periods for prenatal androgen effects than did others (mounting) and that genital masculinization was not necessary for masculinization of behavior with peers.

Seven of the pseudohermaphroditic females described by Goy (1968) and Goy and Resko (1972) were ovariectomized as young adults (5–7 years of age) and, together with a control group of normal ovariectomized females, were treated with testosterone propionate and paired with receptive female partners during 10-min tests once a week (Eaton, Goy, & Phoenix, 1973). Prenatally androgenized females were significantly more aggressive than control females before and during androgen treatment, but there were no significant differences in sexual behaviors between the two groups of females. Compared with normal females, the pseudohermaphrodites had somewhat higher rates of the typical male mounting pattern, which increased with androgen treatment from 0.43 to 0.91 per min, but neither the difference nor the increase was statistically significant. However, 3 of the 7 prenatally androgenized females displayed clear behavioral masculinization: One female obtained intromission with her phallus and exhibited the muscle spasms and rigidity, as well as fluid emission, seen during ejaculation by males, and two others "ejaculated" after masturbation. Ten years later, the same prenatally androgenized females were studied again under similar testing conditions while receiving daily injections of estradiol benzoate and, after estrogen withdrawal, while receiving testosterone propionate. Their behavior was compared with that of gonadectomized, similarly treated normal females and males that were at least 21 years old (Phoenix & Chambers, 1982). Again, irrespective of hormone treatments, proportionally more pseudohermaphrodites than normal females and males were aggressive toward female partners. Erections (not detectable in normal females) increased with estrogen and especially with androgen treatment, but mount latencies and mount and mounting attempt rates more closely resembled those of normal females than of males, and the female that had intromitted and "ejaculated" 10 years earlier now failed to do so. When 6 of the 7 prenatally androgenized females were treated with estradiol benzoate and paired with males 1 year later (Phoenix, Jensen, & Chambers, 1983), their sexual interactions with males did not differ significantly from those of similarly treated normal females, and the authors found no evidence of behavioral defeminization. Indeed, there was little evidence that sexual behavior was either masculinized or defeminized after 7 years of age in this group of pseudohermaphrodites when they were given either androgen or estrogen and paired with appropriate normal partners.

However, behavioral defeminization was demonstrated in studies using younger, intact pseudohermaphrodites (6–9 years old) and different testing conditions (Pomerantz, Roy, Thornton, & Goy, 1985). Experimental subjects were observed for 20 to 30 min three times a week in a large arena containing a tethered vasectomized male. Females were prenatally androgenized from Day 42 of gestation for about 55 or 80 days with either testosterone propionate or dihydrotestosterone propionate. When given subcutaneous estradiol implants, these females displayed fewer proceptive behaviors toward intact males (defeminization) than did estrogen-treated normal females, but more than estrogen-treated males that had been castrated at birth. However, despite the absence of a vagina, pseudohermaphrodites did not differ from normal females in their receptivity to the male partner's mounting attempts. Because there were no differences between females prenatally androgenized with testosterone (which can be aromatized to estradiol) or DHT (which cannot be aromatized), it was concluded that testosterone's effects on defeminization in the primate, unlike in rodents (Baum, 1979), are not mediated by its conversion to estradiol (Pomerantz, Roy, et al., 1985). This theme was revisited in our studies on hormone uptake by the brains of fetal, neonatal, and adult rhesus and cynomolgus monkeys, described in the following section.

Treatment of pregnant female rhesus monkeys with androgens during gestation must have resulted in the birth of some prenatally androgenized males of which no mention was made in any of the studies already cited, presumably because no behavioral or morphological differences could be detected. In a more recent study on Japanese macaques maintained in naturalistic social groups housed in outdoor enclosures, pregnant females were given silastic implants of testosterone between about Days 40 and 100 of gestation, and the behavior of their female and male offspring was studied from birth to 2 years of age (Eaton, Worlein, & Glick, 1990). Like rhesus monkeys, prenatally androgenized female Japanese monkeys displayed more mounting and less grooming than did normal females, but there were no effects of prenatal androgen treatment on either the genital morphology or the behavior of males.

Androgenization during the middle trimester of gestation appears, then, to masculinize the play and mounting behavior of sexually immature genetic females independently of genital virilization. However, play virtually ceases at puberty in macaques, and effects of prenatal androgenization on sexual behavior seem to disappear with increasing age and experience, requiring sophisticated observations for their detection when animals are given activational doses of gonadal hormones in adulthood. This might be related to the timing, duration, or amount of androgen actually reaching the fetus, and it would help to understand these matters if the ontogeny of androgen and estrogen receptors in primate brain and peripheral tissues were studied throughout the embryonic period.

DEVELOPMENTAL CHANGES IN HORMONE UPTAKE BY THE PRIMATE BRAIN

The level of androgens in the plasma of the rhesus monkey fetus was first systematically studied by Resko and colleagues (see the following section). The fetal testes become active as the Leydig cells develop at 40 to 50 days of gestation (Van Wagenen & Simpson, 1965), and between 50 and 80 days of gestation plasma testosterone can attain adult male levels (about 800 ng/100 ml). Between about 100 and 130 days they appear to decline, which coincides with interstitial cell regression, but again increase to high levels from about 140 days gestation until after birth (Resko & Ellinwood, 1984): The timing of these changes is remarkably similar in many respects to that in humans (Reyes, Boroditsky, Winter, & Faiman, 1974; Van Wagenen & Simpson, 1965; Winter, Hughes, Reyes, & Faiman, 1976). The hypothalamic–gonadal axis then remains quiescent until its activation at puberty. In female fetuses, testosterone and estradiol levels are low throughout gestation and the ovaries remain quiescent. In line with the behavioral work already cited, testosterone or its metabolites seemed likely candidates for masculinizing the behavior of genetic males, and this could be due to an action of the steroids on the brain. Evidence supporting this view can be summarized: (a) Cytoplasmic androgen and estrogen receptors are present in the fetal macaque brain during the critical period (Handa, Connolly, & Resko, 1988; Pomerantz, Fox, Sholl, Vito, & Goy, 1985); (b) aromatase and 5α-reductase are also present in the fetal brain, and are involved in the actions of testosterone in the adult brain (Resko, Connolly, & Roselli, 1988; Resko & Ellinwood, 1984; Roselli & Resko, 1986); (c) throughout gestation, plasma testosterone is considerably higher in male fetuses than in female fetuses (Resko & Ellinwood, 1984); and (d) male fetuses show the adult type of castration effect on luteinizing hormone (LH) levels; testosterone subsequently becomes ineffective in suppressing LH levels in males, whereas it remains effective in reducing LH levels in the female fetus (Resko & Ellinwood, 1984). Nevertheless, direct evidence for an effect of testicular hormones on neurons in the fetus was lacking.

Hormone Uptake by the Fetal Brain: Testosterone and Its Metabolites

We used autoradiography to map sites in the primate brain where testosterone may have sexual differentiating actions on brain function and behavior during fetal development (Michael & Rees, 1986). This required accurately timed pregnancies produced by mating female rhesus (*Macaca mulatta*) or cynomolgus (*M. fascicularis*) monkeys with a male daily for 1 hr during the middle 7 days of their menstrual cycles. The timing of conceptions was further narrowed by measuring plasma levels of estradiol and progesterone using radioimmunoassays. At 112 to 114 days of gestation, abdominal and uterine incisions were made, the sex of the fetus was determined (female fetuses were used), and 275 µCi of tritiated testosterone ([^{3}H]T) in 0.5 ml 15% ethanol:saline was injected into the fetal rump. The fetus was returned to the uterus, which was then closed, and the pregnancies were maintained for 30 to 60 min, when they were terminated by cesarean section. Fetal body weights were about 200 g. The brains were immediately prepared for thaw-mount autoradiography on emulsion-coated slides and, after 20 to 60 weeks exposure at $-19°$ C in the dark, gave quite good autoradiograms. A cell was considered labeled if it had a silver grain density more than twice that of background, and an X–Y recorder mounted on a microscope stage was used to plot the location of labeled cells on drawings of brain sections. All labeled cells appeared to be neurons, and the highest percentages of labeled neurons were in the ventromedial hypothalamic nucleus, accessory basal amygdaloid nucleus, medial preoptic nucleus, premammillary nucleus, anterior hypothalamic nucleus, and cortical amygdaloid nucleus. Somewhat lower labeling indices were seen in the arcuate nucleus, bed nucleus of the stria terminalis, medial amygdaloid nucleus, and lateral septal nucleus. Occasional individual neurons had silver grain densities five times that of the neuropil background. The pattern of labeled neurons in these female fetuses was in good agreement with that following the administration of [^{3}H]T to ovariectomized adult females, but the percentages of labeled neurons in most brain regions were less than one third those in adults (Michael & Rees, 1986). This study did not provide any information about the chemical form of the radioactivity in the brain, but it did provide evidence for an active steroid uptake (receptor) system at this stage of gestation.

Because the first studies using autoradiography were performed on female rhesus monkey fetuses, a subsequent study (Michael, Bonsall, & Rees, 1989) used both male and female fetuses, and was augmented by high-performance liquid chromatography (HPLC) to identify the chemical nature of the ligands. One hour after injection of 250 µCi of [^{3}H]T via the umbilical vein at about Day 120 of gestation, purified pellets of neuronal nuclei were prepared, and radioactivity in ether extracts was fractionated by HPLC and identified by coelution with internal standards. Concentrations of radioactivity were significantly higher in the hypothalamus–preoptic area than elsewhere in the brain, and about 75% of the radioactivity in the hypothalamus–preoptic area coeluted with 17β-estradiol. In contrast, 80% of the radioactivity extracted from pituitary gland nuclei coeluted with testosterone. Quantitative data from autoradiograms using stringent Poisson criteria (Arnold, 1981) are shown in Figure 1. There was well-marked labeling of neurons

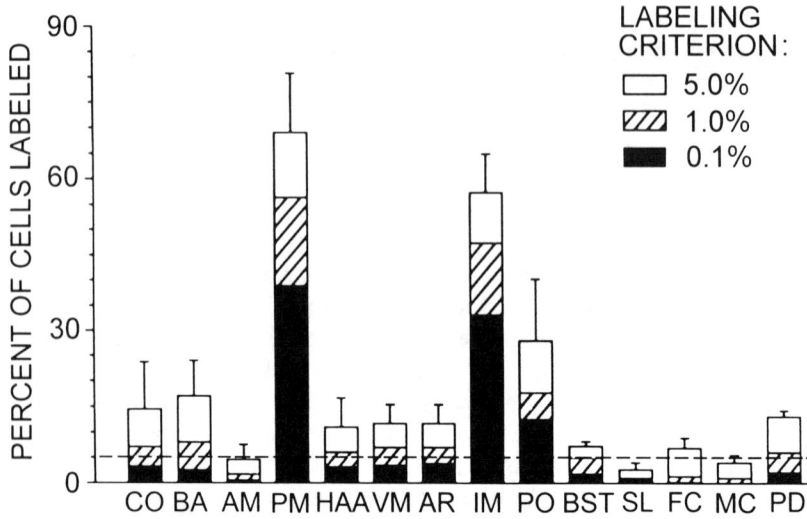

FIGURE 1 Mean percentages of brain neurons and pars distalis cells labeled according to three Poisson criteria after the administration of 250 µCi [^{3}H]T to three fetal macaques. The horizontal interrupted line gives the percentage expected by chance at the 5% criterion. Highest labeling indexes occurred in the premammillary and intercalated mammillary nuclei and, to a lesser extent, in preoptic area. Abbreviations: CO = cortical amygdaloid nucleus (n); BA = accessory basal amygdaloid n; AM = medial amygdaloid n; PM = premammillary n; HAA = anterior hypothalamic n; VM = ventromedial n; AR = arcuate n; IM = intercalated mammillary n; PO = medial preoptic n; BST = bed n of stria terminalis; SL = lateral septal n; FC = dorsolateral frontal cortex; MC = dorsal anterior central gyrus (motor cortex); PD = pars distalis. Vertical bars give standard error of mean. From "The Uptake of [^{3}H]Testosterone and its Metabolites by the Brain and Pituitary Gland of the Fetal Macaque," by R. P. Michael, R. W. Bonsall, and H. D. Rees, 1989, *Endocrinology, 124,* pp. 1319–1326. Copyright 1989 by The Endocrine Society. Reprinted with kind permission from The Endocrine Society.

in the preoptic area and, to a lesser extent, in ventromedial and arcuate nuclei, and in the cortical amygdaloid nucleus. However, the most striking and intense labeling occurred in two nuclei we had previously overlooked, namely, the premammillary and intercalated mammillary nuclei (Figures 1 and 2). The relative abundance of [^{3}H]estradiol ([^{3}H]E$_2$; about 75% of radioactivity) in cell nuclei from the hypothalamus–preoptic area was consistent with aromatase activity and the presence of estrogen receptors. The form of radioactivity in the premammillary and intercalated mammillary nuclei could not be reliably established in the fetus, as samples were very small, but it was [^{3}H]T and [^{3}H]DHT in the adult (Bonsall, Rees, & Michael, 1989).

A further study was aimed at comparing the nuclear uptake of [^{3}H]T and its metabolites by the brains of intact male and female fetuses at around 120 days of

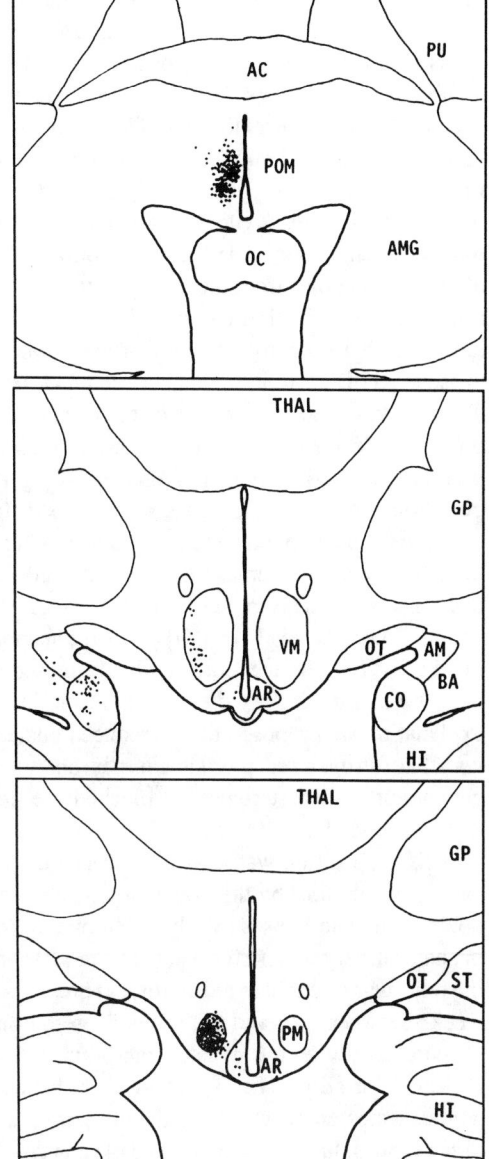

FIGURE 2 Maps of the brain of a female cynomolgus monkey fetus (Day 119 of gestation) showing labeled neurons 60 min after the administration of 250 µCi [^{3}H]T. Each dot represents one labeled neuron. Note heavy labeling in preoptic and premammillary areas. Abbreviations: AC = anterior commissure; AM = medial amygdaloid nucleus (n); AMG = amygdala; AR = arcuate n; BA = accessory basal n; BST = bed n of stria terminalis; CD = caudate n; CL = claustrum; CO = cortical amygdaloid n; GP = globus pallidus; HI = hippocampus; OC = optic chiasm; OT = optic tract; PM = premammillary n; PO = medial preoptic n; PU = putamen; SL = lateral septal n; ST = stria terminalis; THAL = thalamus; VM = ventromedial n. From "The Uptake of [^{3}H]Testosterone and its Metabolites by the Brain and Pituitary Gland of the Fetal Macaque," by R. P. Michael, R. W. Bonsall, and H. D. Rees, 1989, *Endocrinology, 124*, pp. 1319–1326. Copyright 1989 by The Endocrine Society. Reprinted with kind permission from The Endocrine Society.

243

gestation (Bonsall, Zumpe, & Michael, 1990). Animals received either 250 μCi [^{3}H]T via the umbilical vein or 500 μCi [^{3}H]T subcutaneously. We preferred the subcutaneous route of administration because ethanolic injections into the umbilical vein sometimes provoked fetal distress. Purified nuclear and supernatant fractions from brain, pituitary gland, and genital tissue were analyzed by HPLC, as previously described. Concentrations of radioactivity extracted from cell nuclei were significantly higher ($p < .01$) in the hypothalamus–preoptic area than in other brain regions. Nuclear concentrations of [^{3}H]T did not differ significantly between males and females in any brain region, but in the pituitary gland they were 48% lower in males than in females ($p < .001$; Figure 3, top). [^{3}H]E$_2$ represented about 65% of the extracted radioactivity, and nuclear concentrations were 73% lower in males than in females ($p < .001$; Figure 3, bottom). Unchanged [^{3}H]T was detectable in all nuclear samples from the male genital tract, but represented less than 4% of the radioactivity. DHT, the 5α-reduced metabolite of T, was not detected in nuclei from any brain region or from the pituitary gland, but in the penis, seminal vesicles, and prostate [^{3}H]DHT represented between 84% and 94% of the radioactivity present. There was no evidence of a sex difference in the tissue uptake of radioactivity from blood, but levels of endogenous plasma testosterone were significantly higher in males (600 ng/100 ml) than in females (40 ng/100 ml). Thus, at about 120 days of gestation, there was a highly significant sex difference in the nuclear accumulation of [^{3}H]E$_2$ in the hypothalamus–preoptic area following the administration of [^{3}H]T to intact male and female fetuses. The reduced uptake in males could not be explained in terms of reduced availability of [^{3}H]T, because there were no differences of note in levels of [^{3}H]T in supernatants. Nor could the reduced nuclear uptake of [^{3}H]E$_2$ be accounted for by decreased aromatization because, again, there were no significant sex differences in the levels of [^{3}H]E$_2$ in supernatants. The explanation we proposed for the reduced nuclear uptake of [^{3}H]E$_2$ in male fetuses was that estrogen receptor sites in neurons were substantially occupied by endogenous, unlabeled steroids that blocked the uptake of labeled steroids (Bonsall, Zumpe, & Michael, 1990).

This proposition was examined in a study that compared the uptake of [^{3}H]T and its metabolites by the brains of castrated male, intact male, and intact, sham-operated female fetuses (Michael, Zumpe, & Bonsall, 1992). Fetal orchidectomy or sham surgery was performed between 110 and 121 days of gestation, after which the fetus was returned to the uterus and pregnancy was maintained for about 1 more week. Between 120 and 125 days of gestation, fetuses received 500 μCi [^{3}H]T subcutaneously and, 1 hr later, the brain, pituitary gland, and genital tract were collected for HPLC. Fetal castration abolished both the sex differences in endogenous testosterone levels and the nuclear uptake of labeled steroids by hormone-target tissues. Intact fetal males had plasma testosterone levels (570 ng/100 ml) that were significantly higher ($p < .05$) than those in females (34 ng/100 ml) and castrated males (15 ng/100 ml). Moreover, intact males had significantly lower (p

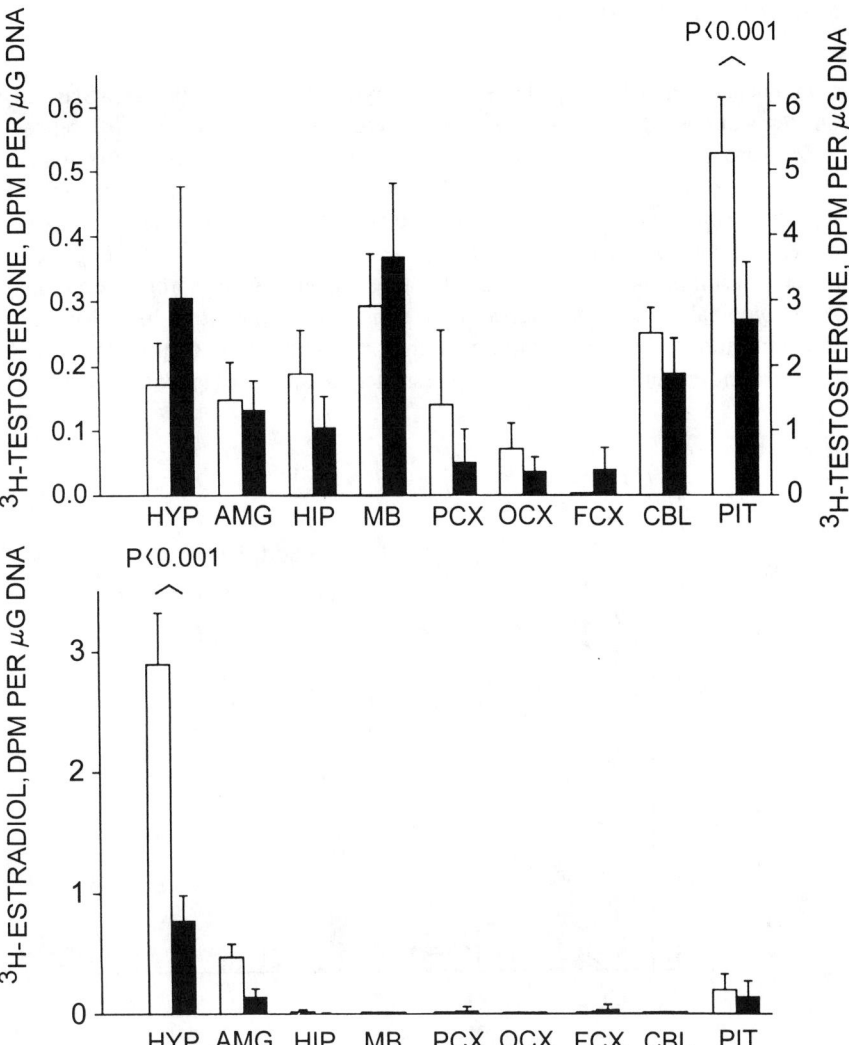

FIGURE 3 Mean concentrations of [^{3}H]T (top) and [^{3}H]E$_2$ (bottom) in cell nuclear fractions from the brains and pituitary glands of 7 intact female (open bars) and 5 intact male (solid bars) macaque fetuses 60 min after the administration of [^{3}H]T on about Day 122 of gestation. Top: There were no significant differences in [^{3}H]T concentrations between males and females in any brain region. In the anterior pituitary gland, levels were significantly lower ($p < .01$) in males than in females. Bottom: There was a significant difference ($p < .001$) in [^{3}H]E$_2$ concentrations between males and females in the hypothalamus–preoptic area, but not elsewhere in the brain or pituitary gland. Abbreviations: HYP = hypothalamus–preoptic area; AMG = amygdala; HIP = hippocampus; MB = midbrain; PCX = parietal cortex; OCX = occipital cortex; FCX = frontal cortex; CBL = cerebellar cortex. Vertical bars give standard error of mean. From "Comparison of the Nuclear Uptake of [^{3}H]-Testosterone and its Metabolites by the Brains of Male and Female Macaque Fetuses at 122 Days of Gestation," by R. W. Bonsall, D. Zumpe, and R. P. Michael, 1990, *Neuroendocrinology, 51*, pp. 474–480, 1990. Copyright 1990 by Karger, Basel. Reprinted with kind permission from Karger, Basel.

< .05) nuclear concentrations of $[^3H]E_2$ in the hypothalamus–preoptic area than did females and castrated males (Figure 4). There were no significant differences between groups of fetuses in nuclear concentrations of $[^3H]E_2$ in other brain regions, nuclear concentrations of unchanged $[^3H]T$ anywhere in the brain, or concentrations of $[^3H]T$ in supernatants. Because orchidectomy abolished the differences between the sexes in the nuclear uptake of $[^3H]E_2$, the hypothesis was strongly supported; namely, that the occupation of estrogen receptors, rather than of androgen receptors, in the hypothalamus–preoptic area of the male fetus is important for behavioral masculinization. The earlier view was that masculinization of the male fetus depended on the androgenic effects of testosterone and, perhaps, of DHT, but it

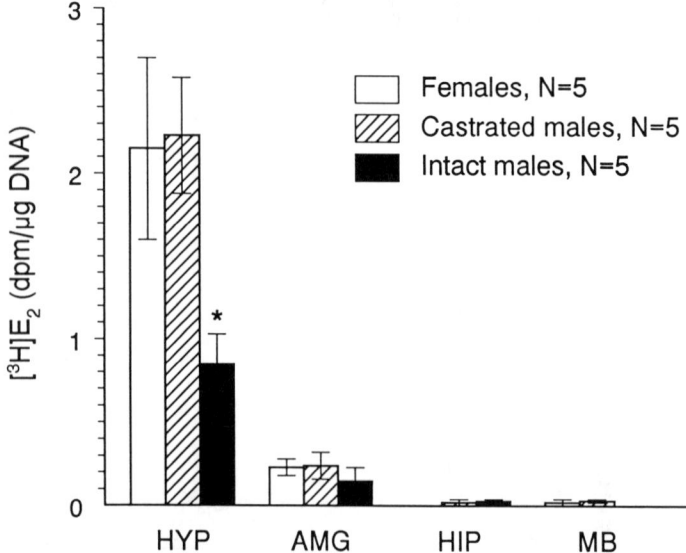

FIGURE 4 Nuclear concentrations of radioactivity identified by HPLC as $[^3H]E_2$ in samples from the brains of macaque fetuses around Day 122 of gestation 60 min after the subcutaneous administration of 500 µCi $[^3H]T$. Fetal castrations were performed 1 week earlier and pregnancies were maintained until the injections. Nuclear concentrations of $[^3H]E_2$ in castrated males were indistinguishable from those in intact, sham-operated females, and significantly higher than in intact males ($p < .05$, indicated by asterisk). Abbreviations: HYP = hypothalamus–preoptic area; AMG = amygdala; HIP = hippocampus; MB = midbrain. Vertical bars give standard error of mean. Reprinted from *Brain Research*, 570, R. P. Michael, D. Zumpe, and R. W. Bonsall, "The Interaction of Testosterone With the Brain of the Orchidectomized Primate Fetus," pp. 68–74, Copyright 1992, with kind permission from Elsevier Science – NL, Sara Burgerhartstraat 25, 1055 KV Amsterdam, The Netherlands.

now seems clear that fetal masculinization depends considerably on the estrogenic effects of testosterone by its aromatization to estradiol locally in the selected brain regions. This brings the primate data more in line with those of other mammals. We would not wish to exclude a role for unchanged testosterone, but the fact that injections of DHT to pregnant females can masculinize aspects of the behavior of female offspring (Pomerantz, Roy, et al., 1985) is not proof of a physiological role, because there was very little nuclear uptake of DHT derived from testosterone locally in the brain. Moreover, there were no differences between males and females in plasma levels of either DHT or androstenedione, neither of which was changed by fetal gonadectomy in either sex (Resko & Ellinwood, 1984).

The Uptake of Diethylstilbestrol by the Fetal Brain

The nonsteroidal, synthetic stilbene, diethylstilbestrol (DES), was the first potent, orally active estrogen to be employed clinically. Its administration to women during pregnancy has been associated with a variety of problems, some serious, in their male and female offspring. These include a reported increase in cervical dysplasia and clear-cell adenocarcinoma of the vagina and cervix in daughters. Sons of DES-treated mothers have been reported to differ from control groups in several measures of maleness (Kester, Green, & Finch, 1980). Daughters were reported to show less interest in infant care and in maternal behavior generally, which was regarded as a defeminizing effect (Ehrhardt et al., 1989), and there are data suggesting that women exposed prenatally to DES are more likely than unexposed women to exhibit bisexual or homosexual orientation (Meyer-Bahlburg, Ehrhardt, Rosen, & Gruen, 1995). These and other reports caused something of a public outcry, fortunately now considerably abated. DES is a potent estrogen and this potency is enhanced because it is not bound to sex hormone-binding protein in the plasma of pregnant women (Sheehan & Young, 1979). Nevertheless, its mechanism of action remained unclear and there were no data on DES's ability to enter the primate brain.

We therefore used autoradiography and HPLC to examine the uptake of DES by the brains and genital tracts of intact male and female macaque fetuses ($N = 11$; Michael & Bonsall, 1990). The results demonstrated that there is a system of neurons in the fetal primate brain at this stage of embryonic development with the capacity to take up [^{3}H]DES after its administration to the fetus. Between 121 and 124 days of gestation, fetuses received either 250 µCi [^{3}H]DES via the umbilical vein or 500 µCi [^{3}H]DES subcutaneously. The location of neurons accumulating radioactivity 60 min later was examined by autoradiography in two males and two females (Figure 5) using a rigorous labeling criterion based on the Poisson distribution: 4,400 neurons were counted. In females there were significantly more labeled neurons than expected by chance ($p < .001$) in hypothalamic regions

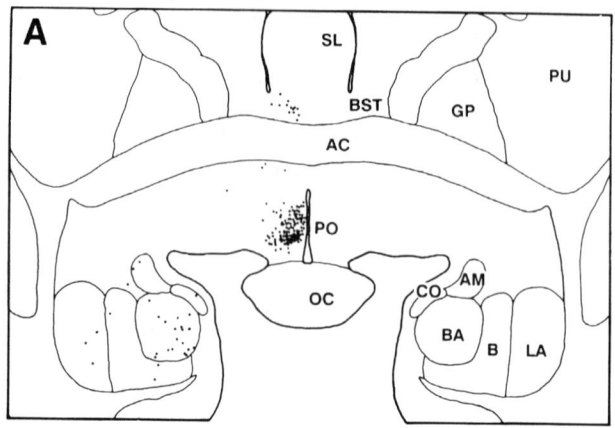
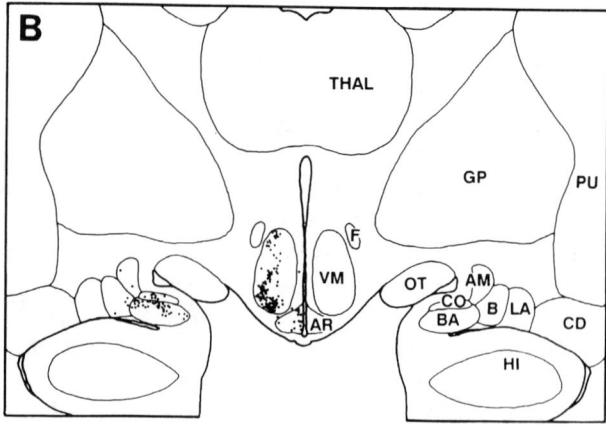

FIGURE 5 Maps of labeled neurons in the brain of a female cynomolgus fetus at 123 days of gestation, 60 min after the administration of 250 µCi [³H]DES via the umbilical vein. Labeled neurons were identified using a twice background criterion, and each dot represents one labeled neuron at the level of the optic chiasm (A) and at the level of the midhypothalamus (B). Abbreviations: AC = anterior commissure; AM = medial amygdaloid nucleus (n); AMG = amygdala; AR = arcuate n; BA = accessory basal n; BST = bed n of stria terminalis; CD = caudate n; CL = claustrum; CO = cortical amygdaloid n; GP = globus pallidus; HI = hippocampus; OC = optic chiasm; OT = optic tract; PM = premammillary n; PO = medial preoptic n; PU = putamen; SL = lateral septal n; ST = stria terminalis; THAL = thalamus; VM = ventromedial n. From "The Uptake of Tritiated Diethylstilbestrol (DES) by the Brain, Pituitary Gland, and Genital Tract of the Fetal Macaque: A Combined Chromatographic and Autoradiographic Study," by R. P. Michael and R. W. Bonsall, 1990, *Journal of Clinical Endocrinology and Metabolism, 71,* pp. 868–874. Copyright 1990 by The Endocrine Society. Reprinted with kind permission from The Endocrine Society.

(ventromedial and arcuate nuclei, bed nucleus of stria terminalis, and anterior hypothalamic area), medial preoptic area, and cortical and basal accessory amygdaloid nuclei, namely, the same brain regions labeled in adult male and female macaques after [^{3}H]E$_2$ administration (Bonsall, Rees, & Michael, 1986; Michael, Bonsall, & Rees, 1986). In three regions—the lateral septum, medial amygdala, and claustrum—there was labeling in the adult after [^{3}H]E$_2$ administration but not in the fetus after [^{3}H]DES administration, and the percentages of neurons labeled were 60% to 80% lower throughout the brain in the fetus than in the adult. In the ventromedial hypothalamus and amygdala, there were significantly fewer labeled neurons in male than in female fetuses, suggesting blockade of receptors by aromatized testosterone in males.

The chemical identity of radioactivity in cell nuclei was determined by HPLC in 3 male and 4 female fetuses. Most of the radioactivity extracted from cell nuclei from hypothalamus–preoptic area samples coeluted with the DES standard (females 61.5%, males 55.4%), and was thought to be unchanged [^{3}H]DES. Nuclear concentrations of [^{3}H]DES were highest in the hypothalamus–preoptic area and also relatively high in the amygdala, hippocampus, and midbrain, but there were no significant differences between males and females. Thus, although the autoradiographic and chromatographic data were largely in agreement, the significant male–female differences in autoradiograms were not confirmed by the HPLC results. Nuclear concentrations of radioactivity were higher in the pituitary gland and in male and female genital tracts (including gonads) than in the brain. The best documented abnormalities in DES-exposed children were structural changes in the uterus and vagina, and these high concentrations of radioactivity in nuclear fractions from the genital tract tissues of both males and females suggested a direct action on these structures. We were unable to identify the metabolites eluting before and after the [^{3}H]DES peak, which comprised up to half the total radioactivity, and these metabolites may have an important role in the overall effects of DES in the fetus. Blood samples were taken from the fetal hearts at the time of cesarean delivery for analysis by HPLC and for measurement of testosterone levels. Plasma concentrations of [^{3}H]DES were similar in males and females. About 90% of this radioactivity could be adsorbed onto Sephadex LH–20 columns and was thought not to bind with high affinity to plasma proteins, in agreement with findings in the human. It therefore appears that a physiological mechanism exists in the brain and genital tract of the fetal primate that could help account for some of the observed behavioral and structural deficits reported in sons and daughters of women receiving DES during early pregnancy.

Hormone Uptake by the Neonatal Brain: Testosterone and Its Metabolites

In male primates, including the human, plasma testosterone reaches adult levels during the first neonatal weeks (Corbier et al., 1990; Plant, 1982; Robinson &

Bridson, 1978; Winter et al., 1976), dropping thereafter to very low levels until the onset of puberty. In the neonate, as in the adult, there is a well-marked diurnal variation in plasma testosterone levels (high at night), and neonatal castration dramatically increases plasma LH levels (Plant, 1983). For these reasons, the hypothalamic gonadotropin releasing hormone pulse generator that activates the adenohypophysis is thought to be fully active in neonates. To examine hormone uptake and metabolism by the neonatal brain, 9 macaques (4 males, 5 females) were gonadectomized 2 to 5 days after birth and given 500 µCi [^{3}H]T subcutaneously 3 days later. After 60 min, tissue samples from the brain, pituitary gland, and genital tract were collected for analysis by HPLC (Bonsall & Michael, 1992). In both male and female brains, nuclear concentrations of the aromatized metabolite [^{3}H]E$_2$ were almost entirely restricted to, and predominated in, the hypothalamus–preoptic area (52%–55% of total radioactivity) and amygdala (40%–47% of total radioactivity), and there were no significant sex differences. Nuclear concentrations of unchanged [^{3}H]T were up to double those of [^{3}H]DHT in all brain regions, and both androgens were higher in females than in males: [^{3}H]T by 37% ($p = .003$) and [^{3}H]DHT by 68% ($p = .005$). Because this difference was associated with higher levels of [^{3}H]T and [^{3}H]DHT in supernatants, it was thought that it might depend on the lower body weights of females (366 ± 11 g) compared with males (428 ± 49 g) in the period after birth, as doses of [^{3}H]T were not corrected for body weight. In nuclear pellets from pituitary gland and peripheral tissues 6 to 7 days after birth, there was virtually no [^{3}H]E$_2$ in the pituitary gland, adrenal gland, uterus, and liver, whereas in prostate-seminal vesicles and penis, 82% to 86% of total radioactivity was in the form of [^{3}H]DHT. The only clear sex difference was in the genital tract, where high nuclear concentrations of [^{3}H]DHT occurred in males but not in females.

Hormone Uptake by the Adult Brain: Testosterone and Its Metabolites

A series of studies with adult macaques, primarily males, established where [^{3}H]T and its metabolites were taken up by cell nuclei in the brain, pituitary gland, and peripheral target tissues. Adults were gonadectomized and 3 days later were given an intravenous injection of 5 µCi [^{3}H]T: After 60 min, samples from one half of the brain, half the pituitary gland, and peripheral tissues were collected for autoradiography, and those from the other half were collected for HPLC (Bonsall, Rees, & Michael, 1985; Figure 6). After [^{3}H]DHT administration, the majority of radioactivity in cell nuclei from the hypothalamus, amygdala, and anterior pituitary gland was in the form of [^{3}H]DHT, and after [^{3}H]E$_2$ administration it was in the form of [^{3}H]E$_2$. After [^{3}H]T administration, however, all [^{3}H]steroids were present in hypothalamus and amygdala, but only [^{3}H]T and [^{3}H]DHT were present in the anterior pituitary gland.

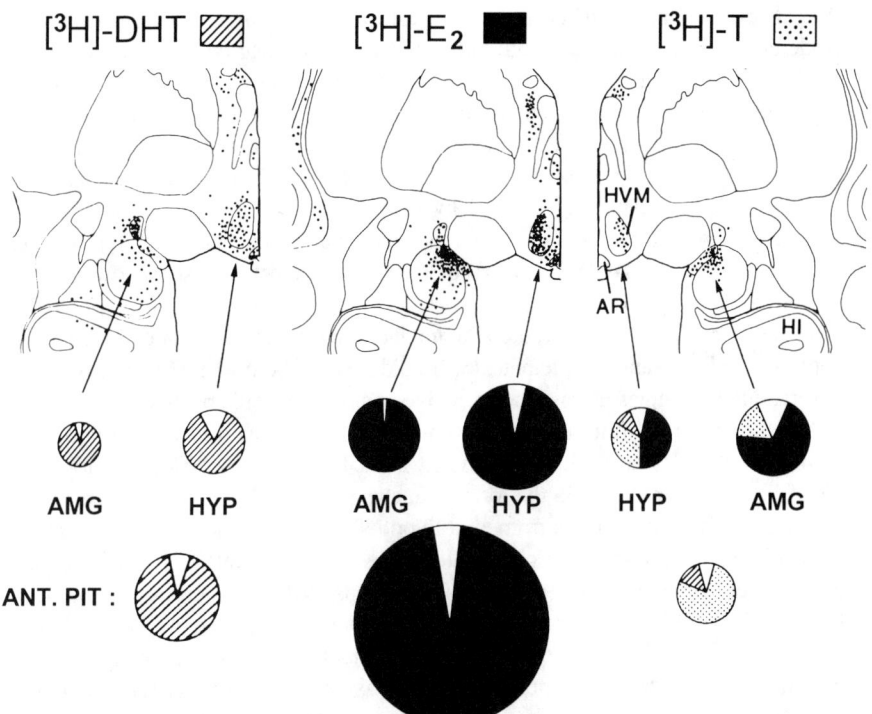

FIGURE 6 Maps of labeled neurons at the level of the midhypothalamus in three adult male rhesus monkeys. Each dot represents six labeled neurons. The radioligand administered 60 min before death is given at the top of each panel. The areas of the circles at the bottom of the figure are proportional to the amounts of ether-extractable radioactivity in cell nuclei from the regions indicated by the arrows. The percentages of the [^{3}H]steroids identified by HPLC in brain nuclei are shown by the areas of the segments within the circles. The white segments represent unknown [^{3}H]steroids. Abbreviations: AMG = amygdala; AR = arcuate nucleus; HI = hippocampus; HVM = ventromedial hypothalamus; ANT.PIT = anterior pituitary gland. Left and right panels reprinted from the *Journal of Steroid Biochemistry*, 23, R. W. Bonsall, H. D. Rees, and R. P. Michael, "The Distribution, Nuclear Uptake and Metabolism of [^{3}H]dihydrotestosterone in the Brain, Pituitary Gland and Genital Tract of the Male Rhesus Monkey," pp. 389–398, Copyright 1985, with kind permission from Elsevier Science Ltd., The Boulevard, Langford Lane, Kidlington OX5 1GB, UK.

Two approaches were used to determine the locations of neurons that accumulated either unchanged [^{3}H]T or its metabolites [^{3}H]E$_2$ and [^{3}H]DHT: (a) One used pretreatments with large doses of unlabeled steroid to block a particular type of receptor before [^{3}H]T was administered, and (b) the other compared these results with data from animals administered either [^{3}H]E$_2$ or [^{3}H]DHT, with or without pretreatments with unlabeled steroid. Although estradiol also binds with measurable affinity to androgen receptors and testosterone-binding globulin, at low to moderate doses pretreatment with unlabeled estradiol selectively blocks estrogen receptors in the brain. For example, pretreatment with cold estradiol would be expected to block all estrogen receptors in the brain, both those in areas with aromatase (where aromatized [^{3}H]T would accumulate) and those in areas without aromatase (where aromatized [^{3}H]T would not accumulate). Autoradiographic labeling after cold estradiol followed by [^{3}H]T administration would therefore be expected to visualize androgen receptors accumulating unchanged [^{3}H]T and its reduced metabolite [^{3}H]DHT; and HPLC would be expected to show low nuclear concentrations of [^{3}H]E$_2$. Thus, areas where [^{3}H]T accumulates in the form of [^{3}H]E$_2$ would be identified by reduced autoradiographic labeling and reduced nuclear concentrations of [^{3}H]E$_2$ in animals pretreated with cold estradiol before [^{3}H]T administration: Several other examples of this type of in vivo competition could be given.

The experimental findings can be summarized briefly as follows. Without any pretreatment, [^{3}H]T accumulated primarily in the form of [^{3}H]E$_2$ (Figure 7, top left) but also, to a lesser extent, in the form of unchanged [^{3}H]T (Figure 7, top right), in the medial preoptic area, ventromedial hypothalamus, and cortical and accessory basal amygdala (Bonsall & Michael, 1989; Bonsall et al., 1989). [^{3}H]DHT concentrations were very low in cell nuclei in these regions. With testosterone pretreatment followed by [^{3}H]T administration, there was a dramatic decrease in [^{3}H]E^2 (almost to zero) and in [^{3}H]T (by 66%–94%) in cell nuclei in these regions (Figure 7, bottom). In contrast, pretreatment with DHT was without effect on [^{3}H]E$_2$ accumulation in cell nuclei from the preoptic area, hypothalamus, and amygdala, and this was also the case for [^{3}H]T accumulation in amygdala (Figure 7, middle). The blockade of [^{3}H]T uptake by pretreatments with testosterone and DHT in the preoptic area and hypothalamus (but not in amygdala) was interpreted to demonstrate an effect on androgen receptors. The blockade of [^{3}H]E$_2$ uptake in the preoptic area, hypothalamus, and amygdala by pretreatment only with testosterone was interpreted as an effect on estrogen receptors. DHT pretreatment failed to decrease [^{3}H]T uptake only in the amygdala, and was also without any effect on [^{3}H]E$_2$ uptake in the preoptic area, hypothalamus, and amygdala. It appeared, therefore, that the amygdala might contain a quantity of testosterone-specific receptors not sensitive to DHT, which we refer to as *amygdaloid tau receptors*. Careful examination of labeling indices in autoradiograms from animals pretreated with DHT (Michael, Rees, & Bonsall, 1989) showed that there were no effects in the accessory basal amygdaloid nucleus, whereas there were significant decreases in the medial amygdaloid ($p < .01$) and cortical amygdaloid ($p < .05$) nuclei (Figure 8). Because of this, it seemed likely that the majority of tau receptors were located in the basal accessory amygdaloid nucleus, which might be unique in this respect.

As anticipated from the androgen pretreatment studies, estradiol pretreatment reduced labeling in these same brain regions (preoptic area, hypothalamus, and amygdala) by 35% to 65% and decreased nuclear concentrations of [^{3}H]E$_2$ by 37%

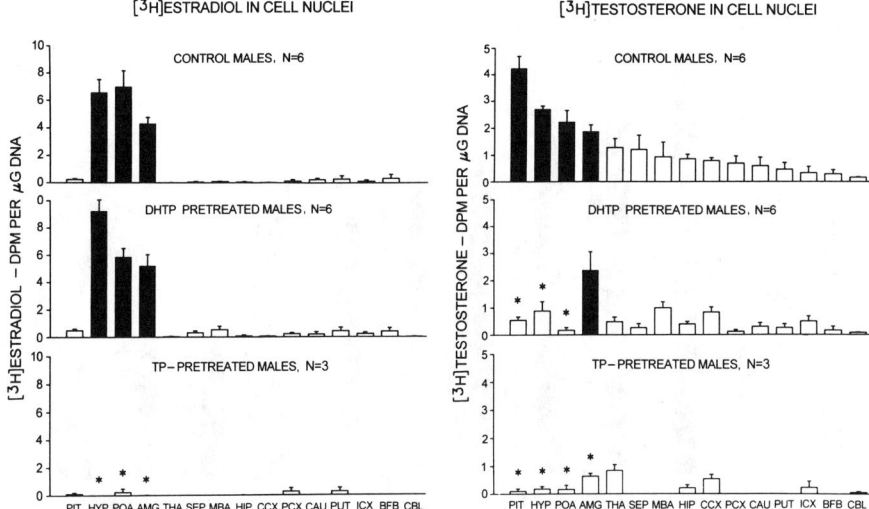

FIGURE 7 Effects of pretreatments with dihydrotestosterone propionate (DHTP) or testosterone propionate (TP) on concentrations of [^{3}H]E$_2$ (left) and [^{3}H]T (right) in cell nuclei from the brains and pituitary glands of castrated male rhesus monkeys 60 min after the intravenous administration of 5 mCi [^{3}H]T. Left: DHTP pretreatment did not change [^{3}H]E$_2$ uptake in hypothalamus, preoptic area and amygdala, which remained similar to that of controls. TP pretreatment significantly reduced [^{3}H]E$_2$ uptake in these regions (bottom). Right: Pretreatments with both DHTP and TP substantially blocked the uptake of [^{3}H]T in all regions except in the amygdala, where it was not blocked by DHTP pretreatment (middle), suggesting the presence of testosterone-specific tau receptors. Solid columns give tissues with significantly elevated radioactivity. Statistically significant ($p < .05$) differences from control males are given by asterisks. Abbreviations: PIT = pituitary gland; HYP = hypothalamus; POA = preoptic area; THA = thalamus; SEP = septal area; MBA = mammillary body area; HIP = hippocampus; CCX = cingulate cortex; PCX = postcentral gyrus; CAU = caudate; PUT = putamen; ICX = inferior temporal gyrus; BFB = basal forebrain; CBL = cerebellar cortex. Vertical bars give standard error of mean. Reprinted from the *Journal of Steroid Biochemistry, 33,* R. W. Bonsall and R. P. Michael, "Pretreatments With 5a-dihydrotestosterone and the Uptake of Testosterone by Cell Nuclei in the Brains of Male Rhesus Monkeys," pp. 405–411, Copyright 1989, with kind permission from Elsevier Science Ltd., The Boulevard, Langford Lane, Kidlington OX5 1GB, UK.

to 55% compared with controls (Rees, Bonsall, & Michael, 1988a). Moreover, the finding that the preoptic area, hypothalamus, and amygdala accumulate [^{3}H]T largely as its aromatized metabolite [^{3}H]E$_2$ was supported by autoradiographic and HPLC data from animals given [^{3}H]E$_2$ after pretreatment with testosterone (Michael, Bonsall, & Rees, 1987). In the preoptic area, ventromedial hypothalamus, and amygdala, then, containing both androgen and estrogen receptors as well as aromatase activity, testosterone can act both as an androgen and as an estrogen in male and female.

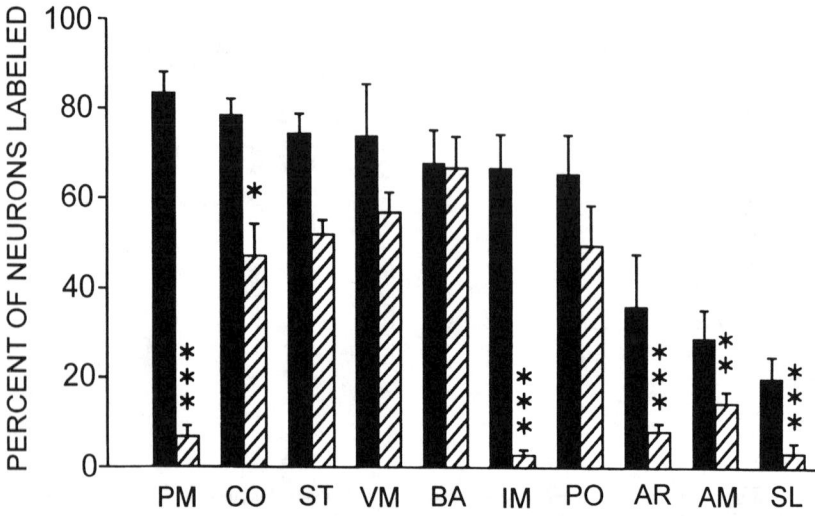

FIGURE 8 Mean percentages of neurons labeled according to the 1% Poisson criterion following the administration of [^{3}H]T to control (solid columns) and to DHTP-pretreated (hatched columns) castrated male rhesus monkeys. Significant reductions in DHTP-pretreated males are indicated by asterisks: *$p < .05$. **$p < .01$. ***$p < .001$. Note the lack of any blocking effect in the accessory basal amygdaloid nucleus, in contrast to other amygdaloid nuclei. Abbreviations: PM = premammillary nucleus (n); CO = cortical amygdaloid n; ST = bed n of stria terminalis; VM = ventromedial hypothalamic n; BA = accessory basal amygdaloid n; IM = intercalated mammillary n; PO = medial preoptic n; AR = arcuate n; AM = medial amygdaloid n; SL = lateral septal n. Vertical bars give standard error of mean. Reprinted from *Brain Research, 502*, R. P. Michael, H. D. Rees, and R. W. Bonsall, "Sites in the Male Primate Brain At Which Testosterone Acts As an Androgen," pp. 11–20, Copyright 1989, with kind permission from Elsevier Science – NL, Sara Burgerhartstraat 25, 1055 KV Amsterdam, The Netherlands.

These and other studies have helped to characterize the hormone uptake mechanisms in other brain regions. Some areas, such as the arcuate nucleus and lateral septum (and pituitary gland), contain both androgen- and estrogen-concentrating neurons, but in them testosterone acts largely as an androgen (Michael et al., 1987) because these regions lack sufficient aromatase to produce estradiol (Roselli, Stadelman, Horton, & Resko, 1987). These areas might respond to peripheral aromatization in males and could accumulate estradiol in females at midcycle and during pregnancy. In other regions, most notably the premammillary nucleus and intercalated mammillary nucleus, testosterone acts exclusively as an androgen, as these regions contain androgen but not estrogen receptors. In male genital tract tissues, the situation is simple because [^{3}H]T accumulates in nuclei almost exclusively in the form of [^{3}H]DHT (Rees, Bonsall, & Michael, 1988b), whereas in the female genital tract [³H]T accumulates primarily as unchanged [³H]T in the uterus and as [³H]DHT in the clitoris (Michael et al., 1986).

From these studies, as far as they have gone, it appears that there are no detectable differences between the receptor systems in the brains of adult males and females but, of course, as in the fetus and neonate, the hormonal milieu differs vastly in the two sexes. Because we were unable to identify any sex differences in steroid receptor distributions and numbers in the macaque brain, one is left to assume that it is the brain's hormonal milieu, which differs vastly in the two sexes, that is a major source of the sex differences in behavior, although it is clearly not sufficient in itself: not a very satisfying conclusion. We do not have any data from in vivo competition studies in fetuses and neonates. As they would be difficult to perform, it would be valuable to use immunocytochemistry to study the ontogeny of different classes of steroid receptors in the brains of both sexes from fetus to maturity. Immunocytochemistry offers the best means for doing this, particularly now that double (and triple) labeling techniques are available for nonprimate mammals. Immunocytochemistry has an advantage over autoradiography in that labeling is restricted to the particular type of receptor (androgen, estrogen, or progestin) against which the antibody is raised, whereas autoradiography simply demonstrates steroid uptake by the neuronal nucleus. We used this method to map the distribution of androgen receptors in the brains of male and female macaques (Michael, Clancy, & Zumpe, 1995). Labeling distributions were very similar to those using autoradiography after [³H]T administration, but areas of immunocytochemical labeling were generally more restricted, and no sex differences were observed.

Comparisons of Hormone Uptake in Fetuses, Neonates and Adults: Testosterone and Its Metabolites

Although there are very large gaps in our knowledge, it is worthwhile to attempt to make some comparisons between different stages of primate development; this is difficult because it is impossible to match accurately doses of [³H]T on a body weight basis. Both body weights and body composition change dramatically during development, and so does the rate of steroid metabolism. In the fetus, of course, the placenta greatly enhances clearance rates.

Endogenous plasma testosterone levels were all remarkably similar (about 600–800 ng/100 ml) in male fetuses at 120 days of gestation, in male neonates during the 1st week of life, and in fully adult males. Fetuses and adults had approximately the same levels of radioactivity in supernatants, and levels were about double those in neonates (Bonsall & Michael, 1992): We think they were overdosed with radioactivity relative to the other age groups. In the hypothalamus–preoptic area, nuclear concentrations of [³H]T after [³H]T administration were more than sixfold higher in gonadectomized adults (males and females) than in fetuses (castrated males and intact females), probably due to increased concentrations of androgen receptors, and levels in gonadectomized neonates were intermediate between those in fetuses and in adults; nevertheless, the major increase in the uptake of [^{3}H]T occurred between the neonatal period and adulthood (Figure 9). In the amygdala, the nuclear uptake of [^{3}H]T after [^{3}H]T administration was considerably higher in adults than in fetuses (Bonsall & Michael, 1992). In the hypothalamus, nuclear concentrations of [^{3}H]E$_2$ after [^{3}H]T administration were 2.7 times higher in adults than in fetuses, although the proportion of aromatized metabolite, compared with unchanged [^{3}H]T, was twice as high in fetuses as in adults. In the amygdala, the nuclear uptake of [^{3}H]E$_2$ was massively increased between fetus and adult, but a substantial increase (fourfold) occurred between the neonatal period and adulthood. This postnatal increase might be related to the long period of prepubertal development in primates and to the ontogeny of behavioral patterns. In the premammillary area, it was noteworthy that autora-

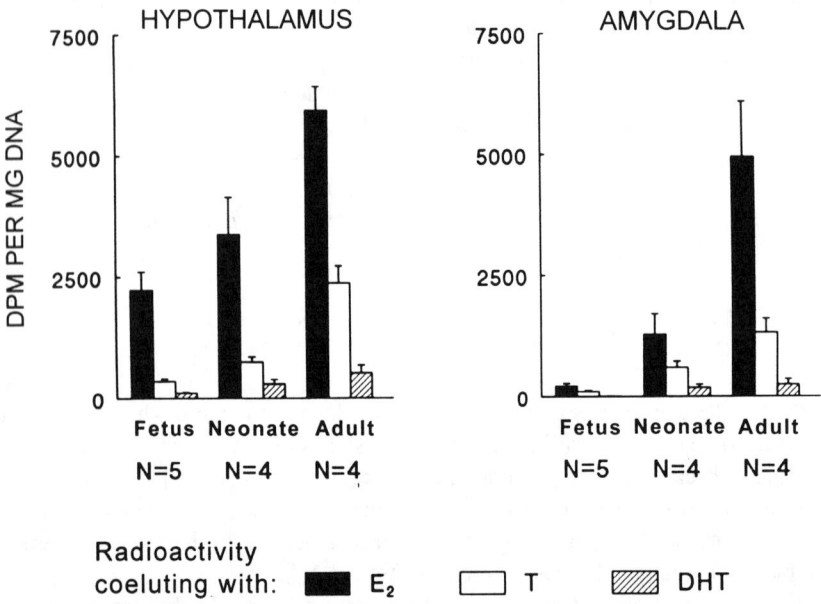

FIGURE 9 Nuclear pellets from the macaque brain at three stages of development. Radioactivity identified by HPLC in samples from castrated males 60 min after the administration of [^{3}H]T to fetuses (122 days of gestation), neonates (6–8 days old), and adults. In the hypothalamus, there was a progressive increase in [^{3}H]E$_2$ uptake with age but, in the amygdala, the major increase was between neonate and adult. From "Developmental Changes in the Uptake of Testosterone by the Primate Brain," by R. W. Bonsall and R. P. Michael, 1992, *Neuroendrocrinology, 55*, pp. 84–91. Copyright 1992 by Karger, Basel. Reprinted with kind permission from Karger, Basel.

diographic labeling indices (percentage of neurons labeled) after [^{3}H]T administration were quite similar (50%–60%) in fetuses and adults of both sexes. Although lower, labeling indices in the medial preoptic area were also similar (about 30%–40%) in fetuses (Michael, Bonsall, & Rees, 1989) and adults (Rees et al., 1988a). In the male fetus, of course, plasma testosterone levels are high at 120 days of gestation so receptors would presumably be occupied, unlike in the female fetus in which plasma testosterone levels remain very low throughout gestation.

ACKNOWLEDGMENTS

The original work reported here was supported by U.S. Public Health Service Grants MH 40420 and MH 19506.

REFERENCES

Arnold, A. P. (1981). Quantitative analysis of steroid autoradiograms. *Journal of Histochemistry and Cytochemistry, 29,* 207–211.

Baum, M. J. (1979). Differentiation of coital behavior in mammals: A comparative analysis. *Neuroscience and Biobehavioral Reviews, 3,* 265–284.

Bonsall, R. W., & Michael, R. P. (1989). Pretreatments with 5a-dihydrotestosterone and the uptake of testosterone by cell nuclei in the brains of male rhesus monkeys. *Journal of Steroid Biochemistry, 33,* 405–411.

Bonsall, R. W., & Michael, R. P. (1992). Developmental changes in the uptake of testosterone by the primate brain. *Neuroendocrinology, 55,* 84–91.

Bonsall, R. W., Rees, H. D., & Michael, R. P. (1985). The distribution, nuclear uptake and metabolism of [^{3}H]dihydrotestosterone in the brain, pituitary gland and genital tract of the male rhesus monkey. *Journal of Steroid Biochemistry, 23,* 389–398.

Bonsall, R. W., Rees, H. D., & Michael, R. P. (1986). ^{3}H-Estradiol and its metabolites in the brain, pituitary gland and reproductive tract of the male rhesus monkey: A combined autoradiographic and chromatographic study. *Neuroendocrinology, 43,* 98–109.

Bonsall, R. W., Rees, H. D., & Michael, R. P. (1989). Identification of radioactivity in cell nuclei from brain, pituitary gland and genital tract of male rhesus monkeys after the administration of [^{3}H]testosterone. *Journal of Steroid Biochemistry, 32,* 599–608.

Bonsall, R. W., Zumpe, D., & Michael, R. P. (1978). Menstrual cycle influences on operant behavior of female rhesus monkeys. *Journal of Comparative and Physiological Psychology, 92,* 846–855.

Bonsall, R. W., Zumpe, D., & Michael, R. P. (1990). Comparisons of the nuclear uptake of [^{3}H]-testosterone and its metabolites by the brains of male and female macaque fetuses at 122 days of gestation. *Neuroendocrinology, 51,* 474–480.

Burns, R. K. (1956). Hormones versus constitutional factors in the growth of embryonic sex primordia in the opossum. *American Journal of Anatomy, 98,* 35–67.

Corbier, P., Dehennin, L., Castanier, M., Mebazaa, A., Edwards, D. A., & Roffi, J. (1990). Sex differences in serum luteinizing hormone and testosterone in the human neonate during the first few hours after birth. *Journal of Clinical Endocrinology and Metabolism, 71,* 1344–1348.

Dantchakoff, V. (1936). Réalisation du sexe à volonté par inductions hormonales. I. Inversion du sexe dans un embryon génétiquement mâle [Sex determination at will by hormonal induction. I. Sex reversal in a genetically male embryo]. *Bulletin Biologique de la France et de la Belgique, 70,* 241–307.

Eaton, G. G., Goy, R. W., & Phoenix, C. H. (1973). Effects of testosterone treatment in adulthood on sexual behavior of female pseudohermaphrodite rhesus monkeys. *Nature New Biology, 242,* 119–120.

Eaton, G. G., Worlein, J. M., & Glick, B. B. (1990). Sex differences in Japanese macaques (*Macaca fuscata*): Effects of prenatal testosterone on juvenile social behavior. *Hormones and Behavior, 24,* 270–283.

Ehrhardt, A. A., Meyer Bahlburg, H. F., Rosen, L. R., Feldman, J. F., Veridiano, N. P., Elkin, E. J., & McEwen, B. S. (1989). The development of gender-related behavior in females following prenatal exposure to diethylstilbestrol (DES). *Hormones and Behavior, 23,* 526–541.

Goy, R. W. (1968). Organizing effects of androgen on the behaviour of rhesus monkeys. In R. P. Michael (Ed.), *Endocrinology and human behaviour* (pp. 12–31). London: Oxford University Press.

Goy, R. W., Bercovitch, F. B., & McBrair, M. C. (1988). Behavioral masculinization is independent of genital masculinization in prenatally androgenized female rhesus macaques. *Hormones and Behavior, 22,* 552–571.

Goy, R. W., & Resko, J. A. (1972). Gonadal hormones and behavior of normal and pseudohermaphroditic nonhuman female primates. *Recent Progress in Hormone Research, 28,* 707–733.

Greene, R. R. (1942). Hormonal factors in sex inversion: The effects of sex hormones on embryonic sexual structures of the rat. *Biological Symposia, 9,* 105–123.

Hammarbäck, S., Damber, J.-E., & Bäckström, T. (1989). Relationship between symptom severity and hormone changes in women with premenstrual syndrome. *Journal of Clinical Endocrinology and Metabolism, 68,* 125–130.

Handa, R. J., Connolly, P. B., & Resko, J. A. (1988). Ontogeny of cytosolic androgen receptors in the brain of the fetal rhesus monkey. *Endocrinology, 122,* 1890–1896.

Harlow, H. F., & Zimmerman, R. R. (1959). Affectional responses in the infant monkey. *Science, 130,* 421–432.

Jost, A. (1953). Problems of fetal endocrinology: The gonadal and hypophysial hormones. *Recent Progress in Hormone Research, 8,* 379–418.

Keller, K., & Tandler, J. (1916). Über das Verhalten der Eihäute bei der Zwillingsträchtigkeit des Rindes [On the behavior of the chorion in twin pregnancies of cattle]. *Wiener tierärztliche Wochenschrift, 3,* 513–526.

Kester, P., Green, R., & Finch, S. J. (1980). Prenatal female hormone administration and psychosexual development in human males. *Psychoneuroendocrinology, 5,* 269–285.

Lillie, F. R. (1916). The theory of the freemartin. *Science, 43,* 611–613.

Lillie, F. R. (1917). The freemartin: A study of the action of sex hormones in the foetal life of cattle. *Journal of Experimental Zoology, 23,* 371–452.

Meyer-Bahlburg, H. F. L., Ehrhardt, A. A., Rosen, L. R., & Gruen, R. S. (1995). Prenatal estrogens and the development of homosexual orientation. *Developmental Psychology, 31,* 12–21.

Michael, R. P., & Bonsall, R. W. (1977). Peri-ovulatory synchronisation of behaviour in male and female rhesus monkeys. *Nature, 265,* 463–465.

Michael, R. P., & Bonsall, R. W. (1990). The uptake of tritiated diethylstilbestrol (DES) by the brain, pituitary gland and genital tract of the fetal macaque: A combined chromatographic and autoradiographic study. *Journal of Clinical Endocrinology and Metabolism, 71,* 868–874.

Michael, R. P., Bonsall, R. W., & Rees, H. D. (1986). The nuclear accumulation of [^{3}H]testosterone and [^{3}H]estradiol in the brain of the female primate: Evidence for the aromatization hypothesis. *Endocrinology, 118,* 1935–1944.

Michael, R. P., Bonsall, R. W., & Rees, H. D. (1987). Sites at which testosterone may act as an estrogen in the brain of the male primate. *Neuroendocrinology, 46,* 511–521.
Michael, R. P., Bonsall, R. W., & Rees, H. D. (1989). The uptake of [^{3}H]testosterone and its metabolites by the brain and pituitary gland of the fetal macaque. *Endocrinology, 124,* 1319–1326.
Michael, R. P., Clancy, A. N., & Zumpe, D. (1995). Distribution of androgen receptor-like immunoreactivity in the brains of cynomolgus monkeys. *Journal of Neuroendocrinology, 7,* 713–719.
Michael, R. P., & Rees, H. D. (1986). Neurons in the brain of fetal rhesus monkeys accumulate ^{3}H-testosterone or its metabolites. *Life Sciences, 38,* 1673–1677.
Michael, R. P., Rees, H. D., & Bonsall, R. W. (1989). Sites in the male primate brain at which testosterone acts as an androgen. *Brain Research, 502,* 11–20.
Michael, R. P., & Zumpe, D. (1993). A review of hormonal factors influencing the sexual and aggressive behavior of macaques. *American Journal of Primatology, 30,* 213–241.
Michael, R. P., Zumpe, D., & Bonsall, R. W. (1992). The interaction of testosterone with the brain of the orchidectomized primate fetus. *Brain Research, 570,* 68–74.
Money, J., & Erhardt, A. A. (1972). *Man & woman, boy & girl.* Baltimore: The Johns Hopkins University Press.
Phoenix, C. H. (1974). Prenatal testosterone in the nonhuman primate and its consequences for behavior. In R. C. Friedman, R. M. Richart, & R. L. Vande Wiele (Eds.), *Sex differences in behavior* (pp. 19–32). New York: Wiley.
Phoenix, C. H., & Chambers, K. C. (1982). Sexual behavior in adult gonadectomized female pseudohermaphrodite, female, and male rhesus macaques (*Macaca mulatta*) treated with estradiol benzoate and testosterone propionate. *Journal of Comparative and Physiological Psychology, 96,* 823–833.
Phoenix, C. H., Jensen, J. N., & Chambers, K. C. (1983). Female sexual behavior displayed by androgenized female rhesus macaques. *Hormones and Behavior, 17,* 146–152.
Plant, T. M. (1982). A striking diurnal variation in plasma testosterone concentration in infantile male rhesus monkeys (*Macaca mulatta*). *Neuroendocrinology, 35,* 370–373.
Plant, T. M. (1983). Ontogeny of gonadotropin secretion in the rhesus macaque. In R. L. Norman (Ed.), *Neuroendocrine aspects of reproduction* (pp. 133–147). New York: Academic.
Pomerantz, S. M., Fox, T. O., Sholl, S. A., Vito, C. C., & Goy, R. W. (1985). Androgen and estrogen receptors in fetal rhesus monkey brain and anterior pituitary. *Endocrinology, 116,* 83–89.
Pomerantz, S. M., Roy, M. M., Thornton, J. E., & Goy, R. W. (1985). Expression of adult female patterns of sexual behavior by male, female, and pseudohermaphroditic female rhesus monkeys. *Biology of Reproduction, 33,* 878–889.
Rees, H. D., Bonsall, R. W., & Michael, R. P. (1988a). Estrogen binding and the actions of testosterone in the brain of the male rhesus monkey. *Brain Research, 452,* 28–38.
Rees, H. D., Bonsall, R. W., & Michael, R. P. (1988b). Localization and identification of nuclear radioactivity in the pituitary gland and genital tract after administering ^{3}H-testosterone, ^{3}H-dihydrotestosterone or ^{3}H-estradiol to male rhesus monkeys. *Cell and Tissue Research, 254,* 139–146.
Resko, J. A., Connolly, P. B., & Roselli, C. E. (1988). Testosterone 5a-reductase activity in neural tissue of fetal rhesus macaques. *Journal of Steroid Biochemistry, 29,* 429–434.
Resko, J. A., & Ellinwood, W. E. (1984). Sexual differentiation of the brain of primates. In M. Serio, M. Motta, M. Zanisi, & L. Martini (Eds.), *Sexual differentiation: Basic and clinical aspects* (pp. 79–91). New York: Raven.
Reyes, F. I., Boroditsky, R. S., Winter, J. S. D., & Faiman, C. (1974). Studies on human sexual development: II. Fetal and maternal serum gonadotropin and sex steroid concentrations. *Journal of Clinical Endocrinology and Metabolism, 38,* 612–617.
Robinson, J. A., & Bridson, W. E. (1978). Neonatal hormone patterns in the macaque: I. Steroids. *Biology of Reproduction, 19,* 773–778.
Roselli, C. E., & Resko, J. A. (1986). Effects of gonadectomy and androgen treatment on aromatase activity in the fetal monkey brain. *Biology of Reproduction, 35,* 106–112.

Roselli, C. E., Stadelman, H., Horton, L. E., & Resko, J. A. (1987). Regulation of androgen metabolism and luteinizing hormone-releasing hormone content in discrete hypothalamic and limbic areas of male rhesus macaques. *Endocrinology, 120,* 97–106.

Sheehan, D. M., & Young, M. (1979). Diethylstilbestrol and estradiol binding to serum albumin in pregnancy plasma of rat and human. *Endocrinology, 104,* 1442–1446.

Van Wagenen, G., & Simpson, M. E. (1965). *Embryology of the ovary and testis, Homo sapiens and Macaca mulatta.* New Haven, CT: Yale University Press.

Wells, L. J., & Van Wagenen, G. (1954). Androgen-induced female pseudohermaphroditism in the monkey (*Macaca mulatta*): Anatomy of the reproductive organs. *Contributions to Embryology, 35,* 93–106.

Westermarck, E. (1891). *The history of human marriage.* New York: Macmillan.

Wilkins, L., Jones, H. W., Holman, G. H., & Stempfel, R. S. (1958). Masculinization of the female fetus associated with administration of oral and intramuscular progestins during gestation: Non-adrenal female pseudohermaphroditism. *Journal of Clinical Endocrinology and Metabolism, 18,* 559–585.

Winter, J. S. D., Hughes, I. A., Reyes, F. I., & Faiman, C. (1976). Pituitary-gonadal relations in infancy: 2. Patterns of serum gonadal steroid concentrations in man from birth to two years of age. *Journal of Clinical Endocrinology and Metabolism, 42,* 679–686.

Young, W. C. (1961). The hormones and mating behavior. In W. C. Young (Ed.), *Sex and internal secretions* (pp. 1173–1239). Baltimore: Williams & Wilkins.

Zumpe, D., Clancy, A. N., Bonsall, R. W., & Michael, R. P. (1996). Behavioral responses to Depo-Provera, Fadrozole and estradiol in castrated, testosterone-treated cynomolgus monkeys (*Macaca fascicularis*): The involvement of progestin receptors. *Physiology and Behavior, 60,* 531–540.

Zumpe, D., & Michael, R. P. (1996). Social factors modulate the effects of hormones on the sexual and aggressive behavior of macaques. *American Journal of Primatology, 38,* 233–261.

Sex Differences in the Auditory System

Dennis McFadden
Department of Psychology and Institute for Neuroscience
University of Texas, Austin

A number of sex differences have been documented in the human auditory system. Females as a group have greater hearing sensitivity, greater susceptibility to noise exposure at high frequencies, shorter latencies in their auditory brain-stem responses, more spontaneous otoacoustic emissions (SOAEs), and stronger click-evoked otoacoustic emissions than males as a group. Males are better at sound localization, detecting binaural beats, and detecting signals in complex masking tasks than are females. During the first half of the menstrual cycle, several aspects of female hearing move in the male direction. The sex difference normally present in SOAEs is absent in females from opposite-sex twin pairs. The implication is that their auditory systems have been masculinized prenatally by exposure to high levels of androgens produced by their male cotwins, analogous to an effect well established in other mammals. This suggests that some of the other sex differences in hearing are also attributable to differences in exposure to hormones. Thus, the SOAE findings suggest an organizational effect of hormones on the human auditory system, and the menstrual findings suggest an activational effect. Said differently, the auditory system appears to be among those brain structures that are altered by hormones pre- and postnatally, implying that some auditory measures may eventually prove valuable as windows onto other hormone-driven processes, characteristics, and abilities.

The human auditory system exhibits a number of sex differences. These are generally small, and their origin and evolutionary significance, if any, are still unknown. There is accumulating evidence, however, both that prenatal hormones contribute to some of these auditory sex differences, and that auditory sex differences have the potential to shed light on other sex differences as well as on other topics. Some of the basic facts are summarized here, but it must be emphasized at

---

Requests for reprints should be sent to Dennis McFadden, Department of Psychology, Mezes Hall 330, University of Texas, Austin, TX 78712–1189. E-mail: mcfadden@psy.utexas.edu

the outset that there is still far more ignorance than knowledge on the topics of sex differences and hormonal influences in the auditory system. Accordingly, this article has about as many promissory notes and speculations as established facts. The hope was that by getting the facts assembled in one place my colleagues in audition would be better able to locate the gaps in our knowledge, and readers from other disciplines would be alerted to possible connections with their own research areas. It does not require careful reading to see a number of research possibilities nearly guaranteed to yield interesting, relevant results.

Surely, we should not be surprised to find evidence of sex differences in the human auditory system, for it, like the other senses, is an important part of a nervous system that is now known to exhibit many sex differences in structure and function. Yet many outsiders to auditory research are surprised, or at least nonplussed, on first hearing of their existence. Perhaps the reason is that simple intuition handles well the idea that complex behaviors and structures—higher order functions—can differ between the sexes, but it stumbles over the existence of sex differences in what are regarded to be simple, low-level functions and structures. Why this counterintuition? Perhaps because the existence of sex differences in simple, low-level abilities carries the implication that they—both the sex differences and the abilities—have, all along, been more important than has been appreciated. As a lifelong psychoacoustician who has been accused of spending (read: wasting) my life studying simple (read: less important) phenomena, I personally revel in the implication that the sensory periphery is more important than others have appreciated.

In this article, physiological and psychophysical (behavioral) evidence of sex differences in the auditory system are intermixed. For some readers, it is behavior that is ultimately more important, but having some knowledge of the underlying physiology could provide a valuable guide to their thinking about the possible processes underlying the behavioral differences. For other readers, the physiological evidence may be of greater interest because of its ability to suggest relations with the physiology in other systems. Mentioned along the way are ear differences, when such are known to exist. The reason is that various other lateral asymmetries are known to exist in the brain, and some of those appear to differ across sex (e.g., Nordeen & Yahr, 1982). Whether or not differential actions of hormones are responsible for any of these asymmetries and differences in asymmetry is unknown to me, but their ubiquity suggested that the story on the auditory system was at risk of being incomplete without mention of the known ear differences. Perhaps for some readers, the existence of ear differences will be persuasive that what is being discussed is relevant to other brain differences.

By way of background, the reader should recall that the job of the inner ear, or cochlea, is to transform the fluctuating patterns in air pressure that are present at the eardrum into neural activity in the eighth cranial nerve. The cochlea accomplishes this task by producing traveling waves of displacement that propagate along the 35-mm length of the basilar membrane, and, in the process, stimulate the relevant receptor cells, which, in turn, stimulate the relevant nerve fibers. Because the basilar membrane is continuously changing in mass, stiffness, and coupling along its length, it is able to perform a mechanical frequency analysis of the complex waveform present at the eardrum, with the result that the highest frequency components maximally activate the basal end of the membrane and successively lower frequencies maximally activate successively more apical locations. That is, the basilar membrane is tonotopically organized, and as a consequence, the receptors and neurons serving different basilar membrane locations are maximally responsive (tuned) to different bands of acoustic frequencies. Tonotopic segregation of information persists throughout the auditory chain, meaning that frequency channels and the "place" principle play important roles in the functioning of the auditory system.

To help the reader follow the discussion, Table 1 summarizes the basic points from this review.

TABLE 1
Summary of Topics Covered in This Review

Type of Measurement	*Outcome*
Physical differences	Male heads, pinnas, external ear canals, and middle-ear volumes larger, and cochleas longer
Psychophysical differences	
Hearing sensitivity	Females more sensitive, at least above 2 kHz
Binaural tasks	
Sound localization	Males more sensitive to differences in both interaural time and intensity
Binaural beats	Males hear them up to higher frequency
Right-ear advantage (REA)	Females have smaller REA (are less asymmetric)
Noise-induced hearing loss	
Permanent	Males have more
Temporary	Females have less below about 1.5 kHz and more above about 3 kHz
Complex masking tasks	
Profile analysis	Males more sensitive
Lateral suppression	Males have more
Overshoot	Females have more
Gap detection	Females more sensitive
Physiological differences	
Auditory brain-stem response (ABR)	Females have greater amplitude and shorter latency in Wave V
Otoacoustic emissions (OAEs)	Females have more SOAEs and stronger CEOAEs
Prenatal masculinization	Females with a male cotwin have OAEs more like males
Menstrual effects	See Table 2

Note. SOAE = spontaneous otoacoustic emissions; CEOAE = click-evoked otoacoustic emissions.

PHYSICAL SIZE

To the layman, surely the most obvious sex difference in the auditory system is the same as that for most other bodily parts—physical size. Male heads, pinnas, external ear canals, and middle-ear volumes are all, on the average, slightly larger than those of females (Burkhard & Sachs, 1975; Ward, 1966), and these differences matter acoustically. The effective sound-pressure level (SPL) at the eardrum in each frequency region can differ depending on these various physical dimensions, especially for sounds in the real world. There is also some evidence for sex differences in certain other middle-ear characteristics (Jerger, Jerger, & Mauldin, 1972; Margolis & Heller, 1987). Further, the basilar membranes of males are about 13% longer than those of females (Don, Ponton, Eggermont, & Masuda, 1993; Sato, Sando, & Takahashi, 1991; also see Kimberley, Brown, & Eggermont, 1993), which could affect various measures, such as those involving latency, either directly or indirectly.

To my view, any psychophysical or physiological sex difference in the auditory system that can be explained wholly on the basis of physical size differences at the periphery is much less interesting than a difference that arises from non-size-related differences of structure or function in the cochlea or auditory brain. The reason is that differences attributable to sex only as a secondary consequence of differences in peripheral size offer no prospects of insights into underlying mechanisms, and will not even exist when people are matched on size of head, ear canal, or whatever. It may be that some of the sex differences noted here will eventually prove to stem, in part, from peripheral size differences, but it seems highly unlikely that all will. Clearly, though, it will be necessary for everyone concerned with sex differences in the auditory system to continue to consider physical size differences, and their consequences, before reaching for other explanations. Examples of sex differences that are attributable simply to differences in body size can be found in Larkin, Reilly, and Kittler (1986) and Lautenbacher and Strian (1991).

HEARING SENSITIVITY

Perhaps the most elementary auditory ability is the detection of weak sounds in the quiet, so it seems an appropriate topic with which to begin this discussion. Further, hearing sensitivity in the quiet is surely the best established sex difference in the auditory system. Females as a group are more sensitive than males as a group by about 3 dB, at least for audiometric test frequencies of 2000 Hz and above (Chung, Mason, Gannon, & Willson, 1983), and this sex difference exists in children as well as adults (Roche, Siervogel, Himes, & Johnson, 1978). Stelmachowicz, Beauchaine, Kalberer, and Jesteadt (1989) found females to be about 4 dB more sensitive than males at test frequencies between 8 and 20 kHz, which lie above the standard audiometric range (compare Matthews, Lee, Mills, & Dubno, 1997). Differences of 3 to 4 dB are admittedly small relative to the approximately 120- to 140-dB range between the weakest and most intense sounds heard, yet (logarithmic scales being what they are) every 3 dB does amount to a halving (or doubling) of the power of the sound. Overlaid on the sex difference in hearing sensitivity is an ear difference, with right ears being about 2 to 3 dB more sensitive than left ears, at least in adults (see McFadden, 1993b, for a review of ear and sex differences in sensitivity). This ear asymmetry in sensitivity is greater in males than in females (Chung et al., 1983), and there is some evidence that the right-ear superiority is reduced in left-handed males (Emmerich, Harris, Brown, & Springer, 1988; Ward, 1957).

To the outsider, it might seem that these sex and ear differences in sensitivity would be even better established than they are, for, after all, hundreds of thousands—even millions—of measures of hearing sensitivity are made annually in the United States alone. Unfortunately, those audiometric measures are generally inappropriate for the purpose of determining sex and ear differences, for several reasons. Often the ears are being tested because of some medical problem, including complaints of hearing loss; order effects (the ear and frequencies tested first) are generally not controlled; the psychophysical methods typically used confound sensitivity with the criterion for response (Green & Swets, 1966); and, generally, the grain of the measurement steps is quite coarse relative to the size of the sex and ear differences, meaning that the differences easily can be missed.

The basis for the sex difference in hearing sensitivity is not clear, but Previc (1991) ingeniously suggested that ear differences in hearing sensitivity, among other lateral asymmetries in humans, may originate in asymmetric prenatal stimulation caused by asymmetries in the forward and backward acceleration forces during maternal locomotion. Also relevant may be the efferent fibers that synapse in the cochlea and exert an inhibitory influence (McFadden, 1993b).

BINAURAL ABILITIES

There are a number of two-eared auditory tasks for which sex differences have been demonstrated. The process of localizing sound sources in three-dimensional space involves the use of two cues—interaural differences in the time of arrival of the sound at the two ears, and interaural differences in the intensity of the sound at the two ears. When the sound source is located on the midsaggital plane that bisects the body into left and right halves, the time and intensity differences are both zero, but when the sound is off that median plane, there are varying combinations of time and intensity differences, depending on the location of the sound source. Langford (1994; personal communication, 1995) showed that males are better at discriminating both small differences in interaural time and intensity than are females. For 67%

correct decisions in a forced-choice oddity task, the 24 males required 86 µs or 3.1 dB of difference, and the 26 females required 113 µs or 4.0 dB (see Figure 1). For both tasks, Langford used noise bands and slow rise-decay times to reduce onset effects.

Sound-localization tasks such as these (technically, they are lateralization tasks when headphones are used) require that details of the waveforms at the two ears be accurately compared. This can only be done once the neural information from the two ears has been brought together, and that occurs for the first time in the brain stem, where different subnuclei appear to be concerned with the two cues (Pickles,

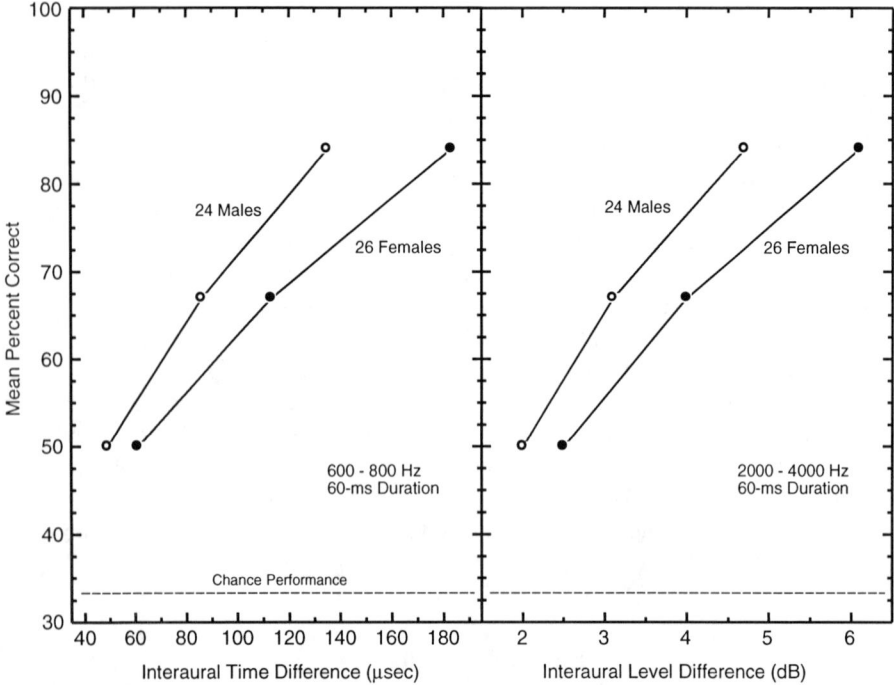

FIGURE 1 Average psychometric functions for discriminating interaural differences in time (left) or intensity (right) from no difference. The psychophysical task was oddity—on each trial, the narrow-band waveform was presented during each of the three observation intervals but only during one of the intervals did it contain the relevant interaural difference, and the participant indicated which interval by pressing the appropriate response key. Thus, chance performance was 33% correct. During each block of 100 trials, two sequences were interleaved, one estimating the interaural value for 50% correct and the other for 84% correct. The values shown for 67% correct were read from ogives fitted to the two obtained values. The band of noise used to measure sensitivity to interaural time differences was 600 to 800 Hz, and that for intensity differences was 2000 to 4000 Hz. Data from "Individual Differences in Sensitivity to Interaural Disparities of Time and Level," by T. L. Langford, 1994, *Journal of the Acoustical Society of America, 96*(Suppl. 1), p. 3256. Copyright 1994 by American Institute of Physics. Adapted with permission.

1988). The existence of separate, parallel pathways concerned with interaural differences of time and intensity creates the opportunity for individual differences in performance on the two tasks (McFadden, Jeffress, & Russell, 1973), including sex differences. In this context, the Langford results suggest that male auditory systems are able to encode more precisely the neural concomitants of the two cues for sound localization.

The phenomenon of binaural beats is of long-standing interest to psychoacousticians. They can be heard when a low-frequency pure tone is delivered to one earphone, and a second tone of slightly different frequency is delivered to the other earphone. Under the appropriate stimulus conditions, most people will report the experience of a single (fused) sound waxing and waning in loudness and moving from side to side inside the head—the rate of fluctuation in both loudness and location being directly related to the difference in frequency between the two primary tones (e.g., Licklider, Webster, & Hedlun, 1950). Binaural beats are interesting, in part, because—unlike monaural beats—they do not exist in the physical stimulus, but must be a product of the processing of the separate sounds at the two ears. Specifically, the existence of binaural beats strongly suggests that the temporal periodicities of the tones at the two ears are being preserved in their individual neural encodings, and, further, that the two neural streams are interacting at some central site(s) to produce the experience of a beat. Logic strongly suggests that the same site(s) responsible for sound localization are responsible for binaural beats, implying that the male superiority Langford (1994) showed for sound localization ought to exist for binaural beats as well, and the data of Tobias (1965) confirm this. For the majority of Tobias's 20 female listeners, the ability to hear binaural beats failed when the frequencies of the primary tones were in the range of 600 to 800 Hz, whereas for the majority of his 20 male listeners, the ability persisted up to about 800 to 1000 Hz. The implication is that the temporal periodicities of the tonal stimuli were not being preserved as well by the female auditory systems as acoustic frequency was increased.

The existing sex difference in head size (Burkhard & Sachs, 1975) means that the interaural time and intensity differences generally will be larger in males for any given degree of displacement of a real-world sound source off the median plane. Also, to the extent that there are systematic sex differences in pinna size, the magnitudes of the interaural intensity differences in certain frequency regions could differ across the sexes. No such stimulus differences existed in the experiments just discussed because the participants wore earphones. However, differences in head size and pinna size may have created, developmentally, a neural substrate having greater resolution for the two cues in males than in females. For example, in males, more neural elements may be operating per degree of change in stimulus location, making discrimination of such changes in location easier. Accordingly, a physical size difference ultimately may prove to underlie the sex differences in processing the cues used for localization and binaural beats (but see the discussion on p. 285).

There is one dichotic-listening task that has received more attention from traditional experimental psychologists than from psychoacousticians. It involves the simultaneous presentation of two words, one to each ear, and the participant is asked to report what was heard. The standard finding is that the words presented to the right ear are more accurately reported (particularly in right-handed participants) than are those presented to the left ear—thus, a right-ear advantage (REA). The effect is small, and accordingly is best seen when large numbers of participants are tested. The differences in the acoustics of different words make it impossible to specify with certainty what role interaural differences in time and intensity might play in these dichotic tasks, but Divenyi and Efron (1979) argued that the REA originates in a right-ear superiority in the processing and ordering of temporal information. A sex difference can exist in the standard REA task (see Kimura & Harshman, 1984); namely, females can show a smaller REA (less asymmetry) than males. A common interpretation of this finding is that male brains (specifically, their cortices) are functionally more asymmetric than female brains, although Kimura and Harshman (1984) argued that alternative explanations do exist and should be considered. They also reported that when the stimuli are melodic patterns or environmental sounds, females appear more asymmetric than males. When the ear-superiority issue is discussed in this literature, it is invariably implicit that the structural and functional differences being considered (between the "ears" or the sexes) reside in the cortex; differences in the peripheral auditory system are not commonly considered—which may prove to be a serious oversight.

For completeness, it should be noted that there is some evidence for an ear (side) asymmetry in certain binaural-localization tasks using loudspeakers rather than headphones. The suppression of echoes is greater when the first wavefront activates the right ear before the left (see Clifton & Freyman, 1989; Grantham, 1996). Although the asymmetry was greater in the female participants in one experiment (Grantham, 1996), this sex difference was not significant.

HEARING LOSS FROM INTENSE SOUNDS

Following exposure to intense sounds, hearing sensitivity can be reduced by an amount that varies with the intensity and duration of the exposure—and with individual susceptibility. Under many circumstances, the hearing loss recovers to normal over the course of minutes, hours, or days spent in a quiet or less noisy environment. Under other circumstances, recovery is incomplete and a permanent hearing loss results. The component of such exposure-induced hearing losses that recovers is known as *temporary threshold shift* (TTS), and the other is *permanent threshold shift* (PTS). There is little doubt from industrial noise-exposure databases that males end up with more PTS than do females (e.g., Royster, Royster, & Thomas, 1980), but the issue of why is a complex one. It may be that males are inherently more susceptible to noise-induced hearing loss. Alternatively, males may simply be exposed more often, to more intense, and to longer duration, sounds than females, both on the job and off. Laboratory research has reduced some of these uncertainties.

In an experiment with young listeners with nominally normal hearing, Ward (1966) found that females showed about 30% less TTS than males when the exposure sound was low frequency (700–1400 Hz), about 30% more TTS when the exposure was high frequency (2800–5600 Hz), and about the same as males in the region of 2000 Hz. Apparently, then, there is a sex difference in TTS, but not a simple one. Ward argued convincingly against any inherent differences in fragility of cochlear structures in the two sexes, choosing instead to emphasize presumed differences in the middle-ear muscles. He suggested that females had faster acting and stronger middle-ear muscles that better protected the inner ear from the large-amplitude displacements associated with intense sounds, at least at low frequencies. If Ward's interpretation has been tested directly, the results are unknown to me (see also p. 286).

COMPLEX MASKING TASKS

Auditory masking occurs when the presence of one sound, the masker, diminishes the detectability of a second sound, the signal. For decades, experiments on masking have been a source of considerable information about the mechanisms of hearing. Neff was able to test for a sex difference in a particular masking task by looking retrospectively at conditions common to several individual experiments (Neff, Kessler, & Dethlefs, 1996). The auditory task was to detect the presence of one fixed-frequency tone of 1000 Hz in the presence of an array of 10 other masker tones, the frequencies of which ranged from 300 to 3000 Hz. Because the 10 masker tones were changed at random from observation interval to observation interval, there was tremendous listener uncertainty about the details of the masker. An interesting fact about the auditory system is that even quite high uncertainty about the frequency of the signal leads to only small declines in detectability relative to the no uncertainty condition, but uncertainty about the background masking sound can produce substantial declines in detectability of the signal (Neff & Green, 1987). When the Neff et al. participants are put in rank order depending on their sensitivity in this task, the function in Figure 2 (left) results. Males (open circles) and females (solid circles) are both represented at both ends of this function, but not equally so. When the data are partitioned into 10-dB ranges, the histogram in Figure 2 (right) results. Males, as a group, were better at this task than were females, as a group; the difference of 7.6 dB was significant. An effect size for this sex difference was estimated by dividing the difference in the means by the overall standard deviation, using values read from a magnified version of Figure 2 (left). The result was 0.73. Note the extraordinary range of individual differences in Figure 2.

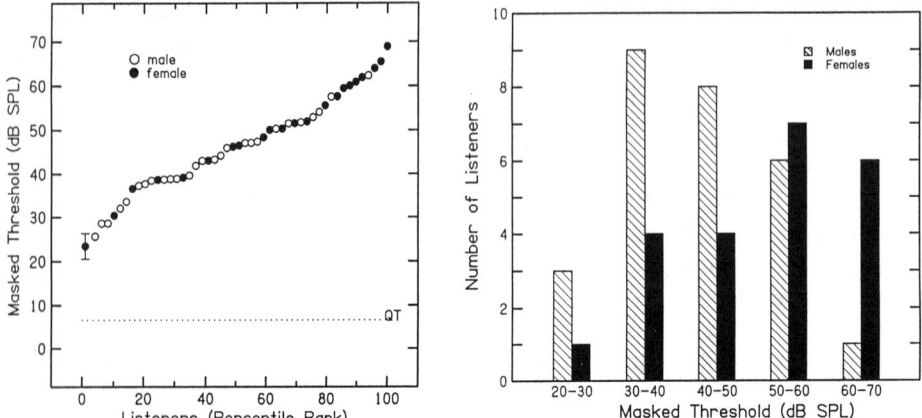

FIGURE 2 Left: Rank ordering of the performance of 49 individuals in a complex masking task, with different symbols used for the 27 males and 22 females. Small ordinate numbers indicate better performance. The task involved detecting a 1000-Hz signal under high uncertainty about the spectral composition of the 10-component masker. The dotted line indicates the average sensitivity for the 1000-Hz signal in the quiet (QT), averaged across the sexes. The error bar indicates the average standard deviation within participants across replications. Right: Histograms constructed from the rank-order data shown at the left. Data from "Sex Differences in Simultaneous Masking With Random-Frequency Maskers," by D. L. Neff, C. J. Kessler, and T. M. Dethlefs, 1996, *Journal of the Acoustical Society of America, 100*, pp. 2547–2550. Copyright 1996 by American Institute of Physics. Adapted with permission.

Wright (1994) studied sex and ear differences in two psychophysical tasks. One is the auditory analog of lateral inhibition in vision, but, for a number of reasons, is referred to as *lateral suppression*. The task is forward masking of a tonal signal, and two conditions are compared. In the first condition, the masker is a single tone of the same frequency as the signal; in the second condition, the masker is a two-tone complex, where one tone is again at the frequency of the signal and the other tone is more intense and higher in frequency than the first. Curiously, there is less forward masking (the signal is easier to hear) when there are two tones in the masker interval than when there is only one. This result is often counterintuitive on first telling but is easily explained by assuming that the second, higher frequency masker is producing a suppression of the on-frequency masking tone, thereby causing it to be less effective as a forward masker. Thus, the difference in masking effectiveness when the higher frequency suppressing tone is present and absent is taken as the magnitude of suppression. Wright used a signal and masker of 1000 Hz and a suppressor of 1150 Hz. She found significantly less suppression in her 20 female than in her 20 male participants. The implication is that inhibitory strength differs in the two sexes, and a consequence of this difference (see Moore & O'Loughlin, 1986) is that the frequency-resolving power of females should be somewhat less than that of males.

Wright's (1994) second task involved simultaneous masking of a tone by a noise band. Many listeners find it much harder to detect a brief tonal signal when it is presented at the onset of a burst of wideband noise than when its presentation is delayed by a couple of hundred milliseconds relative to masker onset. This difference in detectability is known as *overshoot,* and one possible explanation for overshoot is that time is required for the auditory filters to narrow to their operating width following the onset of a sound. (A wider filter at masker onset would allow a greater range of frequency components in the noise to contribute to the masking of the signal than would be possible once the filter had narrowed to its minimum width.) Wright used a 1000-Hz signal and a wideband noise masker (that happened to have a range of frequencies filtered out around the signal frequency). The signal was presented at the onset of the 500-msec masker or 400 msec later, in different blocks of trials. The difference in detectability averaged 7 dB, but it was significantly greater in the female participants than in the males. An unpublished study of my own produced the same result with fewer, but more highly trained, individuals. (Also, masked sensitivity was significantly greater in right ears than in left ears.) The implication is that males attempting to detect brief, narrow-band signals are bothered less by the simultaneous onset of other sounds than are females.

In passing, it is worth noting that the sex differences Wright (1994) found did not exist in the initial testing sessions, but emerged only with training, a commodity in short supply in some of the psychophysical experiments discussed here. That is, the claimed presence or absence of a sex difference on some task should always be examined with an eye to whether or not the participants had a reasonable opportunity to reach asymptotic performance.

GAP DETECTION

In some unpublished work, G. L. Dykstra and I studied the ability of males and females to detect the presence of a brief temporal gap in a band of noise centered at 2500 Hz. For all SPLs of the noise band except the highest, the females were able to detect temporal gaps several milliseconds smaller than those needed by the males. This difference existed only for the left ear; in the right ear, the sexes were equally sensitive. Other temporal-resolution tasks exist and should be studied, including retrospective examinations (à la Neff et al., 1996).

AUDITORY BRAIN-STEM RESPONSE

There are also some physiological measures showing sex differences in the auditory system. A gross potential called the *auditory brain-stem response* (ABR) can be recorded using scalp electrodes, recurring click stimuli, and averaging techniques. The ABR waveform is a series of five waves, commonly attributed to successive waystations in the auditory nervous system from cochlea to midbrain (inferior colliculus). The latency and amplitude of Wave V, typically attributed to the midbrain, is commonly used as an objective measure of the integrity of the auditory periphery in individuals for whom standard audiometric testing is impractical or impossible. The way the ABR is typically collected, the result can be thought of as the summed response across populations of neurons carrying information from different frequency regions. However, a clever technique developed by Teas, Eldredge, and Davis (1962) allows information about specific frequency regions to be extracted from gross potentials of this sort. The technique involves presenting, along with the click stimuli, high-pass masking noises with successively lower cutoff frequencies, and taking the difference between pairs of potentials so evoked as the contribution from the frequency region between the two cutoff frequencies.

ABRs evidence a sex difference—Wave V has greater amplitude and shorter latency in females, and this is true for both the unmasked and masked ABRs (Don et al., 1993). This sex difference remains even when the differences in head size and hearing sensitivity are taken into account (Don et al., 1993; Trune, Mitchell, & Phillips, 1988). This sex difference was originally attributed to faster conduction velocity, and less variability in conduction velocity, in female than male auditory neurons, but recent work calls this interpretation into question. Don et al. (1993) argued compellingly that the latency and amplitude differences in ABR arise primarily from the difference in the length of male and female cochleas. Specifically, the shorter length in females results in a shorter response time to the acoustical stimulus (and thus the shorter latency in Wave V), and in better synchrony across responding elements (and thus the greater amplitude). From their ABR data, Don et al. calculated that male cochleas are about 13% longer than female cochleas, which is in excellent agreement with the anatomical measurements of Sato et al. (1991). Don et al. also examined the possibility that the slightly higher core body temperature in females than males (about 0.3°C) could account for the difference in ABR latency, and concluded that it could not. If the Don et al. interpretation is correct, then the sex differences in ABR will be attributable to a difference in physical size, and will thereby become uninteresting using the criterion described at the beginning of this article (but see p. 284).

For completeness, it should be noted that there is some evidence that one early wave of the ABR (Wave III) is stronger for the right ear than the left, at least in right-handed individuals (Levine, Liederman, & Riley, 1988), and one report suggests that the asymmetry may be greater in *females* than males (Kamenkovich & Alekseenko, 1991). This early wave is commonly believed to originate from brain-stem structures involved with sound localization, specifically with the interaural time cue (Levine et al., 1988), which makes this right-ear asymmetry in ABR interesting relative to the previously mentioned right-side asymmetry reported for echo suppression (Clifton & Freyman, 1989; Grantham, 1996). Also, handedness has similar effects on the ABR and echo-suppression asymmetries.

As this summary reveals, there are a number of sex differences in hearing. Apart from physical size, what factors might be responsible for these various sex differences? At this point, no one knows, but there is a tantalizing suggestion that at least part of the story lies in differential prenatal development. To understand that link, it is necessary to know about yet another characteristic of the human auditory system.

OTOACOUSTIC EMISSIONS

It is now known that, contrary to traditional belief (and common sense), normal cochleas do not just receive, process, and analyze sounds; they also make sounds. These sounds are known as otoacoustic emissions (OAEs), and they come in a number of forms, depending on the acoustic stimulation used to elicit them.[1] For all types of OAEs, a miniature microphone system is inserted into the external ear canal, with or without miniature earphones, and the waveforms recorded by this microphone are processed to reveal the OAEs.

One type of OAE is known as the *click-evoked otoacoustic emission,* or CEOAE. This emission is like an echo coming back out of the fluid-filled cochlea into the air-filled middle- and outer-ear spaces in response to a very brief acoustic event such as a 100-µs click. This echolike response is from 20 to 40 msec in duration and is so weak that the responses to hundreds of clicks are typically averaged to reveal it. The CEOAE has a number of interesting characteristics such as being frequency dispersed (high frequencies echo back with shorter latency than low frequencies) and being more prominent at weak SPLs than at high ones (see Probst, Lonsbury-Martin, & Martin, 1991, for a review), but these are facts for another discussion. For present purposes, it is sufficient to know that essentially every normal-hearing ear produces a highly individualistic echolike waveform (the CEOAE) in response to a weak click.

The second form of OAE of interest here requires no acoustic stimulation to elicit it. Simply recording the ambient sounds in external ear canals reveals that one or more tonal sounds is being continuously produced by the majority of normal-hearing ears; hence, their name—*spontaneous otoacoustic emissions* (SOAEs). Interestingly, SOAEs are rarely heard by their owners, presumably because of some form of perceptual adaptation to a steady, long-term stimulus; accordingly, SOAEs are not the basis for chronic tinnitus (McFadden, 1982). Numerous demonstrations offer convincing evidence of the cochlear origin of both SOAEs and CEOAEs (Probst et al., 1991). Two ears having differing numbers of SOAEs are illustrated in Figure 3.

---

[1] The discussion here concentrates on OAEs in humans, but OAEs of various sorts have been found in other mammals, and in birds, reptiles, and frogs (see Köppl, 1995, for a review). Thus, they seem to be a fundamental characteristic of vertebrate hearing organs.

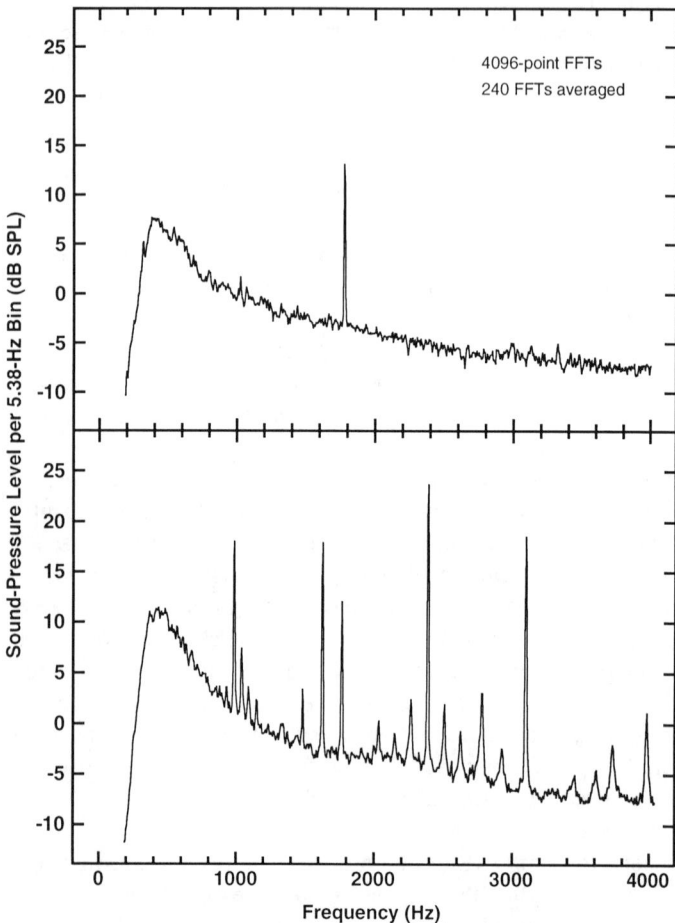

FIGURE 3 The spectra of the sounds measured in the external ear canals of two participants quietly lying supine. Plotted is the SPL in each 5.38-Hz bin over the range of about 200 to 4000 Hz (as determined by averaging 240 Fast Fourier Transforms; FFTs). The ragged baselines represent a combination of the electronic noise floor of the recording system and the resting noise level of the individual (respiration, pulse, involuntary muscle contractions, etc.). Participant noise has been reduced to some extent by filtering out the frequency components below about 400 Hz. The peaks in the two spectra are the spontaneous otoacoustic emissions (SOAEs), which are similar to continuous pure tones. The participant at the top has one prominent SOAE, and the participant at the bottom has about two dozen over the same frequency range. Some of the latter are what are known as combination tones or distortion products—the result of nonlinear interactions between pairs of strong SOAEs.

OAEs, in and of themselves, have been of considerable interest to hearing scientists ever since their discovery by Kemp (1978, 1979) because they provide a noninvasive tool for studying some of the fundamental operating characteristics of the human inner ear. OAEs are also interesting because of their potential to provide objective measures of the integrity of an individual inner ear, where the most common forms of hearing loss reside. This is because OAEs can originate only from sections of basilar membrane that are structurally and functionally normal (Probst et al., 1991). Objective tests of hearing have obvious value with various specialized populations such as infants and brain damaged people, and for this reason, it is likely that the repertoire of standard audiometric tests will soon be augmented with one or more tests based on OAEs (Norton, 1994). However, it is the potential of OAEs to inform us about matters other than the ear itself that is of primary interest here.

OAEs in humans show sex and ear differences that are remarkably similar to those seen in hearing sensitivity. There are more SOAEs and stronger CEOAEs in females than in males. According to the most recent surveys, something like 75% to 85% of females and 45% to 65% of males have at least one SOAE (Talmadge, Long, Murphy, & Tubis, 1993), and CEOAEs are 2 to 3 dB stronger in females than males (McFadden, Loehlin, & Pasanen, 1996). There are also more SOAEs and stronger CEOAEs in right ears than in left ears. That is, the same subsets of ears that have good hearing sensitivity also have high prevalence and strength of OAEs. These same patterns of sex and ear differences are evident in newborns (e.g., Burns, Arehart, & Campbell, 1992), and, although truly long-term longitudinal studies have yet to be conducted, SOAEs have been monitored for over a decade in some ears (Burns, Campbell, & Arehart, 1994; Burns, Campbell, Arehart, & Keefe, 1993), where they have proved to be highly stable. The number and strength of SOAEs, and the strength of CEOAEs, are all greater in infants than in adults (Burns et al., 1992; Norton, 1992), but this may not be attributable to any inherent change in cochlear structures. Rather, maturational changes in middle-ear structures may make it more difficult for emission energy to pass from the cochlea to the external ear canal. To be sure, OAEs are not immutable; they can be diminished or lost because OAEs can originate only from regions of cochlea that are normal, and localized cochlear damage and its attendant hearing loss are common in modern society. Additional study of the OAEs of infants, plus truly longitudinal studies, could provide additional evidence on the issue of OAE stability, but the best working hypothesis seems to be that high stability exists at least until the onset of hearing loss. In passing, it is worth noting that the seeming constancy of OAEs through life makes this a human characteristic that is apparently exempt from the interpretation that some or all sex differences exist only because of differential treatment or experience given to the two sexes postnatally (e.g., Caplan, MacPherson, & Tobin, 1985).

Effect sizes for the sex and ear differences in OAEs have been calculated for the data reported by McFadden and Loehlin (1995) and McFadden, Loehlin, and Pasanen (1996). When the data were pooled across ears, the effect sizes for sex in the CEOAE data were 0.51, 0.65, and 0.88 for nontwins, same-sex dizygotic twins, and monozygotic twins, respectively. The corresponding values for the SOAE data were 0.57, 0.73, and 0.74. When the data were pooled across sex, the effect sizes for ears in the CEOAE data were 0.34, 0.01, and 0.16 for the nontwins, same-sex dizygotics, and monozygotics, respectively. The corresponding values for the SOAE data were 0.44, 0.24, and 0.26.

To better understand the presumed substrate for OAEs, additional background on the inner ear is necessary. The mammalian cochlea contains two types of receptor cells. In humans, there are about 11,000 to 16,000 outer hair cells arrayed in three rows along the length of the basilar membrane, and about 2,800 to 4,400 inner hair cells arrayed in a single row (Pickles, 1988). The less numerous inner hair cells actually receive about 90% to 95% of the afferent innervation from the 30,000 nerve fibers comprising the auditory nerve, leaving only about 5% to 10% for the outer hair cells. This simple fact of neuroanatomy suggests that the outer hair cells do not make a major direct contribution to the afferent flow to higher auditory centers, and this suggestion is supported by evidence from a number of sources. Without getting into details, the evidence is that the primary job of the outer hair cells is to alter the local micromechanics of the cochlea in such a way as to increase the magnitude of displacement—and hence the magnitudes of depolarization and hyperpolarization—experienced by the inner hair cells. Because each individual outer hair cell is called into action only by a relatively narrow band of frequencies, the outer hair cells are often described as being like an array of sharply tuned amplifiers—components in what is known as the cochlear-amplifier system (Davis, 1983). When the outer hair cells are locally inactivated by such manipulations as exposure to intense sound, ototoxic drugs, and anoxia, the tuning curves of the inner hair cells and the primary auditory fibers in that frequency region lose their characteristically extremely sharp tips, and their absolute sensitivity is thereby reduced by about 30 dB. The behaviorally measured hearing sensitivity of animals having inactivated outer hair cells, but intact inner hair cells, is also decreased by about 30 to 40 dB. Evidence of this sort is the basis for the belief that the outer hair cells are crucial elements in the cochlear-amplifier system.

Most relevant to this discussion is the fact that ears with inactivated or absent outer hair cells exhibit weak, or no, OAEs (Probst et al., 1991). Thus, the outer hair cells and the cochlear-amplifier system with which they are involved are generally regarded to be the source of OAEs. (In the case of SOAEs, the idea is that one or more local cochlear amplifiers is defective and has gone into cyclic self-stimulation.) It is not a major leap from these facts to thinking about differences in OAEs across individuals, sexes, ears, and so forth, as being attributable to differences in the strengths of the cochlear amplifiers. And because the cochlear amplifiers are responsible for the most sensitive 30 to 40 dB of hearing, it is not unreasonable to expect that OAEs and hearing sensitivity will covary. Unfortunately, there are no large-scale studies comparing OAEs and hearing sensitivity in the same participants, in part because precise measurements of hearing sensitivity are extremely time consuming and OAE equipment is expensive. However, in one experiment, the hearing sensitivity of 14 individuals with no SOAEs was compared with that of 11 individuals with at least four SOAEs in one ear, and the result was that the participants with SOAEs were about 3 dB more sensitive than those with none (McFadden & Mishra, 1993). This difference in sensitivity was present in the data for both ears and both sexes. (In accord with past research—e.g., Chung et al., 1983—right ears were about 2.5 dB more sensitive than left ears.) Dividing the differences in the means by the corresponding standard deviations revealed effect sizes of 0.47 for the SOAE factor (calculated across sexes and ears), and 0.33 for the ear difference (calculated across sexes and presence and absence of SOAEs).

Of special interest here is the fact that, contrary to past research, there was no difference in hearing sensitivity between the sexes for the participants in the McFadden and Mishra (1993) experiment. The way to think about this fact is that the fundamental sex difference operating here is the strength of the cochlear amplifiers, and that both hearing sensitivity and the prevalence and strength of OAEs follow from that difference. Because females, as a group, have stronger cochlear amplifiers than males as a group, a sex difference in hearing sensitivity can be evident when individuals are selected without knowledge of their cochlear amplifiers (as, e.g., in Chung et al., 1983), but not when a variable related to the cochlear amplifier, like number of SOAEs, is controlled (as in McFadden & Mishra, 1993). When viewed this way, the implication is that the evolutionary pressure at work to produce strong cochlear amplifiers was driven by its effect on hearing sensitivity. By this view, OAEs are presumably epiphenomena resulting from the specific mechanisms that evolved to achieve high sensitivity. Exactly why females, as a group, ended up with stronger cochlear amplifiers and greater hearing sensitivity than males as a group stands as a mystery to be solved.

HERITABILITY OF OAES

Recent work with twins has revealed that there is a substantial genetic contribution to the expression of OAEs. Both the number of SOAEs and the strength of CEOAEs were more similar in monozygotic (MZ) cotwins than in same-sex dizygotic (SSDZ) cotwins. Something on the order of 75% of the individual variation in the expression of both SOAEs and CEOAEs can be attributed to the genes (McFadden & Loehlin, 1995; McFadden et al., 1996; Russell, 1992). (The two variables of SOAE number and CEOAE power were themselves correlated about 0.6–0.7, meaning that it was not pointless to obtain estimates of heritability from both sets of data from the same individuals.) This is among the first demonstrations of a genetic contribution to a characteristic of the auditory system that is not related to a pathology. In the data available, there was a weak tendency for the specific acoustic frequencies of the SOAEs in corresponding ears of MZ cotwins to be more similar than those in corresponding ears of SSDZ cotwins, but the prevalence of SOAEs was inadequate to determine whether this was a real effect. Consequently, the safest conclusion seems to be that what is inherited is the general tendency to have cochlear amplifiers of a particular strength, and the specific expression of SOAEs and CEOAEs follows from that.

PRENATAL MASCULINIZATION OF OAES

In the twins experiment conducted to study the issue of heritability of OAEs (McFadden & Loehlin, 1995; McFadden et al., 1996), data were collected for opposite-sex dizygotic (OSDZ) twins as well as for SSDZ and MZ twins. In both cases, the data for the OSDZ females were more like those for males than for other females. That is, females having a male cotwin had fewer SOAEs and weaker CEOAEs than all other females (see Figure 4). When the data from OSDZ females were compared with those from SSDZ females, the difference was statistically significant for SOAEs (McFadden, 1993a), but not for CEOAEs (McFadden et al., 1996). (The most appropriate comparison is between OSDZ and SSDZ females because both had cotwins, only the sex of that cotwin differed.) Effect sizes were calculated by dividing the difference in the means for OSDZ and SSDZ females by the common standard deviation. They were 0.49 and 0.43 for the SOAE and CEOAE data, respectively. (The values for MZ females shown in Figure 4 are clearly extreme; possible explanations for this outcome are discussed later.)

A parsimonious way to account for male-like OAEs in OSDZ females is to presume that it is an example, in humans, of the prenatal masculinizing effects that have been reported in litter-bearing mammals (e.g., Clark & Galef, this issue; vom Saal, 1989; vom Saal et al., 1990). If correct, this interpretation sheds light on the possible ontogenetic origin of the auditory sex differences discussed so far, and it raises a number of additional interesting questions about the auditory system (and the brains of OSDZ females).

Specifically, the suggestion is that—in much the same way that prenatal exposure to androgens is presumed to alter higher brain structures (e.g., Collaer & Hines, 1995; Witelson, Glezer, & Kigar, 1995, for reviews)—it also alters cochlear structures in the direction of diminishing the strength of the cochlear amplifiers, which leads in turn to reduced hearing sensitivity, fewer SOAEs, and weaker CEOAEs. According to this account, the reductions in strength of the cochlear amplifiers (and the concomitant auditory effects) occur in human males in the normal course of prenatal exposure to the androgens they themselves produce, and

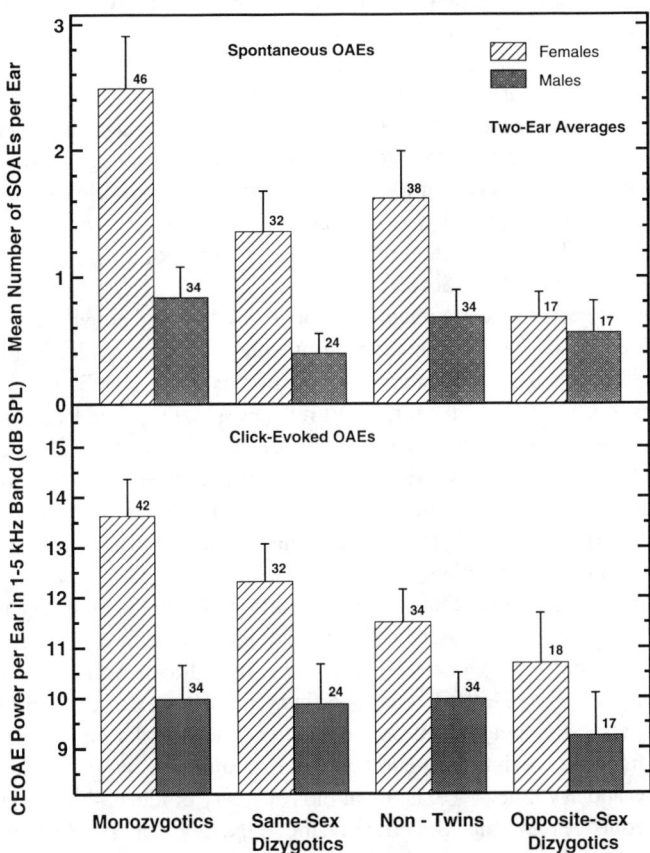

FIGURE 4 The average number of spontaneous otoacoustic emissions (SOAEs) per ear and the average power in the click-evoked otoacoustic emissions (CEOAEs) in individuals of various types. Shown are two-ear averages, but both the number of SOAEs and the power of CEOAEs were significantly greater in the right ear than in the left. The numbers above the individual bars indicate the number of participants contributing to each mean, and the flags on the bars indicate the standard errors. CEOAE power was calculated from 1 to 5 kHz in 20-msec samples beginning 6 msec after click onset. The difference in CEOAE power between OSDZ and SSDZ females did not achieve statistical significance ($p < .07$), but the difference in SOAE number between those two groups did ($p < .03$). Data from McFadden and Loehlin (1995); McFadden, Loehlin, and Pasanen (1996).

similar reductions occur in OSDZ females presumably as a result of prenatal exposure to the androgens produced by their male cotwins. Note that comparative measures of hearing sensitivity have yet to be made for OSDZ females, but the prediction is that their hearing will be more like that of males than other females (another prediction from Figure 4 is that the sensitivity of MZ females will be the best of any group ever measured). This prenatal interpretation of the OSDZ results is made possible, in part, by the fact that infants have the same patterns of OAEs as adults, and that OAEs appear to be highly constant through life (see preceding).

If this offered interpretation is correct, we appear to have an example of an organizational effect of prenatal hormones on structures of the inner ear.[2] For me, this carries a number of implications.

First, it suggests that certain auditory measures have the potential to provide a noninvasive window onto prenatal developmental processes, with all of the attendant ramifications that implication carries. For example, OAEs or some other measure of cochlear-amplifier function might eventually prove useful for establishing—after the fact—whether some disorder originated from some particular prenatal hormonal upset. With time, it might even be determined that the critical period(s) for development of the cochlear amplifiers pre- or postdate the critical periods for certain other effects, again making cochlear measurements potentially useful as a supplementary diagnostic tool.

A second implication is that sex and ear differences in the auditory periphery may play a role in sex and lateral differences higher in the brain. The remarkable plasticity of higher cortical centers, especially early in life, is well established (e.g., Daw, 1995). To a large extent, what one finds in the cortex of a juvenile or adult animal depends to a great extent on the nature of the stimulation received by that cortex from more peripheral neural structures. Intuition suggests that the sex differences and asymmetries existing at the periphery of the auditory system must have consequences centrally. Specifically, the suggestion is that some of the cortical differences in auditory function that have been reported for the two sexes and two hemispheres might be—at least in part—differences driven from below. It may be that some cortical sex differences are not simply the result of prenatal hormones operating (or not operating) at those specific sites, but are the result of both direct hormonal effects on those cortical sites and indirect effects of biasing at peripheral

---

[2]To be precise, the OSDZ effect suggests an organizational effect of androgens, but the normal sex difference in OAEs in adults could have both organizational and activational components. The reason for the latter ambiguity is that adult males do have high levels of circulating androgens that could be partially responsible for weakening the cochlear amplifiers and diminishing OAEs. The ambiguity could be resolved by studying adult males having markedly reduced levels of androgens. Soon after birth, there is no sex difference in circulating androgens (Reyes, Boroditsky, Winter, & Faiman, 1974; Smail, Reyes, Winter, & Faiman, 1981), yet there is a sex difference in OAEs (Burns et al., 1992), clearly implying an organizational effect.

sites that contribute to the activation of those cortical sites. Of course, both the direct and indirect effects might be produced by the same prenatal hormones. Fitch, Brown, O'Connor, and Tallal (1993), Levine et al. (1988), and Previc (1991) also argued for a bottom-up contribution to cortical function and malfunction in the auditory system, and elsewhere I have suggested that the parallel sex and ear differences in sensitivity and OAEs may arise from differential asymmetries in the efferent fibers that innervate the cochlea and modulate afferent flow from it (McFadden, 1993b). Over the years, high-level lateral asymmetries have most often been presented as causes rather than results, and because logically they must be both, it is time that both roles are acknowledged and examined.

A third implication—actually fundamental to the others, but probably notable only to fellow students of the auditory system—is that the micromechanics of the cochlea appear to be under the direct control of prenatal hormones. This continues to be an extraordinary fact to someone who has spent his life studying the adult auditory system for its own sake, without much thought to the developmental processes giving rise to cochlear function or to their consequences for higher centers.

MENSTRUAL EFFECTS ON THE AUDITORY SYSTEM

Some strength is added to the suggestion that the auditory system is under the control of hormones by the fact that a number of auditory characteristics appear to fluctuate with the menstrual cycle. Unfortunately, the same problems that plague the study of menstrual effects in other topic areas (Kimura & Hampson, 1994; Parlee, 1983) exist for hearing research as well, making it an extremely difficult literature from which to extract generalizations. This is because different investigators have not taken measurements at the same times in the cycle, often data have been obtained only during one cycle, hormone levels have rarely been measured or ovulation confirmed, generally few individuals have been studied and the individual differences have been large, learning effects may have been confounded with menstrual effects, and so on. Further, when behavioral measures do indicate the presence of menstrual effects, it is necessarily uncertain whether the reason is direct hormonal action or intermediate mechanisms such as temperature, metabolism, blood pressure, or cerebrospinal fluid pressure, all of which are affected by the hormones. Fortunately, there is a general appreciation that oral contraceptives can reduce or eliminate certain oscillations in both physiology and behavior, and recent experimenters have been careful about studying normal-cycling women separately from those using oral contraceptives. Ideally, experimenters would monitor the individuals' hormone levels and take data at at least four times in the cycle: (a) during menstruation; (b) near the first estrogen peak, but prior to the sharp rise in follicle-stimulating hormone (FSH) and luteinizing hormone (LH); (c) at ovulation during the first small peak in progesterone; and (d) near the simultaneous peaks for estrogen and progesterone in the second half of the cycle. However, it is rare to find experiments in which this has been done.

With all that said, there are some indications that the menstrual cycle can alter certain aspects of hearing, just as it does a wide array of other perceptual-motor and cognitive abilities (Hampson, 1990a, 1990b; Parlee, 1983). Table 2 is an attempt to summarize the discussion that follows, and to compare the auditory results with the known fluctuations in the hormones that are thought to be most relevant to the monthly cycle. For what follows, when there were discrepancies in the literature, I emphasize what appear to be the best data, but indicate experiments in which contradictory outcomes have been obtained. Again, the reader is cautioned that multiple interpretations are possible for essentially every experiment considered because of the experimental inconsistencies and weaknesses already mentioned.

One finding is that hearing sensitivity appears to vary through the monthly cycle. Sensitivity can be 5 dB or more worse at menstruation than later in the cycle (e.g., Davis & Ahroon, 1982; Swanson & Dengerink, 1988; but compare Baker & Weiler, 1977). Recall that the nominal dynamic range of hearing is about 120 to 140 dB, so, again, these are modest changes, but they do bolster the idea of activational hormonal effects on the auditory system as well as organizational effects. Note that the decline in hearing sensitivity at the time of menstruation constitutes a move in the male direction, and this occurs at a time when all the relevant hormones except FSH are at a minimum. These fluctuations in hearing sensitivity are greatly reduced by birth-control drugs (Swanson & Dengerink, 1988). As an example, in the McFadden and Mishra (1993) experiment described earlier on the relation between SOAEs and hearing sensitivity, the data were kept separate for the 12 women on birth-control pills and the 6 normal-cycling women. The sensitivity differences between people having SOAEs and those having none, and between the ears, were significant whether or not the normal-cycling women were included, but their inclusion considerably reduced the decibel difference for both factors (presumably because some of the normal-cycling women experienced a menses-induced loss of sensitivity during the 2-week course of measurements).

At this time, it is unclear how much of the monthly change in hearing sensitivity can be attributed to changes inside the cochlea itself. SOAEs can oscillate slightly in frequency through the monthly cycle, with the nadir being just before menses and the zenith just before ovulation in the majority of women (Bell, 1992; Haggerty, Lusted, & Morton, 1993; Wilson, 1986), and with multiple SOAEs in the same ear (or individual) showing similar patterns of oscillation. However, the range of the oscillation is typically less than 1%, and no corresponding, systematic change in the magnitude of the SOAEs has been found. This makes it appear as if there is some fluctuation in the tuning of the cochlea through the menstrual cycle, but no major change in the strength of the cochlear amplifiers, although measures of OAEs

TABLE 2
A Summary of Menstrual Effects on Various Auditory Tasks and Characteristics

	Nominal 28-Day Menstrual Cycle						
	Follicular Phase		Ovulation	Luteal Phase			
Substance or Task	Menstruation Days 1–5	Preovulation 10–14	13–15	Midluteal 19–23	Premenstrual 25–27	Range of Effect	Source
Estrogen (E2)	Low	High	Low	Moderate			Ferin, Jewelewicz, & Warren (1993)
Progesterone	Low	Low	Moderate	High			
Follicle-stimulating hormone	Moderate	Low	High	Low			
Luteinizing hormone	Low	Low	High	Low			
Auditory sensitivity	Worst[a]		Best	Near best		5 dB	Swanson & Dengerink (1988)
Temporary threshold shift	Least[a]		Most	Near most		3–6 dB	Swanson & Dengerink (1988); Davis & Ahroon (1982)
Binaural beats		Worst	Intermediate		Best[a]	200 Hz	Tobias (1965)
Click lateralization	Best[a]		Intermediate	Worst		CND	Haggard & Gaston (1978)
Interaural intensity difference	Worst[b]	Best				0.3 dB	ns; Langford (personal communication, 1995)
Absolute pitch settings	Low	High	Low	High		6 Hz	Wynn (1972)
Octave matching	Intermediate		Best	Worst		CND	Haggard & Gaston (1978)
Monaural beats	Best		Worst	Intermediate		CND	ns; Haggard & Gaston (1978)
Right-ear advantage	Less strong	More strong[a]			Less strong	5%	Altemus et al. (1989); Hampson (1990a)
ABR latency (Wave V)	Short	Long[a]		Short		0.13 msec	Elkind-Hirsch et al. (1992), Elkind-Hirsch et al. (1994)
ABR amplitude (Wave V)						No effect	Elkind-Hirsch et al. (1992), Elkind-Hirsch et al. (1994)
SOAE frequency	Lowest	Intermediate	Highest	Intermediate	Intermediate	0.4–0.8%	Bell (1992); Haggerty et al. (1993); cf. Wilson et al. (1986)
SOAE amplitude						No effect	Bell (1992)

Note. The ranges of days shown were determined to some extent by the ranges used in the experiments surveyed. ns = not significant; CND = could not determine; ABR = auditory brain-stem response; SOAE = spontaneous otoacoustic emissions.
[a]Corresponds, or presumably corresponds, to a shift toward male performance. [b]Corresponds to a shift away from male performance.

other than SOAEs would be helpful in settling this important matter. The implication is that the menstrual effect on hearing sensitivity resides in postcochlear structures.

Additional evidence also suggests that the primary locus of the menstrual effect is postcochlear. Elkind-Hirsch, Stoner, Stach, and Jerger (1992) collected ABR data at four points during the menstrual cycles of 9 normal-cycling women. The result was that Wave I (attributed to the auditory nerve fibers) showed no changes with the menstrual cycle—in accord with the minimal changes in SOAEs—but Wave V (attributed to the inferior colliculus) did. Specifically, on the day after serum estradiol (E_2) reached a criterion value during midcycle (Days 12-15, but presumably prior to ovulation), Wave V latency was longer by about 0.13 msec (about 2.3%) than at all three other points in the cycle sampled. There was no significant change in the amplitude of Wave V, progesterone levels and basal body temperature confirmed that ovulation did occur in all these women, and body temperature itself did not covary with Wave V latency. This increase in Wave V latency during midcycle is a move toward typical male values (Don et al., 1993; Trune et al., 1988). For the 9 women taking oral contraceptives and for the male controls, there were no significant changes through time in either the latency or amplitude of Waves I or V, nor were there changes in progesterone levels or body temperatures. Women with preovarian failure who were receiving hormone replacement therapy (Estrace and Provera) also showed an increase in Wave V latency during the phase of the cycle when only estrogen was being administered, and a return to baseline when estrogen and progesterone were being administered (Elkind-Hirsch, Wallace, Malinak, & Jerger, 1994). Elkind-Hirsch et al. (1994) apparently collected data separately from the two ears of their participants, but used two-ear averages for publication, and I am unaware of any attempts to monitor changes in the degree of ear asymmetry in the early waves of the ABR (observed by Kamenkovich & Alekseenko, 1991; Levine et al., 1988) during the monthly cycle.

There are several implications of these ABR results. First, the Don et al. (1993) conclusion attributing the sex difference in the latency and amplitude of ABR Wave V to the physical difference in the lengths of male and female cochleas may not be the whole story. Although it is possible that the menstrual effects on ABR latency are due only to changes in cochlear tuning—as would be suggested by the Don et al. explanation—it is also possible that changes in neural conduction time are involved. If so, the implication is that neural conduction time is slowed by the midcycle estrogen peak that occurs prior to ovulation, and that progesterone has an antagonistic action on this slowing effect of estrogen. Also, the general agreement between the temporal patterns for the ABR results and those for hearing sensitivity and estrogen levels (see Table 2) suggests that the fluctuations in hearing sensitivity through the menstrual cycle may be attributable, at least in part, to effects acting at a site beyond the cochlea or auditory nerve and prior to the inferior colliculus. Elkind-Hirsch et al. (1992) suggested that estrogen may produce changes in ABR latency by modulating the action of the neurotransmitter GABA (gamma-aminobutyric acid), a suggestion that is in agreement with demonstrated effects of sex steroids on neurons in the central nervous system (e.g., McEwen et al., 1984).

The implication that central locations in the auditory system can be affected by the menstrual cycle is in accord with some of the other menstrual effects that have been reported. As noted, the experience of binaural beats must originate from interactions between the neural streams flowing from each ear, and, thus, its site of origin lies in the central nervous system. Tobias (1965) showed that the magnitude of the sex difference for binaural beats varied through the monthly cycle. Specifically, the data for women became like those for men in the days just preceding menses, which is when both estrogen and progesterone levels are low. Performance then declined to the baseline level through menses and the preovulatory phase but showed a second, smaller peak about 15 days after the first, when estrogen is again low. Note that this result can be understood easily by assuming that there are changes in the precision of temporal following in auditory neurons, but not by assuming only that there are changes in cochlear tuning (à la Don et al., 1993). Traditionally, binaural beats have been studied using low-frequency tones (Licklider et al., 1950), but they can also be obtained with certain high-frequency stimuli (Bernstein & Trahiotis, 1996; McFadden & Pasanen, 1975); to my knowledge, no sex or menstrual effects have yet been studied with these latter waveforms.

Another binaural task for which there is some evidence of change in sensitivity through the monthly cycle is sound localization. Haggard and Gaston (1978) asked 9 women to determine whether pairs of clicks (one to each ear) either did or did not have an interaural time difference, and found that this ability was best at menses and worst in the midluteal phase. As noted earlier, Langford (1994) demonstrated that males as a group are better than females as a group at lateralization on the basis of interaural time differences, so the improvement shown by Haggard and Gaston's participants at menses is a movement in the male direction. Langford (personal communication, 1995) also attempted to measure differences in lateralization through the monthly cycle, and although the data for interaural intensity differences were better during the preovulatory phase than during menses, that difference was not significant (and the two sets of data for interaural time differences were superimposed). Pertinent to an issue discussed earlier is the obvious fact that female head size does not change with the menstrual cycle, suggesting that physical size differences are not the sole basis for the sex differences in sound localization discussed earlier.

Haggard and Gaston (1978) found menstrual effects for another auditory task—accuracy at judging the octave frequency for a 203-Hz tone. Performance was best around the time of ovulation and worst in the midluteal phase. There was no menstrual fluctuation when the standard frequency was 1530 Hz. I am not aware of any evidence for a sex difference on this task. However, it is not uncommon for psychoacousticians to see differences in performance above and below about 1300 Hz, and the common (sometimes too glib) explanation invokes the suggestion of two codes used by the auditory system—only place of stimulation for high-frequency tones and both place and temporal (periodicity) information for low-frequency tones.

Worth noting for the reader familiar with experimental psychology is the fact that Haggard and Gaston (1978) reported and analyzed separately measures of both discriminability and response bias. Although the latter did show significant variation through the monthly cycle for some tasks, the discriminability measures revealed that changes in criterion were not the sole reason for the behavioral changes reported by other investigators who did not use criterion-free measures.

Apparently the susceptibility to noise-induced hearing loss also fluctuates through the monthly cycle. Both Swanson and Dengerink (1988) and Davis and Ahroon (1982) found that TTS for a fixed-intensity exposure was less at menses that at other times in the cycle. That is, the time of poorest hearing sensitivity corresponds to the time of least loss in sensitivity from exposure to intense sounds, and for both measures, the change at menses represents a movement toward the male data (because Swanson & Dengerink measured TTS at high frequencies where females typically show greater TTS than males). In the Swanson and Dengerink (1988) study, women using oral contraceptives had essentially constant TTS across the cycle, as did the males. A covariation between poorer sensitivity and lesser TTS has been observed before (e.g., Pirilä, 1991; Ward, 1963). The existence of a menstrual effect on TTS in the high-frequency region calls into question Ward's (1966) suggestion that the sex difference in TTS and PTS is attributable to a difference in middle-ear musculature because that musculature should have little effect at high frequencies. If direct measures of menstrual effects on middle-ear musculature have been made, I am unaware of the result.

Altemus, Wexler, and Boulis (1989) observed changes in REA across the menstrual cycle. The stimuli were pairs of nonsense words, real words, and emotion-laden words that differed only in a single consonant. The REA was less strong in the week prior to menses than in the second week or so following, at least for four of the five stimulus sets used. That is, the female REA moved in the male direction during the preovulatory phase of the cycle. Altemus et al. interpreted their results in terms of cyclic shifts in the relative contribution to processing made by the two hemispheres. Unfortunately, there was no explicit statement that the women in this experiment were normal cycling. Hampson (1990a) did a similar study with similar results (except one of her two measurement points was at menses), so the entry in Table 2 reflects both reports.

Finally, Wynn (1972) studied menstrual effects in a unique group—women having absolute pitch. The task for the two women tested was to sing the A (440 Hz) above middle C, and their accuracy was measured using a digital frequency meter. For the best studied woman, there was a sliding constant error of about 20

Hz across time, but the day-to-day range of fluctuation was small. Only the results for the participant providing data over eight periods are summarized in Table 2, but the settings for both women studied showed the two full cycles of fluctuation per monthly cycle. The lowest settings occurred at the onset of menses and between Days 11 and 15. Curiously, a single male participant also showed cyclic fluctuations having a period of about 20 days. Questions about long-term and diurnal fluctuations in cochlear tuning have a long history (e.g., Jeffress, 1949), and absolute pitch might provide a window onto the underlying processes, which may have a hormonal component.

It would be assuring to be able to conclude this section with a summary that tied together all of the reported menstrual effects on hearing with a simple explanation at the level of the hormone cycles involved. Unfortunately, the data do not permit that (recall the caveats about differences in methodology noted at the beginning of this section), but there do seem to be some consistencies across the data shown in Table 2. Perhaps most obvious is the fact that, for several of the tasks tested, there was a shift toward male values (the entries with superscripts) during the first half of the cycle. (During this time, progesterone levels are low, and estrogen levels are initially low and build to a peak.) This pattern has some similarity to the one seen with various nonauditory tasks. For example, over a series of three experiments testing various verbal, spatial, and motor skills, Kimura and Hampson (1994) observed that, at menses, performance was more male-like on tasks that normally favor men, and less male-like on tasks that normally favor females. Sometimes Kimura and Hampson used as their control condition measurements made at the preovulatory phase of the cycle (when estrogen levels are high), and sometimes they used measurements made in the midluteal phase (when both estrogen and progesterone levels are elevated). In both cases, the participants performed better on tasks at which females typically excel and worse on tasks at which males typically excel. Thus, there is general agreement with the data shown in Table 2.

The intent of emphasizing the menstrual data here was to strengthen the implication that hormones have the potential to alter the auditory system, meaning conversely that the auditory system may provide a valuable window onto hormonal processes primarily affecting other structures. Personally, I hope the topic of menstrual effects receives renewed attention from psychoacousticians because it appears to have the potential to contribute to our general knowledge about activational effects of hormones on the brains of humans.

In the context of possible activational effects of hormones on the auditory system, it should be noted that Burns et al. (1993) monitored the SOAEs in one woman through the course of a pregnancy. Hormone levels were not measured, but estrogen levels are known to be greatly elevated during pregnancy. Four of this woman's five SOAEs did show a monotonic decline in frequency, with the nadir at the last measurement session prior to birth (about 1 month antepartum), presumably when estrogen levels were approaching their peak. The frequency shifts were only about 0.7% to 1.3%, or about 12 to 60 Hz, which is in the same range observed in the studies on menstrual effects on SOAEs, but there is an inconsistency. In the pregnant woman, the nadir in SOAE frequency occurred at a presumed estrogen peak, whereas the nadir in the menstrual data occurred at an estrogen minimum (Table 2). Perhaps the apparent inconsistency is attributable to the markedly higher levels of estrogen present during pregnancy than during the menstrual cycle. Whatever the correct explanation, these pregnancy measurements support the implication that, in adults, changes in hormone levels can activate small changes in cochlear tuning.

DIURNAL AND SEASONAL EFFECTS

For readers wondering whether there are also diurnal effects on the auditory system, the answer appears to be yes, at least for OAEs (see Bell, 1992; Haggerty et al., 1993; Wilson, 1986; Wit, 1985). However, the number of individuals studied so far is small, and the individual differences large. It appears that SOAE frequency is lowest during the late-night or early-morning hours, but beyond that, generalizations are impossible. In the absolute pitch experiment of Wynn (1972), no relation was found between pitch accuracy and the diurnal fluctuations in body temperature. In a related phenomenon, Kimura and Hampson (1994) demonstrated activational hormonal effects in human males (testosterone levels are generally higher in the fall than in the spring), but, to my knowledge, this male cycle has not been studied with auditory measures.

PIGMENTATION AND THE AUDITORY SYSTEM

Not mentioned to this point is a variable that might prove of interest to some readers. Pigmentation appears to be involved in cochlear mechanics in some way (e.g., Jastreboff, Issing, Brennan, & Sasaki, 1988; Meyer zum Gottesberge, 1988). Melanocytes are found throughout the cochleo-vestibular system, their density appears to vary directly with pigmentation of the skin and eye, and various drugs that have effects on the auditory system bind to this cochlear melanin. For decades there have been reports of auditory differences between the races in such measures as hearing sensitivity, susceptibility to noise exposure, and incidence of tinnitus, among other measures. The general direction of effect is that light-skinned, light-eyed people tend to have less-sensitive hearing, are more susceptible to noise-induced hearing loss, and have greater problems with severe tinnitus than dark-skinned, dark-eyed people (reviewed by McFadden & Wightman, 1983). More recently, it has been shown that SOAEs are significantly less numerous in lightly pigmented people than in more heavily pigmented people (Russell, 1992; Whitehead, Kamal, Lonsbury-Martin, & Martin, 1993). Further, many genetic defects of the auditory system are accompanied by anomalies of pigmentation (Spillman, 1994; Steel & Brown, 1994). In this context, it is commonly pointed out that, embryologically, the neural crest cells give rise both to the sense organs, including the auditory periphery, and to all pigmented cells in the body. Thus, disorders contained within, or acting on, neural crest cells could have implications for both audition and pigmentation. The lesser hearing loss in more heavily pigmented people following exposure to intense sounds (e.g., Royster et al., 1980) suggests that the inner-ear melanocytes may play a role in restorative functions and dissipation of energy, but the mechanism for none of these pigment-related differences has been established.

ANIMAL MODELS

There would be considerable scientific value to having a suitable animal model of the sex differences mentioned here on which to perform some of the more extreme hormonal manipulations that come to mind. Unfortunately, the topics of sex (and ear) differences have historically not been of much interest to auditory scientists studying mammals other than humans. As a consequence, (to my knowledge, at least) there is no evidence of sex or ear differences in "simple" behavioral measures such as hearing sensitivity, or in physiological measures such as OAEs in any of the small mammals commonly studied in auditory research—chinchillas, guinea pigs, gerbils, mice, rats, and cats. In large part, this absence of knowledge stems simply from failures of experimenters to analyze their data along these dimensions, for auditory physiologists and animal psychophysicists often do test both sexes and both ears, although generally not in a systematic way. Thus, there is the possibility that reanalyses of data already collected for other purposes could reveal either sex or ear differences, at least for some of the species noted and for some physiological measures. For other species and phenomena, however, data adequate for a reanalysis that would be informative probably do not yet exist. One reason is that often there has been systematic exclusion of females in the work done on higher primates, largely because of the pragmatic difficulties associated with maintaining mixed-sex colonies. A second reason is that it would have been highly unusual for auditory scientists to have noted the state of estrus of their female animals at the time of testing (let alone to have collected full sets of data in the different stages), meaning that sex differences could be underestimated. Other reasons are familiar by now: Animal psychophysicists often have not had time to use criterion-free (but inefficient) forced-choice procedures for measuring hearing tasks, meaning that small effects could be lost in criterion differences (see Green & Swets, 1966). As we have seen, even in humans, sex and ear differences are small and require precise, time-consuming measurements to emerge. Also, the grain of the steps in stimulus strength have sometimes been so coarse that a small effect could escape notice.

This is not to say that no relevant demonstrations of sex or ear differences exist for nonhuman mammals. They do, but, unfortunately, the auditory tasks were typically rather more complex than those discussed earlier—in part because the experiments were often done by scientists whose primary interests were not the mechanisms of hearing per se. As a consequence, the results are typically difficult to interpret in the current context. For example, Fitch et al. (1993) demonstrated sex and ear differences for a tonal-sequence task in rats, a finding they believed demonstrates continuity across species with the functional cortical asymmetry that is well established in humans. Clearly, it would be easier to accept these results as being attributable solely to cortical differences if there were information available about simple detectability, and so forth, of these stimuli in the two sexes and ears. With such data, the across-species parallels might be even more striking than Fitch et al. appreciated. Similar comments apply to many of the other demonstrations of lateral asymmetries and sex differences in nonhumans reviewed by Fitch et al.

Little is known about sex and ear differences in OAEs in nonhuman species, but one report does suggest that higher primates have emission patterns like those of humans. Lonsbury-Martin and Martin (1988) surveyed 102 macaque monkeys for SOAEs (which are extremely rare in the small mammals typically used in auditory research). They found SOAEs only in the females, and more of those were in right ears than in left ears—just like the human pattern. This finding is encouraging, and it is hoped that others will look for sex and ear differences in OAEs of other types in this and other species.

SUMMARY AND COMMENTS

In summary, even though sex and ear differences have not been a primary topic of interest to students of the human auditory system, there is a reasonable amount of evidence suggesting their existence. Some of these differences are in characteristics that are apparently present at birth and remain reasonably constant through life. Thus, there is a strong implication that they originate ontogenetically in some of the same prenatal hormonal processes that produce other sex differences in the morphology and function of body and brain. Further, there is also evidence that the menstrual cycle affects certain auditory characteristics and abilities, thereby bolstering the idea that the auditory system can be affected by hormones. The existence of sex and ear differences in various auditory characteristics and simple abilities suggests that there may be a considerable contribution made by the periphery to the well-known sex and lateral differences in higher brain structures and cognitive abilities. Such bottom-up influences deserve more experimental and theoretical attention than they have received in the past.

Unfortunately, essentially all of the psychophysical data discussed in this article suffer from one weakness or another—imprecise psychophysical technique, small numbers of participants, small numbers of observations, uncontrolled variables, relatively little training of the participants, and so on. Clearly, replication will be necessary before many of these effects can be accepted as fact. Even with the caution engendered by this realization, however, it seems clear that small differences do exist between the sexes (and ears) in a number of auditory characteristics and tasks. Some of these differences are in features or abilities that seem quite elementary—cochlear characteristics such as length, OAE prevalence and strength, hearing sensitivity, ABR latency—and it is difficult indeed to imagine such differences not having an impact on higher level characteristics and abilities. My hope is that there will be increasing awareness of the existence of these sex and ear differences, and that they will become integral components in the explanations of scientists concerned with both structural differences at higher levels in the brain and functional differences in more complex tasks and behaviors.

An area of profound ignorance about the sex and ear differences discussed here is when in life they arise. For OAEs, it is known that the pattern of sex and ear differences is the same in infants and adults, so it is parsimonious to interpret those differences as having been present at birth and having survived puberty. For the rest of the auditory characteristics and tasks discussed, there is very little evidence for or against the existence of sex or ear differences prior to puberty. Information on this point is important for the evaluation of any explanation offered for any of the auditory sex or ear differences, but especially for explanations that appeal to hormones, prenatal or otherwise. At puberty, hormone levels change enormously and differentially in the two sexes, and there is a need to know what, if any, contribution to the final adult product is made during this time period. Getting from children reliable and valid measures of the various aspects of hearing has been a problem to which considerable attention has been given. The consensus seems to be that nonsensory factors such as attention and memory play a major role in the poorer hearing ability typically observed in children than adults (Werner & Rubel, 1992). With care, however, these nonsensory factors should be controllable, particularly if the emphasis is shifted to preteens rather than children. Also, given that the question is the time course of development, any absolute differences between preteens and adults would be of less interest than relative differences between the sexes and ears within the preteen subpopulation for the tasks studied. The information obtained would unquestionably be of interest to researchers in various fields. Note that there is some evidence that the sex difference in hearing sensitivity, at least, is the same in children as in adults (Roche et al., 1978), but there is less agreement about the direction of the ear effect in children (see McFadden, 1993b, for references). I am hopeful that my fellow psychoacousticians will begin developmental studies using some of the tasks that have shown sex and ear differences in order to document when in development those differences emerge. When possible, this work should include matching on physical size in order to rule out this pervasive variable.

Although it is tempting (to me, at least) to think about both OAEs and hearing sensitivity as being the result of organizational hormonal effects on the cochlea, it is necessary to be cautious. The reason is that there is another factor that surely makes a considerable contribution to the existence of a sex difference in hearing sensitivity—exposure to intense sounds. Indeed, in the past, the most popular explanation for the sex difference in hearing sensitivity was differential exposure to high levels of noise, and the differential hearing loss consequent to such exposures (e.g., Axelsson, Aniansson, & Costa, 1987; Siervogel, Roche, Johnson, & Fairman, 1982). According to this view, boys and men make more noise than girls and women, they are more attracted to activities that involve high sound levels, and, as a result, have more hearing loss than females, at every stage of life. A major contributor to this view was the fact that the sex difference in hearing sensitivity was often seen to increase with age (e.g., Royster et al., 1980; Ward, 1959), especially in the left ear, presumably reflecting the inevitable, cumulative effects of greater noise exposures in males in a predominately right-handed culture. There is almost surely some truth to this explanation. Because hearing loss is gradual, and is tested longitudinally only very infrequently in infants and children, it could take many years before a small exposure-induced hearing loss would be recognized as such. (The nominal range of normal hearing is wide, meaning that an initially highly sensitive ear could lose as much as 20 dB of sensitivity and still be classified as normal.) The evidence that differential noise exposure is not the whole story includes these facts: (a) The sex and ear differences in sensitivity exist even when care is taken to eliminate those individuals exposed to the noisiest occupations and avocations (Chung et al., 1983; Corso, 1959; Royster et al., 1980); and (b) exposure-induced hearing loss invariably leads to deficits in other auditory abilities (McFadden, Plattsmier, & Pasanen, 1984), yet many of the sex differences measured psychophysically favor males. The association between OAEs and hearing sensitivity suggests that, if it could be measured, the sex difference in sensitivity might exist in infants (because the sex difference in OAEs does), and for infants any sex difference in noise exposure should be minimal. The last chapter is yet to be written on this matter.

The OAE data from twins (Figure 4) contain a feature that catches the eye of most viewers. Namely, MZ females stand out from all the other types of participants in terms of prevalence of SOAEs and strength of CEOAEs (also see Russell, 1992). These extreme scores cannot easily be attributed to such factors as the presence of a second female fetus or the process of MZ twinning per se because extreme scores are not shown by SSDZ females or MZ males, respectively. The fact that MZ females are also extreme on the dimension of size of the corpus callosum (S. F. Witelson, personal communication, 1995)—another sexually dimorphic trait—suggests that MZ females may be different in a number of ways that are relevant to the topics at hand. Accordingly, it is interesting to contemplate how MZ females might have become different. Logically, there seem to be two possible ways for the extreme scores in Figure 4 to arise. Either (a) some mechanism acts to increase the strength of the cochlear amplifiers (and thereby adds SOAEs and increases the strength of CEOAEs) in MZ females only, or (b) all ears start out embryologically with strong cochlear amplifiers having the potential to produce numerous SOAEs and strong CEOAEs, but various prenatal mechanisms act to diminish this potential (more so in males than females, etc.), and, for some reason, MZ females are less susceptible to some of these limiting mechanisms than other fetuses—that is, the cochlear amplifiers are diminished less in MZ females. I admit a preference for the latter option, but, preferences aside, two potentially relevant factors deserve consideration.

Whether or not MZ cotwins share chorionic membranes, amniotic membranes, or both, appears to depend on when after conception separation occurs. Separations within the first 5 days are thought to lead to dichorionic diamniotic pairs and separations after Day 8 to monochorionic monoamniotic pairs (e.g., Bomsel-Helmreich & Al Mufti, 1995). Perhaps for MZ females there is something about the permeability characteristics of one or another of these membranes that act either to increase the concentration of some cochlear amplifier-strengthening substance, or to decrease the concentration of some cochlear amplifier-diminishing substance, relative to the concentrations received by other fetuses and pairs of fetuses. If so, there should be some correlation observable between the type of placenta from which pairs of twins originated and their OAEs (and possibly their corpus callosi). A second, not independent, idea is that perhaps the high strength of the cochlear amplifiers in female MZ fetuses is attributable to some substance that they themselves release, and that the production and release of this substance is periodic and at least partially under genetic control. Accordingly, the periodic release of this substance would be highly synchronized in the MZ females, but presumably less so in the DZ females. The better synchronization in the MZ females means that the short-term concentrations of this substance would be higher for them than for the more poorly synchronized DZ females and singleton females. How this idea could be tested in humans is unclear.

Whatever the mechanisms involved, the extreme status of the MZ females stands as an interesting mystery that may prove to have a hormonal solution, and solving this mystery promises to be informative about prenatal developmental processes in general. Also interesting is whether MZ females are extreme in their hearing sensitivity, in accord with the association established between sensitivity and OAEs (McFadden & Mishra, 1993).

It is not difficult to generate plausible speculations on the evolutionary history of the various sex differences in perception and cognition now known to exist. Consider, for example, hearing sensitivity and sound-localizing ability. Perhaps prehistoric females needed high sensitivity because they were both generally more vulnerable prey than males and typically were the primary defenders of the infants. Perhaps prehistoric males needed accurate sound-localizing ability for success in hunting, an activity that also presumably benefits from the male superiority in learning new routes, finding embedded figures, and directing missiles (e.g., Kimura, 1992). However, had these sex differences gone the other way, equally plausible (and difficult-to-test) explanations surely could have been generated, so there appears to be little value in lingering over such speculations. Perhaps some insight into the evolutionary origins of these sex and ear differences will be had once parallel differences are found in other species. Although it would be interesting if the ear and sex differences in hearing were the result of direct selection pressure, realistically they may be simply epiphenomena. That fact should not diminish our interest in these differences, however, because whatever their origin, they still have the potential to inform us about fundamental processes of brain development and sexual differentiation.

For someone who has been a devoted student of the auditory system for its own sake for many years, it is fascinating for me to contemplate the prospect that the auditory system has the potential to serve as a valuable window onto such fundamental processes as human development and human sexual differentiation. At this point, essentially all that exists is promise and speculation, but the promise seems considerable, and the speculation not unreasonable. As always, time will tell. Even if the promise goes unfulfilled, and the speculations prove wrong, I hope that the reader of this article at least will have learned something about the putative sex, ear, and menstrual differences in the auditory system—facts that those of us acquainted with the auditory system easily can find interesting in and of themselves.

ACKNOWLEDGMENTS

Preparation of this article was supported by National Institute on Deafness and other Communication Disorders Research Grant 5 R01 DC00153. I thank Donna L. Neff and Ted L. Langford for permission to use their data. Thanks are also due to many colleagues for their valuable comments on preliminary versions of this article, including David Buss, David Crews, John Loehlin, Donna Neff, Neal Viemeister, Beverly Wright, and Sheri Berenbaum and her three anonymous reviewers. Edward G. Pasanen and William M. Moss prepared the figures.

REFERENCES

Altemus, M., Wexler, B. E., & Boulis, N. (1989). Changes in perceptual asymmetry with the menstrual cycle. *Neuropsychologia, 2,* 233–240.

Axelsson, A., Aniansson, G., & Costa, O. (1987). Hearing loss in school children. *Scandinavian Audiology, 16,* 137–143.

Baker, M. A., & Weiler, E. M. (1977). Sex of listener and hormonal correlates of auditory thresholds. *British Journal of Audiology, 11,* 65–68.

Bell, A. (1992). Circadian and menstrual rhythms in frequency variations of spontaneous otoacoustic emissions from human ears. *Hearing Research, 58,* 91–100.

Bernstein, L. R., & Trahiotis, C. (1996). Binaural beats at high frequencies: Listeners' use of envelope-based interaural temporal and intensitive disparities. *Journal of the Acoustical Society of America, 99,* 1670–1679.

Bomsel-Helmreich, O., & Al Mufti, W. (1995). The mechanisms of monozygosity and double ovulation. In L. G. Keith, E. Papiernik, D. M. Keith, & B. Luke (Eds.), *Multiple pregnancy: Epidemiology, gestation, and perinatal outcome* (pp. 25–40). New York: Parthenon.

Burkhard, M. D., & Sachs, R. M. (1975). Anthropometric manikin for acoustic research. *Journal of the Acoustical Society of America, 58,* 214–222.
Burns, E. M., Arehart, K. H., & Campbell, S. L. (1992). Prevalence of spontaneous otoacoustic emissions in neonates. *Journal of the Acoustical Society of America, 91,* 1571–1575.
Burns, E. M., Campbell, S. L., & Arehart, K. H. (1994). Longitudinal measurements of spontaneous otoacoustic emissions in infants. *Journal of the Acoustical Society of America, 95,* 385–394.
Burns, E. M., Campbell, S. L., Arehart, K. H., & Keefe, D. H. (1993). Long-term stability of spontaneous otoacoustic emissions. *Abstracts of the Association for Research in Otolaryngology, 16,* 98.
Caplan, P. J., MacPherson, G. M., & Tobin, P. (1985). Do sex-related differences in spatial abilities exist? *American Psychologist, 40,* 786–799.
Chung, D. Y., Mason, K., Gannon, R. P., & Willson, G. N. (1983). The ear effect as a function of age and hearing loss. *Journal of the Acoustical Society of America, 73,* 1277–1282.
Clark, M. M., & Galef, B. G., Jr. (1998/this issue). Effects of intrauterine position on the behavior and genital morphology of litter-bearing rodents. *Developmental Neuropsychology, 14,* 197–211.
Clifton, R. K., & Freyman, R. L. (1989). Effect of click rate and delay on breakdown of the precedence effect. *Perception and Psychophysics, 46,* 139–145.
Collaer, M. L., & Hines, M. (1995). Human behavioral sex differences: A role for gonadal hormones during early development? *Psychological Bulletin, 118,* 55–107.
Corso, J. F. (1959). Age and sex differences in pure-tone thresholds. *Journal of the Acoustical Society of America, 31,* 498–507.
Davis, H. (1983). An active process in cochlear mechanics. *Hearing Research, 9,* 79–90.
Davis, M. J., & Ahroon, W. A. (1982). Fluctuations in susceptibility to noise-induced temporary threshold shift as influenced by the menstrual cycle. *Journal of Auditory Research, 22,* 173–187.
Daw, N. W. (1995). *Visual development.* New York: Plenum.
Divenyi, P. L., & Efron, R. (1979). Spectral versus temporal features in dichotic listening. *Brain and Language, 7,* 375–386.
Don, M., Ponton, C. W., Eggermont, J. J., & Masuda, A. (1993). Gender differences in cochlear response time: An explanation for gender amplitude differences in the unmasked auditory brain-stem response. *Journal of the Acoustical Society of America, 94,* 2135–2148.
Elkind-Hirsch, K. E., Stoner, W. R., Stach, B. A., & Jerger, J. F. (1992). Estrogen influences auditory brainstem responses during the normal menstrual cycle. *Hearing Research, 60,* 143–148.
Elkind-Hirsch, K. E., Wallace, E., Malinak, L. R., & Jerger, J. J. (1994). Sex hormones regulate ABR latency. *Otolaryngology—Head and Neck Surgery, 110,* 46–52.
Emmerich, D. S., Harris, J., Brown, W. S., & Springer, S. P. (1988). The relationship between auditory sensitivity and ear asymmetry on a dichotic listening task. *Neuropsychologia, 26,* 133–143.
Ferin, M., Jewelewicz, R., & Warren, M. (1993). *The menstrual cycle: Physiology, reproductive disorders, and infertility.* New York: Oxford University Press.
Fitch, R. H., Brown, D. P., O'Connor, K., & Tallal, P. (1993). Functional lateralization for auditory temporal processing in male and female rats. *Behavioral Neuroscience, 107,* 844–850.
Grantham, D. W. (1996). Left–right asymmetry in the buildup of echo suppression in normal-hearing adults. *Journal of the Acoustical Society of America, 99,* 1118–1123.
Green, D. M., & Swets, J. A. (1966). *Signal detection theory and psychophysics.* New York: Wiley.
Haggard, M., & Gaston, J. B. (1978). Changes in auditory perception in the menstrual cycle. *British Journal of Audiology, 12,* 105–118.
Haggerty, H. S., Lusted, H. S., & Morton, S. C. (1993). Statistical quantification of 24-hour and monthly variabilities of spontaneous otoacoustic emission frequency in humans. *Hearing Research, 70,* 31–49.
Hampson, E. (1990a). Estrogen-related variations in human spatial and articulatory-motor skills. *Psychoneuroendocrinology, 15,* 97–111.
Hampson, E. (1990b). Variations in sex-related cognitive abilities across the menstrual cycle. *Brain and Cognition, 14,* 26–43.

Jastreboff, P. J., Issing, W., Brennan, J. F., & Sasaki, C. T. (1988). Pigmentation, anesthesia, behavioral factors, and salicylate uptake. *Archives of Otolaryngology—Head and Neck Surgery, 114,* 186–191.

Jeffress, L. A. (1949). Interaural phase difference and pitch variation: Day-to-day changes. *American Journal of Psychology, 62,* 1–19.

Jerger, J., Jerger, S., & Mauldin, L. (1972). Studies in impedance audiometry: I. Normal and sensorineural ears. *Archives of Otolaryngology, 96,* 513–523.

Kamenkovich, V. M., & Alekseenko, N. Y. (1991). Asymmetry of auditory evoked potentials in the human brain stem. *Sensory Systems, 4,* 257–262.

Kemp, D. T. (1978). Stimulated acoustic emissions from within the human auditory system. *Journal of the Acoustical Society of America, 64,* 1386–1391.

Kemp, D. T. (1979). Evidence of mechanical nonlinearity and frequency selective wave amplification in the cochlea. *Archives of Otology, Rhinology, and Laryngology, 224,* 37–45.

Kimberley, B. P., Brown, D. K., & Eggermont, J. J. (1993). Measuring human cochlear traveling wave delay using distortion product emission phase responses. *Journal of the Acoustical Society of America, 94,* 1343–1350.

Kimura, D. (1992). Sex differences in the brain. *Scientific American, 267,* 118–125.

Kimura, D., & Hampson, E. (1994). Cognitive pattern in men and women is influenced by fluctuations in sex hormones. *Current Directions in Psychological Science, 3,* 57–61.

Kimura, D., & Harshman, R. A. (1984). Sex differences in brain organization for verbal and non-verbal functions. *Progress in Brain Research, 61,* 423–441.

Köppl, C. (1995). Otoacoustic emissions as an indicator for active cochlear mechanics: A primitive property of vertebrate auditory organs. In G. A. Manley, G. M. Klump, C. Köppl, H. Fastl, & H. Oeckinghaus (Eds.), *Advances in hearing research* (pp. 207–218). London: World Scientific.

Langford, T. L. (1994). Individual differences in sensitivity to interaural disparities of time and level. *Journal of the Acoustical Society of America, 96*(Suppl. 1), 3256.

Larkin, W. D., Reilly, J. P., & Kittler, L. B. (1986). Individual differences in sensitivity to transient electrocutaneous stimulation. *IEEE Transactions on Biomedical Engineering, 33,* 495–504.

Lautenbacher, S., & Strian, F. (1991). Sex differences in pain and thermal sensitivity: The role of body size. *Perception and Psychophysics, 50,* 179–183.

Levine, R. A., Liederman, J., & Riley, W. (1988). The brainstem auditory evoked potential asymmetry is replicable and reliable. *Neuropsychologia, 26,* 603–614.

Licklider, J. C. R., Webster, J. C., & Hedlun, J. M. (1950). On the frequency limits of binaural beats. *Journal of the Acoustical Society of America, 22,* 468–473.

Lonsbury-Martin, B. L., & Martin, G. K. (1988). Incidence of spontaneous otoacoustic emissions in macaque monkeys: A replication. *Hearing Research, 34,* 313–318.

Margolis, R. H., & Heller, J. W. (1987). Screening tympanometry: Criteria for medical referral. *Audiology, 26,* 197–208.

Matthews, L. J., Lee, F.-S., Mills, J. H., & Dubno, J. R. (1997). Extended high-frequency thresholds in older adults. *Journal of Speech, Language, and Hearing Research, 40,* 208–214.

McEwen, B. S., Biegnon, A., Fishette, C. T., Luine, V. N., Parsons, B., & Rainbow, T. C. (1984). Toward a neurochemical basis of steroid hormone action. In L. Martini & W. F. Ganong (Eds.), *Frontiers in neuroendocrinology* (Vol. 8, pp. 153–176). New York: Raven.

McFadden, D. (1984). *Tinnitus: Facts, theories, and treatments.* Washington, DC: National Academy Press.

McFadden, D. (1993a). A masculinizing effect on the auditory systems of human females having male co-twins. *Proceedings of the National Academy of Science, 90,* 11900–11904.

McFadden, D. (1993b). A speculation about the parallel ear asymmetries and sex differences in hearing sensitivity and otoacoustic emissions. *Hearing Research, 68,* 143–151.

McFadden, D., Jeffress, L. A., & Russell, W. E. (1973). Individual differences in sensitivity to interaural differences in time and level. *Perceptual and Motor Skills, 37,* 755–761.

McFadden, D., & Loehlin, J. C. (1995). On the heritability of spontaneous otoacoustic emissions: A twins study. *Hearing Research, 85,* 181–198.
McFadden, D., Loehlin, J. C., & Pasanen, E. G. (1996). Additional findings on heritability and prenatal masculinization of cochlear mechanisms: Click-evoked otoacoustic emissions. *Hearing Research, 97,* 102–119.
McFadden, D., & Mishra, R. (1993). On the relation between hearing sensitivity and otoacoustic emissions. *Hearing Research, 71,* 208–213.
McFadden, D., & Pasanen, E. G. (1975). Binaural beats at high frequencies. *Science, 190,* 394–396.
McFadden, D., Plattsmier, H. S., & Pasanen, E. G (1984). Aspirin-induced hearing loss as a model of sensorineural hearing loss. *Hearing Research, 16,* 251–260.
McFadden, D., & Wightman, F. L. (1983). Audition: Some relations between normal and pathological hearing. *Annual Review of Psychology, 34,* 95–128.
Meyer zum Gottesberge, A. M. (1988). Physiology and pathophysiology of inner ear melanin. *Pigment Cell Research, 1,* 238–249.
Moore, B. C. J., & O'Loughlin, B. J. (1986). The use of nonsimultaneous masking to measure frequency selectivity and suppression. In B. C. J. Moore (Ed.), *Frequency selectivity in hearing* (pp. 179–250). New York: Academic.
Neff, D. L., & Green, D. M. (1987). Masking produced by spectral uncertainty with multicomponent maskers. *Perception and Psychophysics, 41,* 409–415.
Neff, D. L., Kessler, C. J., & Dethlefs, T. M. (1996). Sex differences in simultaneous masking with random-frequency maskers. *Journal of the Acoustical Society of America, 100,* 2547–2550.
Nordeen, E. J., & Yahr, P. (1982). Hemisphere asymmetries in the behavioral and hormonal effects of sexually differentiating mammalian brain. *Science, 218,* 391–393.
Norton, S. J. (1992). The effects of being a newborn on otoacoustic emissions. *Journal of the Acoustical Society of America, 91*(Suppl. 1), 2409.
Norton, S. J. (1994). Emerging role of evoked otoacoustic emissions in neonatal hearing screening. *American Journal of Otolaryngology, 15,* 4–12.
Parlee, M. B. (1983). Menstrual rhythms in sensory processes: A review of fluctuations in vision, olfaction, audition, taste, and touch. *Psychological Bulletin, 93,* 539–548.
Pickles, J. O. (1988). *An introduction to the physiology of hearing* (2nd ed.). New York: Academic.
Pirilä, T. (1991). Left–right asymmetry in the human response to experimental noise exposure: II. Pre-exposure hearing threshold and temporary threshold shift at 4 kHz frequency. *Acta Otolaryngology, 111,* 861–866.
Previc, F. H. (1991). A general theory concerning the prenatal origins of cerebral lateralization in humans. *Psychological Review, 98,* 299–334.
Probst, R., Lonsbury-Martin, B. L., & Martin, G. K. (1991). A review of otoacoustic emissions. *Journal of the Acoustical Society of America, 89,* 2027–2067.
Reyes, F. I., Boroditsky, R. S., Winter, J. S. D., & Faiman, C. (1974). Studies on human sexual development: II. Fetal and maternal serum gonadotropin and sex steroid concentrations. *Journal of Clinical Endocrinology and Metabolism, 38,* 612–617.
Roche, A. F., Siervogel, R. M., Himes, J. H., & Johnson, D. L. (1978). Longitudinal study of hearing in children: Baseline data concerning auditory thresholds, noise exposure, and biological factors. *Journal of the Acoustical Society of America, 64,* 1593–1601.
Royster, L. H., Royster, J. D., & Thomas, W. G. (1980). Representative hearing levels by race and sex in North Carolina industry. *Journal of the Acoustical Society of America, 68,* 551–566.
Russell, A. F. (1992). *Heritability of spontaneous otoacoustic emissions.* Unpublished doctoral dissertation, University of Illinois, Urbana-Champaign.
Sato, H., Sando, I., & Takahashi, H. (1991). Sexual dimorphism and development of the human cochlea. Computer 3-D measurement. *Acta Otolaryngology, 111,* 1037–1040.

Siervogel, R. M., Roche, A. F., Johnson, D. L., & Fairman, T. (1982). Longitudinal study of hearing in children: Cross-sectional studies of noise exposure as measured by dosimetry. *Journal of the Acoustical Society of America, 71,* 372–377.

Smail, P. J., Reyes, F. I., Winter, J. S. D., & Faiman, C. (1981). The fetal hormonal environment and its effect on the morphogenesis of the genital system. In S. J. Kogan & E. S. E. Hafez (Eds.), *Pediatric andrology* (pp. 9–19). Hague, The Netherlands: Martinus Nijhoff.

Spillman, T. (1994). Genetic diseases of hearing. *Current Opinion in Neurology, 7,* 81–87.

Steel, K. P., & Brown, S. D. M. (1994). Genes and deafness. *Trends in Genetics: DNA, Differentiation, and Development, 10,* 428–435.

Stelmachowicz, P. G., Beauchaine, K. A., Kalberer, A., & Jesteadt, W. (1989). Normative thresholds in the 8- to 20-kHz range as a function of age. *Journal of the Acoustical Society of America, 86,* 1384–1391.

Swanson, S. J., & Dengerink, H. A. (1988). Changes in pure-tone thresholds and temporary threshold shifts as a function of menstrual cycle and oral contraceptives. *Journal of Speech and Hearing Research, 31,* 569–574.

Talmadge, C. L., Long, G. R., Murphy, W. J., & Tubis, A. (1993). New off-line method for detecting spontaneous otoacoustic emissions in human subjects. *Hearing Research, 71,* 170–182.

Teas, D. C., Eldredge, D. H., & Davis, H. (1962). Cochlear responses to acoustic transients: An interpretation of the whole-nerve action potential. *Journal of the Acoustical Society of America, 34,* 1438–1459.

Tobias, J. V. (1965). Consistency of sex differences in binaural-beat perception. *International Audiology, 4,* 179–182.

Trune, D. R., Mitchell, C., & Phillips, D. S. (1988). The relative importance of head size, gender and age on the auditory brainstem response. *Hearing Research, 32,* 165–174.

vom Saal, F. S. (1989). Sexual differentiation in litter-bearing mammals: Influence of sex of adjacent fetuses in utero. *Journal of Animal Science, 67,* 1824–1840.

vom Saal, F. S., Quadagno, D. M., Even, M. D., Keisler, L. W., Keisler, D. H., & Khan, S. (1990). Paradoxical effects of maternal stress on fetal steroids and postnatal reproductive traits in female mice from different intrauterine positions. *Biology of Reproduction, 43,* 751–761.

Ward, W. D. (1957). Hearing of naval aircraft maintenance personnel. *Journal of the Acoustical Society of America, 29,* 1289–1301.

Ward, W. D. (1959). Susceptibility and sex. *Journal of the Acoustical Society of America, 31,* 1138.

Ward, W. D. (1963). Auditory fatigue and masking. In J. Jerger (Ed.), *Modern developments in audiology* (pp. 240–286). New York: Academic.

Ward, W. D. (1966). Temporary threshold shift in males and females. *Journal of the Acoustical Society of America, 40,* 478–485.

Werner, L. A., & Rubel, E. W. (1992). *Developmental psychoacoustics.* Washington, DC: American Psychological Association.

Whitehead, M. L., Kamal, N., Lonsbury-Martin, B. L., & Martin, G. K. (1993). Spontaneous otoacoustic emissions in different racial groups. *Scandinavian Audiology, 23,* 3–10.

Wilson, J. P. (1986). The influence of temperature on frequency-tuning mechanisms. In J. B. Allen, J. L. Hall, A. Hubbard, S. T. Neely, & A. Tubis (Eds.), *Peripheral auditory mechanisms* (pp. 229–236). New York: Springer-Verlag.

Wit, H. P. (1985). Diurnal cycle for spontaneous oto-acoustic emission frequency. *Hearing Research, 18,* 197–199.

Witelson, S. F., Glezer, I. I., & Kigar, D. L. (1995). Women have greater density of neurons in posterior temporal cortex. *Journal of Neuroscience, 15,* 3418–3428.

Wright, B. A. (1994). Individual, sex, and ear differences in measures of overshoot and psychophysical two-tone suppression. *Journal of the Acoustical Society of America, 95*(Suppl. 1), 2942–2943.

Wynn, V. T. (1972). Measurements of small variations in "absolute" pitch. *Journal of Physiology, 220,* 627–637.

Spatial Reasoning in Children With Congenital Adrenal Hyperplasia Due to 21-Hydroxylase Deficiency

Elizabeth Hampson
Neuroscience Program and Department of Psychology
University of Western Ontario
London, Canada

Joanne F. Rovet
Department of Psychology and Division of Endocrinology
The Hospital for Sick Children
Toronto, Canada

Deborah Altmann
Department of Psychology
The Hospital for Sick Children
Toronto, Canada

It has been proposed that exposure of the central nervous system to high concentrations of androgens during sensitive periods in early development may facilitate the ability to process spatial information. Most tests of this proposal have been derived from nonhuman species. To test this hypothesis in humans, we evaluated spatial reasoning in preadolescent children with congenital adrenal hyperplasia (CAH), a condition characterized by elevated androgens during gestation. The Primary Mental Abilities (PMA) Spatial Relations test was administered to 12 children with CAH (7 girls, 5 boys) and 10 unaffected sibling controls (6 girls, 4 boys), ranging in age from 8 to 12 years. Results showed a significant interaction between sex and clinical status. Girls with CAH achieved significantly higher spatial scores than control girls, whereas boys with CAH showed significantly lower spatial scores than control boys.

Requests for reprints should be sent to Elizabeth Hampson, Department of Psychology, University of Western Ontario, London, Ontario, Canada N6A 5C2. E-mail: ehampson@uwovax.uwo.ca

On the PMA Perceptual Speed test, given for comparison, girls with CAH scored significantly lower than control girls, producing a double dissociation. The results demonstrate that group differences in spatial proficiency can be detected in preadolescent children with CAH. The findings replicate and extend results reported previously by Resnick, Berenbaum, Gottesman, and Bouchard (1986), and are consistent with an organizing effect of early androgens on brain areas subserving spatial processes.

In the past 30 years, studies in rodents and nonhuman primates have firmly established that the mammalian central nervous system is sensitive during specific periods in early development to androgens and their metabolites. The presence of high levels of androgens at these times induces permanent alterations in the ultrastructural organization of steroid-sensitive brain regions (including the hypothalamus, limbic system, and neocortex: Bachevalier & Hagger, 1991; Breedlove, 1992; Gorski & Jacobson, 1981; Juraska, 1991; Roof & Havens, 1992; Toran-Allerand, 1991), and irreversibly alters the behavioral propensities of the animal (Beatty, 1992; Goy & McEwen, 1980), promoting the emergence of a male-typical pattern of brain and behavior. These events occur in male animals under the influence of endogenous androgens, but can be induced experimentally in females by exogenous manipulations of hormones.

These organizational effects of androgens were originally described for reproductive behaviors in rodents by Phoenix, Goy, Gerall, and Young (1959). Organizational effects on other sexually differentiated behaviors have now been identified, such as rough-and-tumble play (Goy & Resko, 1972; Meaney, 1988) and the tendency toward aggression (see Beatty, 1992, for a recent review). Whether early androgens or other sex steroids also influence central nervous system (CNS) differentiation in humans is not established, but evidence favors a neuroendocrine contribution to the development of sexual orientation, certain childhood play behaviors, and perhaps tendencies toward aggression in humans (for reviews, see Collaer & Hines, 1995; Hampson & Kimura, 1992).

High levels of androgens during critical periods in early development may also promote a brain organization that facilitates the ability to process certain types of spatial information. Spatial ability has evolved as a sexually differentiated function in many mammalian species, with male animals typically showing greater proficiency than females on various tasks that involve processing or remembering spatial information, such as route learning in an unfamiliar environment (Beatty, 1984; Williams & Meck, 1991). This has been conceptualized as a product of sexual selection, resulting from ecological pressures for greater mobility in males (Gaulin & FitzGerald, 1986). Although it can be modified by learning and other sociocultural factors, vestiges of this sex difference are also seen on laboratory spatial tasks in humans (Linn & Petersen, 1985; Voyer, Voyer, & Bryden, 1995), particularly those involving dynamic stimuli (Hunt, Pellegrino, Frick, Farr, & Alderton, 1988), visualization in three dimensions (Sanders, Soares, & D'Aquila, 1982), or targeting accuracy (Watson & Kimura, 1991), tasks that most closely resemble the three-dimensional natural environment in which spatial abilities likely evolved.

In rodents, hormonal manipulations in the neonatal period have been shown to systematically affect rate of learning in adulthood on spatial tasks such as the radial-arm maze or Morris water maze and to alter reliance on geometric versus landmark cues for spatial navigation (Roof & Havens, 1992; Williams, Barnett, & Meck, 1990; Williams & Meck, 1991). In untreated animals, faster maze learning is typically found in males, but this sex difference is eliminated by castration of males, or by administration of masculinizing hormones to females, in the neonatal period (Dawson, Cheung, & Lau, 1975; Roof & Havens, 1992; Stewart, Skvarenina, & Pottier, 1975; Williams et al., 1990). Developmental alterations in neurons in the frontal cortex and hippocampus may be part of the neural substrate for these effects (Williams & Meck, 1991). In primates, spatial abilities per se have not been examined. However, developmental effects of testosterone have been found in rhesus monkeys on object discrimination learning tasks and on maturation rates in the regions of frontal and temporal cortex that subserve these tasks (Bachevalier & Hagger, 1991).

In humans, the evidence for an organizational influence of early androgens on spatial abilities is inconclusive (Collaer & Hines, 1995; Hampson, 1995). Nevertheless, recent studies implicate the prenatal period as a time when the developing CNS might be sensitive to androgens. Grimshaw, Sitarenios, and Finegan (1995), in a group of children from normal pregnancies, found a positive correlation between testosterone measured in amniotic fluid at midgestation and later mental rotation rates in girls. Cole-Harding, Morstad, and Wilson (1988) found better spatial ability and more rapid learning on the Vandenberg Mental Rotations test in female dizygotic twins who had a male as opposed to a female co-twin. Neuroendocrine effects of proximity to male fetuses in utero have been reported in other species for several sexually differentiated traits, including use of space in natural environments and laboratory tests of spatial ability (Clark & Galef, this issue; Galea, Ossenkopp, & Kavaliers, 1994; Williams & Meck, 1991; Zielinski, vom Saal, & Vandenbergh, 1992). But perhaps the strongest evidence that early androgens may help organize neural systems involved in spatial abilities in humans comes from people with congenital adrenal hyperplasia (CAH), a condition in which the developing fetus of both sexes is exposed to high levels of androgens in utero, but in which postnatal upbringing is gender-appropriate.

The classical form of CAH due to 21-hydroxylase deficiency affects approximately 1 in 15,000 live births (New, 1995). A major feature of this condition is the significant overproduction of adrenal androgens, beginning in the 3rd month of fetal life (New, 1985). In genetic females, this is sufficient to cause varying degrees of genital virilization, which is apparent at birth. Approximately 75% of children with CAH have an associated deficiency in aldosterone production (Pang, Levine,

Chow, Faiman, & New, 1979), which results in excessive sodium excretion in the urine (salt-wasting). CAH is typically diagnosed in the newborn period, although individuals with non-salt-wasting CAH may occasionally escape detection until inappropriate signs of virilization become evident in early childhood (White, New, & DuPont, 1987). Once detected, the hormonal abnormalities can be successfully ameliorated through the use of cortisone-replacement therapy (combined with mineralocorticoid replacement in children with salt-wasting disease). Girls with CAH typically undergo surgical correction of the genitalia at the youngest possible age to ensure psychosexual development progresses normally (New, 1995). Thus, in early-diagnosed cases, the hormonal abnormalities can effectively be confined to the prenatal and early infant period, providing optimal treatment is received.

If androgen levels during critical periods in fetal development do influence the differentiation of spatial abilities in humans, females with CAH would be expected to display superior spatial information processing compared with female controls, given their exposure to prolonged high levels of androgens during gestation. So far one study (Resnick, Berenbaum, Gottesman, & Bouchard, 1986) did find enhanced spatial functioning in adolescent girls with CAH. Compared with a control group made up of unaffected female siblings and first cousins, girls with CAH showed better performance on three different tests of spatial ability—the Hidden Patterns test, Card Rotations, and Mental Rotations. Several other studies, however, have reported nonsignificant findings (e.g., Baker & Ehrhardt, 1974; Helleday, Bartfai, Ritzen, & Forsman, 1994; McGuire, Ryan, & Omenn, 1975). This lack of consensus from the CAH literature is surprising given the variety of other evidence of behavioral masculinization that now exists for girls with CAH (Berenbaum & Hines, 1992; Berenbaum & Snyder, 1995; Dittmann et al., 1990; Ehrhardt & Baker, 1974; Hines & Kaufman, 1994; Money, Schwartz, & Lewis, 1984). Methodological factors, including the use in some studies of experimental tasks with only weak spatial demands, might account for the differing findings.

The purpose of this study was to investigate spatial reasoning in a group of preadolescent children with CAH. If an organizational effect of androgens is truly present, it may be detectable even in preadolescent children, in whom adult levels of circulating hormones have not yet been achieved. This possibility is strengthened by recent evidence that sex differences in spatial abilities emerge at an early age (Voyer et al., 1995). On a standardized test of spatial ability, the PMA Spatial Relations Test, it was predicted that girls with CAH would outperform unaffected sibling controls. Predictions for boys with CAH were more difficult, because exposure of males to excessively high doses of androgens in perinatal life has been shown in animal studies to exert either no effects, or demasculinizing effects, on later behavior (e.g., Baum & Schretlen, 1975; Diamond, Llacuna, & Wong, 1973). The Resnick et al. (1986) study of CAH adolescents found patterns consistent with the latter type of effect, in that boys with CAH showed a statistical trend for lower scores than control boys on the Paper Form Board test. Therefore, in this study, we predicted that boys with CAH would perform, if anything, more poorly than control boys on a standardized test of spatial ability.

METHOD

Participants

Eligible participants were identified through the Divisions of Endocrinology and Gynaecology at the Hospital for Sick Children, Toronto, Canada. All families who had a child with the classical form of CAH due to 21-hydroxylase deficiency between the ages of 8 and 12, and who was being followed at the hospital, were contacted and asked to participate as part of a larger study of intellectual abilities and school achievement in children and adolescents with early-treated CAH. Of the 15 families contacted, 12 (80%) agreed to participate in the study, yielding a total of 12 patients with CAH (7 girls, 5 boys). Five out of 12 patients, or 42%, had the salt-wasting form of CAH. Median age at diagnosis was 0 months (range = 0–75 months). All but one girl were diagnosed and had treatment starting in the immediate newborn period. Three of the 5 boys were diagnosed at ages 3, 4, and 6 years, respectively. All patients were taking appropriate, prescribed medications for CAH and were otherwise in good health.

Controls consisted of 10 unaffected, healthy children (6 girls, 4 boys) who had a brother or sister with CAH, and who fell within the designated age range. Because of family constellations, we were unable to match the CAH children with their own same-sex siblings, but all controls nevertheless had a sibling in the larger study with CAH. Participant characteristics are summarized in Table 1.

Cognitive Tests

All participants traveled to the Hospital for Sick Children to complete an extensive battery of age-appropriate cognitive measures. In addition to the tests described here, the battery included a set of neuropsychological and psychoeducational tests to assess general cognitive functioning. The Spatial Relations Test from the PMA battery (Thurstone & Thurstone, 1963) was given as a test of spatial reasoning suitable for 8- to 12-year-olds. On this test, children must discriminate the shape from among four multiple-choice alternatives that forms a square when combined with the first (sample) figure in each row. Six minutes were allowed to complete 25 items. Data from the PMA Perceptual Speed Test were examined for comparison, because it involves similar visual and perceptual demands, but requires no translations or transformations of a spatial nature. This test was additionally of interest because, in adults, a sex difference in favor of women is often found on tests of perceptual speed and accuracy (Maccoby & Jacklin, 1974; Tyler, 1965).

TABLE 1
Demographic Characteristics of Patients and Controls

	Female				Male			
	CAH[a]		Controls[b]		CAH[c]		Controls[d]	
	M	SD	M	SD	M	SD	M	SD
Current age (years)	9.7	1.5	10.5	1.6	10.2	1.6	10.3	1.7
Grade	4.9	1.3	5.5	1.7	5.0	1.4	5.2	1.7
Wechsler VIQ	102.1	19.8	98.3	17.2	94.6	16.3	106.5	7.8
Wechsler PIQ	112.1	14.0	109.2	12.2	109.2	23.5	115.8	3.8
Wechsler FSIQ	107.4	15.9	103.7	13.7	101.4	19.8	111.7	5.9

Note. CAH = congenital adrenal hyperplasia; VIQ = Verbal IQ; PIQ = Performance IQ; FSIQ = Full-Scale IQ.
[a]$n = 7$. [b]$n = 6$. [c]$n = 5$. [d]$n = 4$.

On this test, the task is to identify the two drawings in each set (row) that are exactly alike. Five minutes were allowed to complete 40 items. On both tests, children responded by marking their answers with an X.

To avoid confounding effects of age, the raw scores on each test were converted to standard age-adjusted deviation quotients before analysis.

In addition, all participants completed the full Wechsler Intelligence Scale for Children–Revised (Wechsler, 1974).

Procedure

All tests were administered by experienced psychometrists who were unfamiliar with the hypotheses of the study. Children with CAH and their siblings were assessed in parallel on the same day. All tests were given individually using standard administration procedures.

RESULTS

Data were analyzed using 2 × 2 factorial analysis of variance (ANOVA) with sex and clinical status as factors. Because the primary purpose of the study was to examine whether there was evidence of cognitive masculinization in girls with CAH, the following planned contrasts were carried out on the Perceptual Speed and Spatial Relations scores: (a) CAH girls versus control girls, and (b) control girls versus control boys. Otherwise, post hoc comparisons were done where appropriate using Bonferroni *t* tests with an overall alpha level of .05. To ensure that obtained significance values were accurate despite the small sample sizes in this study, all obtained probabilities were confirmed using exact randomization tests (Edgington,

1987).[1] In no instance was there any substantive disagreement between the conventional and distribution-free probabilities.

Spatial Reasoning

Mean scores on the PMA Spatial Relations Test for the four groups are shown in Figure 1. An ANOVA on the scores revealed that the predicted interaction between sex and clinical status was highly significant, $F(1, 17) = 8.90$, $p < .01$. All means differed in the expected direction. Among controls, boys outperformed girls on the test, $t(8) = 3.04$, $p < .01$, one-tailed. As predicted, girls with CAH achieved significantly higher spatial scores than control girls. The difference between the means was approximately 1 SD in size. This was true with or without the presence of one outlier participant in the female control group, whose Spatial Relations score fell > 4 SDs above the mean for the rest of the group, $t(10) = 2.12$, $p < .05$, one-tailed, including outlier; $t(9) = 3.54$, $p < .01$, one-tailed, with outlier removed. For boys, the difference between the means was also in excess of 1 SD. Boys with CAH achieved significantly lower scores than control boys, although still well within the normal range ($p < .05$ by post hoc test).

Perceptual Speed

Mean scores on the PMA Perceptual Speed Test are shown in Figure 2. An ANOVA on the scores revealed a significant main effect of CAH, $F(1, 17) = 5.13$, $p < .05$. The two-way interaction between sex and clinical status was not significant, $F(1, 17) = 0.41$, ns. Both boys and girls with CAH achieved lower scores on the Perceptual Speed Test than did sibling controls. For girls, this pattern was opposite to that seen on Spatial Relations. A direct comparison of the two female groups confirmed that girls with CAH performed significantly more poorly than control girls on Perceptual Speed, $t(10) = 2.26$, $p < .025$, one-tailed. The difference between the means was in excess of 1 SD in size. Thus, in girls, a double dissociation was seen between the Perceptual Speed and Spatial Relations scores.

A direct comparison of the CAH and control groups in boys was nonsignificant by Bonferroni test, $t(17) = 0.99$, ns. Planned comparisons failed to reveal any detectable sex difference in performance between male and female controls, $t(8) = 0.23$, ns, one-tailed.

---

[1]The exact randomization test is a distribution-free statistical method in which a test statistic (in this case, t) is repeatedly computed for all possible permutations of the observed data set. The p value is the proportion of permutations of the reference set that yield test statistic values greater than or equal to the empirically obtained results (Edgington, 1987). Randomization tests are recommended when the assumptions underlying conventional parametric statistics may not be met.

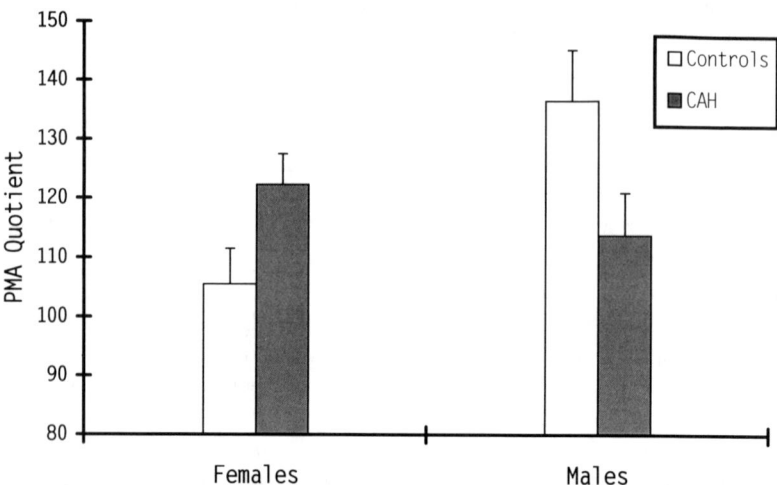

FIGURE 1   Mean performance on the Primary Mental Abilities (PMA) Spatial Relations test in boys and girls with congenital adrenal hyperplasia (CAH) and unaffected sex-matched controls. Error bars represent standard error of the mean.

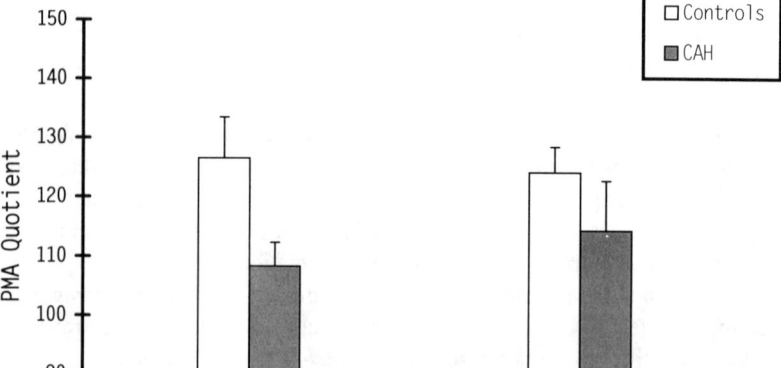

FIGURE 2   Mean performance on the Primary Mental Abilities (PMA) Perceptual Speed test in boys and girls with congenital adrenal hyperplasia (CAH) and unaffected sex-matched controls. Error bars represent standard error of the mean.

Intelligence

Differences among groups in IQ scores did not account for these findings. ANOVA failed to reveal any significant group differences in either Verbal IQ (VIQ), Performance IQ (PIQ), or Full Scale IQ (FSIQ; all $ps > .30$). In all groups, the mean PIQ score was at the top of the average range or greater. PIQ but not VIQ was significantly correlated with both the Spatial Relations and Perceptual Speed scores, for PIQ: $r(19) = .60, p < .01$, and $r(19) = .51, p < .01$, respectively; and for VIQ: $r(19) = .43$, ns, and $r(19) = .35$, ns, respectively. Entering IQ scores as covariates in analyses of covariance (ANCOVAs) did not alter the patterns of results obtained on the Spatial Relations and Perceptual Speed tests; the interactions and main effects described previously remained highly significant when IQ was statistically controlled. In particular, although PIQ was significant as a covariate, $F(1, 16) = 16.43, p < .001$, the Sex × Clinical Status interaction in the Spatial Relations scores was maintained, $F(1, 16) = 10.82, p < .005$, as was the main effect of CAH on Perceptual Speed, $F(1, 16) = 6.30, p < .025$.

A relatively higher PIQ than VIQ was evident in both the CAH children and controls. A 2 × 4 repeated measures ANOVA with IQ Scale as a within-subjects factor and the four participant groups as a between-subject factor confirmed a significant main effect of IQ scale, $F(1, 18) = 9.52, p < .01$. Elevation in PIQ has been observed previously in samples of females with CAH (e.g., Resnick, 1982; Wenzel et al., 1978). All children in this study were proficient in English, but 1 of 12 patients (8%) and 4 of 10 (40%) controls spoke a language other than English in the home. It is possible that this led to some underestimation of VIQ in the controls. The IQ discrepancies in the children with CAH could not be explained on this basis.

Cognitive Profiles

To explore relative cognitive strengths within individuals, each child's perceptual speed quotient was subtracted from his or her spatial quotient. This analysis was possible because all PMA subtests are standardized to a common scale ($M = 100$, $SD = 16$). A positive score therefore denoted relatively stronger spatial than perceptual speed abilities, whereas a negative score denoted relatively stronger perceptual speed than spatial abilities. ANOVA on the resulting difference scores revealed a highly significant Sex × Clinical Status interaction, $F(1, 17) = 19.10, p < .001$. Figure 3 shows the mean difference scores across the four groups. Among controls, girls showed relatively stronger perceptual speed skills, whereas boys showed relatively stronger spatial skills, and this difference was highly significant, $t(8) = 3.90, p < .01$, one-tailed. Girls with CAH closely resembled control boys and differed significantly from control girls, $t(10) = 7.84, p < .005$, one-tailed, in

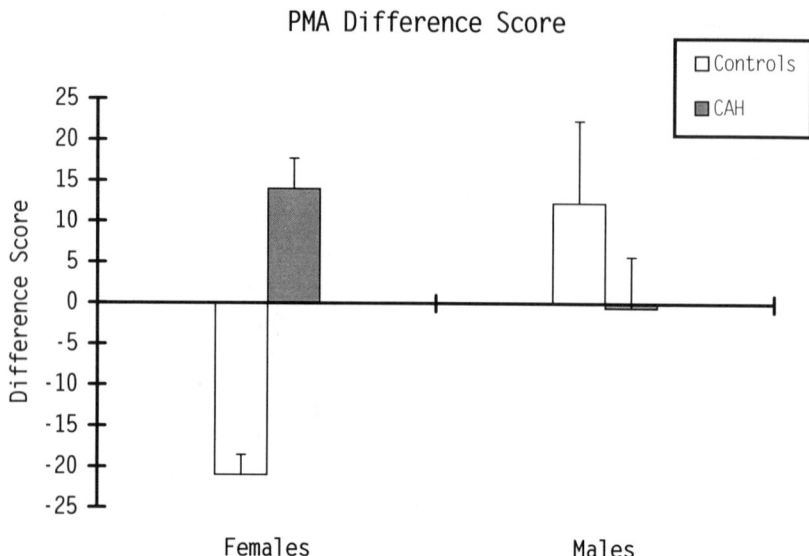

FIGURE 3 Mean intraindividual difference scores reflecting relative strength of spatial versus perceptual speed abilities in the four groups. Difference scores were calculated by subtracting the perceptual speed quotient from the spatial quotient for each child. A positive value indicates relatively greater proficiency in the spatial domain. Error bars represent standard error of the mean.

showing relatively stronger spatial abilities. Boys with CAH, although showing a reduction in the normal male pattern, did not differ significantly from male controls, and continued to be distinct from female controls ($p < .02$ by Bonferroni t test).

DISCUSSION

Recent studies suggest that alterations in sex-typed behaviors are relatively common in children and adults with CAH. For example, compared with female controls, females with CAH reportedly show greater masculinization in patterns of childhood toy and playmate preferences (Berenbaum & Hines, 1992; Berenbaum & Snyder, 1995; Hines & Kaufman, 1994), increased "rough play" and tomboyism (Dittmann et al., 1990; Ehrhardt & Baker, 1974; Hampson, Rovet, & Altmann, 1995; cf. Hines & Kaufman, 1994), more masculine-typical scores on sex-related behavior and personality scales (e.g. Helleday, Edman, Ritzen, & Siwers, 1993), and increased rates of bi- or homosexuality on indexes of sexual orientation (Dittmann, Kappes, & Kappes, 1992; Ehrhardt, Evers, & Money, 1968; Money et al., 1984; Zucker et al., 1996; cf. Mulaikal, Migeon, & Rock, 1987). The nature of the behavioral changes observed and difficulties in accounting for them exclusively through psychosocial explanations have led a number of researchers to the view that these behavioral changes reflect hormonal influences on early brain development, at least to some degree.

In this study, we hypothesized that spatial abilities represent another domain in which early androgens might influence developmental outcome. Consistent with this hypothesis, a group of healthy normal girls with CAH achieved significantly higher scores than control girls on a standardized test of spatial visualization, the PMA Spatial Relations test.[2] The magnitude of the difference between control girls and girls with CAH was large, nearly 1 SD in size. Although some studies have reported significant IQ differences between females with CAH and controls (e.g., Helleday et al., 1994), our groups were well matched on IQ. There was less than 4 points' difference between the CAH girls and controls. Furthermore, controlling for individual differences in IQ using ANCOVAs failed to eliminate the group difference in spatial performance. These results represent the first independent confirmation of Resnick et al.'s (1986) report of enhanced spatial abilities in girls with CAH. Further, we have shown that IQ differences do not account for this effect.

We also found that boys with CAH showed slightly diminished spatial ability relative to age-matched male controls. Our prediction of reduced spatial scores in boys with CAH was based largely on evidence from experimental animals that demasculinization (reduction in male-typical characteristics) can occur in males who are exposed to abnormally high levels of androgens during the early developmental periods critical for sexual differentiation of the nervous system (e.g., Baum & Schretlen, 1975; Diamond et al., 1973; Roof & Havens, 1992; Sherry, Galef, & Clark, 1996). Ours is the first study in which this pattern was statistically significant. However, a similar pattern of means has been reported in at least two other published studies of CAH (McGuire et al., 1975; Resnick et al., 1986). Resnick et al. (1986), for example, reported a statistical trend for CAH males to score lower than control males on the Paper Form Board test, a test of spatial visualization similar to the version of the PMA Spatial Relations used here. Further support for our finding comes from a study of CAH carried out in parallel with our own, in which a significant reduction in spatial scores in boys with CAH has now been observed (Berenbaum, 1992). Despite our small sample size, therefore, this is likely a representative finding. Interestingly, Hines and Kaufman (1994) recently found behavioral demasculinization in 3- to 8-year-old boys with CAH on a measure of rough-and-tumble play, a behavior whose expression has been shown in nonhuman

---

[2]The mean PMA quotients obtained by several CAH and control subgroups in our data were unusually high. This might simply reflect the fact that there is no recent standardization of the PMA battery. Obsolete test norms would affect the CAH group and controls equally, and would not account for the group differences in abilities that we observed. Curiously, however, score inflation has not been noted in other recent research at the Hospital for Sick Children using the PMA tests (e.g., Rovet, Ehrlich, & Czuchta, 1990; Rovet, Ehrlich, & Hoppe, 1987).

primates to be influenced by the level of testosterone or dihydrotestosterone present in the prenatal period (see Meaney, 1988, for review). This suggests that demasculinization in males with CAH might not be limited to spatial functions.

If organizational effects of early androgens predispose children with CAH to better or poorer spatial information processing than their peers, then this difference should be evident from the earliest ages at which spatial ability can reliably be assessed, or at least as early as the sex difference normally emerges among unaffected control children. An important aspect of our data is therefore the demonstration that differences between CAH children and controls are clearly present by middle childhood. The traditional lore is that sex differences in cognitive functions are not expressed or at least not maximally expressed until after puberty. Recent evidence, however, suggests that sex differences in spatial abilities are detectable in the preadolescent age range if age-appropriate and "pure" spatial tests are used (Johnson & Meade, 1987; Kerns & Berenbaum, 1991). A meta-analysis of the spatial abilities literature by Voyer et al. (1995) confirmed that sex differences on the PMA Spatial Relations are reliably found by age 10, the mean age of the participants in our study. Consistent with Voyer's results, we found a significant sex difference between control boys and girls in the Spatial Relations scores. The fact that children with CAH were detectably different from controls even in the preadolescent age range greatly strengthens the case for an organizational influence of hormones.

Despite its failure to elicit a sex difference, the PMA Perceptual Speed test was an effective control task in this study. The patterns we observed on Spatial Relations were not duplicated on Perceptual Speed, a task with relatively complex visual-perceptual requirements but with no spatial processing demands. This increases the likelihood that the effects we found on Spatial Relations reflect the visuospatial demands of the task and not some other extraneous element such as response mode or low-level visual–perceptual processing that the two tasks shared in common. The clearest distinction between the two tasks occurred in girls: CAH girls showed a significant decrement in perceptual speed relative to control girls, in contrast to the superiority they displayed on the spatial task. Thus, a double dissociation was seen. Our observation of reduced perceptual speed in girls with CAH is of particular interest because a female advantage on tests of perceptual speed and accuracy is reliably although not invariably found in adults (Maccoby & Jacklin, 1974; Tyler, 1965) and may also be present in children (Gainer, 1962; Laosa & Brophy, 1972). This raises the possibility of a defeminizing effect of early androgens on cognition (reduction in a female-typical characteristic). In other species, masculinization and defeminization of behavior are distinct organizational processes (e.g., Davis, Chaptal, & McEwen, 1979) although they typically co-occur. Defeminizing effects on cognitive abilities have not previously been seen in girls or women with CAH, but other indications of behavioral defeminization have periodically been reported, including reduced interest in feminine accoutrements (Ehrhardt & Baker, 1974), reduced play with girls' toys (Berenbaum & Hines, 1992), and reduced interest and participation in infant care (Ehrhardt & Baker, 1974; Leveroni & Berenbaum, this issue). In this study, interpretation was complicated by the fact that boys with CAH also showed reduced perceptual speed scores, giving rise to a main effect of CAH. This leaves open the possibility that some other factor associated with having CAH could be responsible for the observed reduction in perceptual speed (e.g., side effects of treatment; cf. Mauri et al., 1993; Naber, Sand, & Heigl, 1996). Further studies will be needed to confirm whether defeminization of cognitive abilities in fact is present in girls with CAH.

Perceptual speed is an ability that is especially vulnerable to the effects of cerebral dysfunction (Aram & Ekelman, 1988). The question therefore arises as to whether the reduction in perceptual speed seen in both CAH groups in this study is reflective of some pathology associated with having CAH. This is unlikely for several reasons. First of all, although scores were reduced relative to controls, the scores for both boys and girls with CAH were in the average range in absolute terms, even if we assume some score inflation on the PMA test due to old test norms. Second, one of our CAH cases had mild electroencephalogram abnormalities at age 3 but otherwise there was no evidence, from medical history, of CNS pathology in our CAH children. Third, as described previously, the average IQ score in our sample was well within the normal range with no discernible difference between CAH patients and sibling controls ($M = 104.9$ for CAH group and $M = 106.9$ for controls). PIQ was above average. Finally, if such pathology did exist, it would be most likely to occur in children with the salt-wasting form of CAH who are at risk of electrolyte crisis in the newborn period before diagnosis takes place. By chance, salt-wasters made up only 42% of our sample, and their PMA Perceptual Speed scores were not remarkably lower than the scores of non-salt-wasters ($M = 108.5$ and $M = 112.5$, respectively). The lack of evidence of CNS pathology in our CAH children suggests that the reductions in perceptual speed that we observed are best regarded as individual variations within the normal range.

The fact that we chose to examine cognitive abilities that are sexually differentiated may help to explain why differences between the CAH and control groups were so salient in this study. Most prior studies of intellectual functioning in CAH have not included measures of spatial ability, but instead focused on general intelligence or neuropsychological functions that exhibit little sexual dimorphism (e.g., Money & Lewis, 1966; Sinforiani, et al., 1994). Past attempts to assess spatial ability in CAH have been subject to a variety of methodological or sampling factors that might have reduced the potential to detect significant differences, including use of spatial tests that elicit only small or no sex differences or that are contaminated by other sources of variance, lack of appropriate control groups, small sample sizes, sampling variations in IQ that might have obscured differences in spatial ability, and progress over time in the treatment and medical management of CAH (Baker & Ehrhardt, 1974; Helleday et al., 1994; McGuire et al., 1975; Perlman,

1973). It is also possible that these effects are more easily detected in children. The study by Resnick et al. (1986), our own study, and the unpublished study by Berenbaum (1992) suggest that judicious choice of spatial tests can reveal spatial processing differences in healthy and well-controlled groups of children with CAH.

Our findings in girls with CAH are consistent with a large body of experimental literature in other species, spanning more than 30 years, showing that masculinization and defeminization of CNS structures and behavioral patterns occurs in female mammals exposed to high levels of androgens pre- or perinatally (Becker, Breedlove, & Crews, 1992; Breedlove, 1992; Goy & McEwen, 1980). The male brain normally masculinizes under the influence of testicular testosterone, or its active metabolites dihydrotestosterone and estradiol. Several studies have now found demasculinization of male-typical behavioral patterns (e.g., Baum & Schretlen, 1975; Diamond et al., 1973; Roof & Havens, 1992) and brain structures (e.g., Sherry et al., 1996) in male animals exposed to excessive androgens, although a few studies have reported no change from male controls (cf. vom Saal, 1979). Roof and Havens (1992), for example, found that gonadally intact male rats given additional testosterone propionate (TP) in the neonatal period showed poorer adult performance on a sexually dimorphic water maze task than control males who did not receive testosterone supplementation. Identical TP treatment of female rats improved maze acquisition to male levels. The mechanisms responsible for demasculinization in males have not been identified. In the case of CAH, an additional complication is that relatively little is known about the regulation of androgen concentrations in the male fetus during gestation. Excess secretion of adrenal sex steroids results in elevated androstenedione in both sexes, and reliable increases in testosterone in females, but in males with CAH, total testosterone in amniotic fluid is more variably elevated beyond the normal male range (Forest, Betuel, & David, 1989; Pang et al., 1980). There is some evidence that the excess adrenal sex steroids may suppress Leydig cell function through hypothalamic–pituitary–gonadal feedback mechanisms (Pang et al., 1979). Postnatally, Pang et al. (1979) reported that testosterone concentrations dropped off rapidly in newborn males with CAH aged 1 to 3 months when glucocorticoid treatment was introduced, and remained below normal for at least 3 to 4 weeks during this period when a surge in testosterone normally occurs in male infants. With prolonged treatment, testosterone levels in the CAH boys were at or only slightly below the normal male range. This report is of interest in light of speculation that the postnatal testosterone surge might be important for sexual differentiation of the human CNS (e.g., Berenbaum, Korman, & Leveroni, 1995; Collaer & Hines, 1995; Hampson, 1995). Which, if any, of these factors contribute to demasculinization of spatial abilities in males is unknown.

This study was undertaken to test an explicit hypothesis raised by animal studies in neuroendocrinology. Although the organizational effects of early androgens provide a parsimonious explanation for our findings, we must consider to what extent differences in socialization, family upbringing, or disease-related factors might explain these results. Any viable alternative must plausibly account for the observed three-way interaction among CAH, sex, and type of cognitive ability, and must recognize the normal overall level of intellectual functioning in these children. Hypothetical disease-related factors such as parental overprotectiveness of chronically ill children, recurrent illnesses and hospitalizations, or untoward effects of salt-wasting, would, if anything, lead to academic underachievement and diminished capabilities, and do not appear to describe the vast majority of children in our sample. This is especially true of girls with CAH who showed not just normal but above-average spatial abilities for their age. These factors would also not be expected to produce opposite effects in the two sexes, and thus do not satisfactorily account for the interaction we observed.

Sex differences in spatial ability are sometimes attributed to the gender-role socialization of boys and girls in Western industrialized societies, but differential socialization practices cannot easily explain our main findings of differences between CAH children and same-sex controls. CAH girls had substantially better spatial ability than female controls despite being raised as girls, and CAH boys had poorer spatial ability than male controls despite being raised as boys. Because all physical indicators of sex (including somatic, genetic, and hormonal) are unambiguously male in boys with CAH, it seems implausible to suggest that they might have been raised in a less masculine fashion than their brothers, resulting in poorer spatial ability. In girls, the presence of genital ambiguity at birth raises the possibility that parents may encourage or enforce more masculine behavioral patterns in their daughters, perhaps because of concerns about the "true" sex of the child (Quadagno, Briscoe, & Quadagno, 1977). We did not directly assess parental attitudes and rearing practices in this study. However, other studies of CAH provide no empirical support for this contention. Parental ambivalence about sex assignment appears to be extremely rare, and parents report that they do not treat girls with CAH in a more masculine fashion (Berenbaum & Hines, 1992; Ehrhardt & Baker, 1974; Resnick, 1982). In fact, a priori, there is at least as much reason to believe that they may, on the contrary, go to extra lengths to ensure gender-appropriate behavior. Several studies have now failed to find any relation between degree of genital virilization at diagnosis and later behavioral masculinization in girls with CAH (Berenbaum & Hines, 1992; Dittmann et al., 1990; Hines & Kaufman, 1994; Slijper, 1984), contrary to what one might expect if behavioral outcome were contingent on parental reactions to external indicators of sex.

Whether we attribute behavioral alterations in girls with CAH to the organizational effects of early androgens or to unidentified social–environmental influences, it seems clear that many girls with CAH do exhibit masculinization of childhood toy and playmate preferences and show greater participation in active outdoor play than control girls (e.g., Berenbaum & Snyder, 1995; Dittmann et al., 1990; Ehrhardt & Baker, 1974; Hines & Kaufman, 1994). Might girls with CAH consequently encounter different childhood learning experiences than their sisters, which lead to enhanced spatial competence? Current evidence suggests that such experiential factors may help to accentuate or diminish any biological predispositions that are present, but are unlikely in themselves to be the primary basis for the large differences in spatial ability we observed. Prior participation in spatial activities has been found in other studies to be minimally related to higher scores on psychometric tests of spatial abilities (e.g., Newcombe & Dubas, 1992). A recent meta-analysis found the magnitude of the relation to be extremely modest, with an average combined $r = .09$ (Baenninger & Newcombe, 1989). The critical early experiential antecedents of later spatial proficiency are unknown, but at present there is little reason to assume that any of the behavioral alterations so far documented in girls with CAH are causally related to better spatial ability. The situation is even more uncertain in boys with CAH, in whom behavioral alterations compared to unaffected boys have yet to be clearly established. Because of our small sample size, we could not meaningfully evaluate the hypothetical relation between childhood experiences and cognitive test scores in this study. In a larger sample of patients with CAH, Resnick et al. (1986) found that females with CAH did show a trend toward greater participation in spatial manipulation activities than female siblings and first cousins on the Early Life Activities Questionnaire. As might be expected from Baenninger and Newcombe's (1989) review, however, scores on the spatial activity scale were not significant predictors of scores on a composite measure of spatial ability $(r = .10)$. In general, examining the relation between childhood experiences and spatial ability presents an inferential problem: If young girls with CAH do show greater participation than their sisters in masculine-typical play behaviors, including spatially demanding activities such as active outdoor play, exploration of surroundings, or play with mechanical or constructional toys, better spatial abilities could as easily be a cause, rather than an effect, of the behavioral differences observed.

Organizational effects of early androgen exposure appear to provide a reasonable and systematic explanation for our findings. Psychosocial factors may contribute to cognitive differences between CAH and healthy control children, but are less likely to be the fundamental basis for the effects reported here. CAH is also characterized by abnormalities in other hormones, especially 17-hydroxyprogesterone. However, in experimental animal studies, progestins have less consistent effects on behavioral development than androgens, and, if anything, seem to prevent masculinization at physiological concentrations (Birke & Sadler, 1983; Diamond et al., 1973; Erpino, 1975; Hull, Franz, Snyder, & Nishita, 1980). This would not explain the enhanced spatial abilities found in girls with CAH, but could contribute to the cognitive demasculinization seen in boys. If so, we can only assume that any protective effect of elevated progestins in girls is insufficient to counteract the masculinizing effects of excess adrenal androgens that also occur.

CONCLUSIONS

Human cognitive abilities are widely considered to be the combined product of genetic and social–environmental forces. This study suggests that androgens in the prenatal or early postnatal period may be another factor that influences the development of spatial functions, perhaps contributing to the sexual differentiation of these abilities. We have hypothesized that the systematic alterations in spatial abilities found in children with CAH to a large degree reflect the organizational effects of early androgens. Support for this view comes from preliminary animal studies suggesting an organizational influence on spatial functions (e.g., Roof & Havens, 1992; Williams et al., 1990), and from emerging evidence that mental rotation ability in humans is correlated with the androgen environment in utero (Cole-Harding et al., 1988; Grimshaw et al., 1995). At least two other CAH studies have reached a similar conclusion (Berenbaum, 1992; Resnick et al., 1986). Our data do not resolve the issue of whether the proposed effects of androgens on spatial information processing are direct (on specific brain systems involved in spatial processing) or indirect (mediated by other behavioral changes induced by androgens, such as differences in exploratory behavior or rough outdoor play in early childhood). Based on current evidence, a direct effect seems probable. Our data thus add to the growing body of evidence that masculinization of behavioral predispositions in girls with CAH reflects hormonal influences on brain development. In turn, finding evidence of organizational effects in humans helps to reinforce the notion that neuroendocrine principles derived from animal studies apply to human brain development as well. Future studies should more clearly address to what extent early endocrine influences are important for the differentiation of other cognitive abilities and try to elucidate whether these influences are direct or secondary to other behavioral changes induced by androgens.

ACKNOWLEDGMENTS

This research was supported by the Medical Research Council of Canada, Grant MA10876. Elizabeth Hampson was the recipient of a New Faculty Research Fellowship from the Ontario Mental Health Foundation.

We thank Robert M. Ehrlich, John D. Bailey, Dennis Daneman, F. Jack Holland, and Kusiel Perlman of the Division of Endocrinology, The Hospital for Sick Children. We are grateful to Joanne Rudolph and Lori Brnjac for assistance in testing participants. We also thank Richard Harshman for statistical advice and programming of MATLAB subroutines.

REFERENCES

Aram, D. M., & Ekelman, B. L. (1988). Scholastic aptitude and achievement among children with unilateral brain lesions. *Neuropsychologia, 26,* 903–916.
Bachevalier, J., & Hagger, C. (1991). Sex differences in the development of learning abilities in primates. *Psychoneuroendocrinology, 16,* 177–188.
Baenninger, M., & Newcombe, N. (1989). The role of experience in spatial test performance: A meta-analysis. *Sex Roles, 20,* 327–344.
Baker, S. W., & Ehrhardt, A. A. (1974). Prenatal androgen, intelligence, and cognitive sex differences. In R. C. Friedman, R. M. Richart, & R. L. VandeWeile (Eds.), *Sex differences in behavior* (pp. 53–76). New York: Wiley.
Baum, M. J., & Schretlen, P. (1975). Neuroendocrine effects of perinatal androgenization in the male ferret. *Progress in Brain Research, 42,* 343–355.
Beatty, W. W. (1984). Hormonal organization of sex differences in play fighting and spatial behavior. *Progress in Brain Research, 61,* 315–329.
Beatty, W. W. (1992). Gonadal hormones and sex differences in non-reproductive behaviors. In A. A. Gerall, H. Moltz, & I. L. Ward (Eds.), *Handbook of behavioral neurobiology: Vol. 11. Sexual differentiation* (pp. 85–128). New York: Plenum.
Becker, J. B., Breedlove, S. M., & Crews, D. (1992). *Behavioral endocrinology.* Cambridge, MA: MIT Press.
Berenbaum, S. A. (1992, May). *Hormonal influences on cognitive abilities.* Paper presented at the Third Annual Meeting of Theoretical and Experimental Neuropsychology/Neuropsychologie Experimentale et Theorique (TENNET), Montreal, Canada.
Berenbaum, S. A., & Hines, M. (1992). Early androgens are related to childhood sex-typed toy preferences. *Psychological Science, 3,* 203–206.
Berenbaum, S. A., Korman, K., & Leveroni, C. (1995). Early hormones and sex differences in cognitive abilities. *Learning and Individual Differences, 7,* 303–321.
Berenbaum, S. A., & Snyder, E. (1995). Early hormonal influences on childhood sex-typed activity and playmate preferences: Implications for the development of sexual orientation. *Developmental Psychology, 31,* 31–42.
Birke, L. I. A., & Sadler, D. (1983). Progestin-induced changes in play behavior of the prepubertal rat. *Physiology and Behavior, 30,* 341–347.
Breedlove, S. M. (1992). Sexual dimorphism in the vertebrate nervous system. *Journal of Neuroscience, 12,* 4133–4142.
Clark, M. M., & Galef, B. G., Jr. (1998/this issue). Effects of intrauterine position on the behavior and genital morphology of litter-bearing rodents. *Developmental Neuropsychology, 14,* 197–211.
Cole-Harding, S., Morstad, A. L., & Wilson, J. R. (1988). Spatial ability in members of opposite-sex twin pairs. *Behavior Genetics, 18,* 710.
Collaer, M. L., & Hines, M. (1995). Human behavioral sex differences: A role for gonadal hormones during early development? *Psychological Bulletin, 118,* 55–107.
Davis, P. G., Chaptal, C. V., & McEwen, B. S. (1979). Independence of the differentiation of masculine and feminine sexual behavior in rats. *Hormones and Behavior, 12,* 12–19.
Dawson, J. L. M., Cheung, Y. M., & Lau, R. T. S. (1975). Developmental effects of neonatal sex hormones on spatial and activity skills in the white rat. *Biological Psychology, 3,* 213–229.
Diamond, M., Llacuna, A., & Wong, C. L. (1973). Sex behavior after neonatal progesterone, testosterone, estrogen or antiandrogens. *Hormones & Behavior, 4,* 73–88.
Dittmann, R. W., Kappes, M. E., & Kappes, M. H. (1992). Sexual behavior in adolescent and adult females with congenital adrenal hyperplasia. *Psychoneuroendocrinology, 17,* 153–170.
Dittmann, R. W., Kappes, M. H., Kappes, M. E., Borger, D., Meyer-Bahlburg, H. F. L., Stegner, H., Willig, R. H., & Wallis, H. (1990). Congenital adrenal hyperplasia II: Gender-related behavior and

attitudes in female salt-wasting and simple-virilizing patients. *Psychoneuroendocrinology, 15,* 421–434.

Edgington, E. S. (1987). *Randomization tests* (2nd ed.). New York: Marcel Dekker.

Ehrhardt, A. A., & Baker, S. W. (1974). Fetal androgens, human central nervous system differentiation, and behavior sex differences. In R. C. Friedman, R. M. Richart, & R. L. VandeWiele (Eds.), *Sex differences in behavior* (pp. 33–51). New York: Wiley.

Ehrhardt, A. A., Evers, K., & Money, J. (1968). Influence of androgen and some aspects of sexually dimorphic behavior in women with the late-treated adrenogenital syndrome. *Johns Hopkins Medical Journal, 123,* 115–122.

Erpino, M. J. (1975). Androgen-induced aggression in neonatally androgenized female mice, inhibition by progesterone. *Hormones and Behavior, 6,* 149–158.

Forest, M. G., Betuel, H., & David, M. (1989). Prenatal treatment in congenital adrenal hyperplasia due to 21-hydroxylase deficiency: Update 88 of the French multicentric study. *Endocrine Research, 15,* 277–301.

Gainer, W. L. (1962). The ability of the WISC subtests to discriminate between boys and girls of average intelligence. *California Journal of Educational Research, 13,* 9–16.

Galea, L. A. M., Ossenkopp, K.-P., & Kavaliers, M. (1994). Performance (reacquisition) of a water-maze task by adult meadow voles: Effects of age of juvenile acquisition and in utero environment (litter sex-ratio). *Behavioral Brain Research, 63,* 177–185.

Gaulin, S. J. C., & FitzGerald, R. W. (1986). Sex differences in spatial ability: An evolutionary hypothesis and test. *American Naturalist, 127,* 74–88.

Gorski, R. A., & Jacobson, C. D. (1981). Sexual differentiation of the brain. In S. J. Kogan & E. S. E. Hafez (Eds.), *Pediatric andrology* (pp. 109–134). Boston: Martinus Nijhoff.

Goy, R. W., & McEwen, B. S. (1980). *Sexual differentiation of the brain.* Cambridge, MA: MIT Press.

Goy, R. W., & Resko, J. A. (1972). Gonadal hormones and behavior of normal and pseudohermaphroditic nonhuman female primates. *Recent Progress in Hormone Research, 28,* 707–733.

Grimshaw, G. M., Sitarenios, G., & Finegan, J. K. (1995). Mental rotation at 7 years: Relations with prenatal testosterone levels and spatial play experiences. *Brain and Cognition, 29,* 85–100.

Hampson, E. (1995). Spatial cognition in humans: Possible modulation by androgens and estrogens. *Journal of Psychiatry and Neuroscience, 20,* 397–404.

Hampson, E., & Kimura, D. (1992). Sex differences and hormonal influences on cognitive function in humans. In J. B. Becker, S. M. Breedlove, & D. Crews (Eds.), *Behavioral endocrinology* (pp. 357–398). Cambridge, MA: MIT Press.

Hampson, E., Rovet, J. F., & Altmann, D. (1995, May). *Sports participation and physical aggressiveness in children and young adults with congenital adrenal hyperplasia.* Presented at the International Behavioral Development Symposium on the Biological Basis of Sexual Orientation and Sex-Typical Behavior, Minot, ND.

Helleday, J., Bartfai, A., Ritzen, E. M., & Forsman, M. (1994). General intelligence and cognitive profile in women with congenital adrenal hyperplasia (CAH). *Psychoneuroendocrinology, 19,* 343–356.

Helleday, J., Edman, G., Ritzen, E. M., & Siwers, B. (1993). Personality characteristics and platelet MAO activity in women with congenital adrenal hyperplasia (CAH). *Psychoneuroendocrinology, 18,* 343–354.

Hines, M., & Kaufman, F. R. (1994). Androgen and the development of human sex-typical behavior: Rough-and-tumble play and sex of preferred playmates in children with congenital adrenal hyperplasia (CAH). *Child Development, 65,* 1042–1053.

Hull, E. M., Franz, J. R., Snyder, A. M., & Nishita, J. K. (1980). Perinatal progesterone and learning, social and reproductive behavior in rats. *Physiology and Behavior, 24,* 251–256.

Hunt, E., Pellegrino, J. W., Frick, R. W., Farr, S. A., & Alderton, D. (1988). The ability to reason about movement in the visual field. *Intelligence, 12,* 77–100.
Johnson, E. S., & Meade, A. C. (1987). Developmental patterns of spatial ability: An early sex difference. *Child Development, 58,* 725–740.
Juraska, J. M. (1991). Sex differences in "cognitive" regions of the rat brain. *Psychoneuroendocrinology, 16,* 105–120.
Kerns, K. A., & Berenbaum, S. A. (1991). Sex differences in spatial ability in children. *Behavior Genetics, 21,* 383–396.
Laosa, L. M., & Brophy, J. E. (1972). Effects of sex and birth order on sex-role development and intelligence among kindergarten children. *Developmental Psychology, 6,* 409–415.
Leveroni, C. L. & Berenbaum, S. A. (1998/this issue). Early androgen effects on interest in infants: Evidence from children with congenital adrenal hyperplasia. *Developmental Neuropsychology, 14,* 321–340.
Linn, M. C., & Petersen, A. C. (1985). Emergence and characterization of gender differences in spatial abilities: A meta-analysis. *Child Development, 56,* 1479–1498.
Maccoby, E. E., & Jacklin, C. N. (1974). *The psychology of sex differences.* Stanford, CA: Stanford University Press.
Mauri, M., Sinforiani, E., Bono, G., Vignati, F., Berselli, M. E., Attanasio, R., & Nappi, G. (1993). Memory impairment in Cushing's disease. *Acta Neurologica Scandinavica, 87,* 52–55.
McGuire, L. S., Ryan, K. O., & Omenn, G. S. (1975). Congenital adrenal hyperplasia: II. Cognitive and behavioral studies. *Behavior Genetics, 5,* 175–188.
Meaney, M. J. (1988). The sexual differentiation of social play. *Trends in Neuroscience, 11,* 54–58.
Money, J., & Lewis, V. (1966). IQ, genetics and accelerated growth: Adrenogenital syndrome. *Bulletin of the Johns Hopkins Hospital, 118,* 365–373.
Money, J., Schwartz, M., & Lewis, V. G. (1984). Adult erotosexual status and fetal hormonal masculinization and demasculinization: 46,XX congenital virilizing adrenal hyperplasia and 46/XY androgen insensitivity syndrome compared. *Psychoneuroendocrinology, 9,* 405–414.
Mulaikal, R. M., Migeon, C. J., & Rock, J. A. (1987). Fertility rates in female patients with congenital adrenal hyperplasia due to 21-hydroxylase deficiency. *New England Journal of Medicine, 316,* 178–182.
Naber, D., Sand, P., & Heigl, B. (1996). Psychopathological and neuropsychological effects of 8-days' corticosteroid treatment. A prospective study. *Psychoneuroendocrinology, 21,* 25–31.
New, M. I. (1985). Clinical and endocrinological aspects of 21-hydroxylase deficiency. *Annals of the New York Academy of Sciences, 458,* 1–27.
New, M. I. (1995). Congenital adrenal hyperplasia. In L. J. DeGroot, M. Besser, H. G. Burger, J. L. Jameson, D. L. Loriaux, J. C. Marshall, W. D. Odell, J. T. Potts, & A. H. Rubenstein (Eds.), *Endocrinology* (Vol. 2, pp. 1813–1835). Philadelphia: Saunders.
Newcombe, N., & Dubas, J. S. (1992). A longitudinal study of predictors of spatial ability in adolescent females. *Child Development, 63,* 37–46.
Pang, S., Levine, L. S., Cederqvist, L. L., Fuentes, M., Riccardi, V. M., Holcombe, J. H., Nitowsky, H. M., Sachs, G., Anderson, C. E., Duchon, M. A., Owens, R., Merkatz, I., & New, M. I. (1980). Amniotic fluid concentrations of delta-5 and delta-4 steroids in fetuses with congenital adrenal hyperplasia due to 21-hydroxylase deficiency and in anencephalic fetuses. *Journal of Clinical Endocrinology and Metabolism, 51,* 223–229.
Pang, S., Levine, L. S., Chow, D. M., Faiman, C., & New, M. I. (1979). Serum androgen concentrations in neonates and young infants with congenital adrenal hyperplasia due to 21-hydroxylase deficiency. *Clinical Endocrinology, 11,* 575–584.
Perlman, S. M. (1973). Cognitive abilities of children with hormone abnormalities: Screening by psychoeducational tests. *Journal of Learning Disabilities, 6,* 26–34.

Phoenix, C. H., Goy, R. W., Gerall, A. A., & Young, W. C. (1959). Organizing action of prenatally administered testosterone propionate on the tissues mediating mating behavior in the female guinea pig. *Endocrinology, 65,* 369–382.

Quadagno, D. M., Briscoe, R., & Quadagno, J. S. (1977). Effects of perinatal gonadal hormones on selected nonsexual behavior patterns: A critical assessment of the nonhuman and human literature. *Psychological Bulletin, 84,* 62–80.

Resnick, S. M. (1982). *Psychological functioning in individuals with congenital adrenal hyperplasia: Early hormonal influences on cognition and personality.* Unpublished doctoral dissertation, University of Minnesota, Minneapolis.

Resnick, S. M., Berenbaum, S. A., Gottesman, I. I., & Bouchard, T. J. (1986). Early hormonal influences on cognitive functioning in congenital adrenal hyperplasia. *Developmental Psychology, 22,* 191–198.

Roof, R. L., & Havens, M. D. (1992). Testosterone improves maze performance and induces development of a male hippocampus in females. *Brain Research, 572,* 310–313.

Rovet, J. F., Ehrlich, R. M., & Czuchta, D. (1990). Intellectual characteristics of diabetic children at diagnosis and one year later. *Journal of Pediatric Psychology, 15,* 775–788.

Rovet, J. F., Ehrlich, R. M., & Hoppe, M. (1987). Intellectual deficits associated with early onset of insulin-dependent diabetes mellitus in children. *Diabetes Care, 10,* 510–515.

Sanders, B., Soares, M. P., & D'Aquila, J. M. (1982). The sex difference on one test of spatial visualization: A nontrivial difference. *Child Development, 53,* 1106–1110.

Sherry, D. F., Galef, B. G., & Clark, M. M. (1996). Sex and intrauterine position influence the size of the gerbil hippocampus. *Physiology and Behavior, 60,* 1491–1494.

Sinforiani, E., Livieri, C., Mauri, M., Bisio, P., Sibilla, L., Chiesa, L., & Martelli, A. (1994). Cognitive and neuroradiological findings in congenital adrenal hyperplasia. *Psychoneuroendocrinology, 19,* 55–64.

Slijper, F. M. E. (1984). Androgens and gender role behavior in girls with congenital adrenal hyperplasia (CAH). *Progress in Brain Research, 61,* 417–422.

Stewart, J., Skvarenina, A., & Pottier, J. (1975). Effects of neonatal androgens on open-field behavior and maze learning in the prepubescent and adult rat. *Physiology and Behavior, 14,* 291–295.

Thurstone, L. L., & Thurstone, T. G. (1963). *Primary mental abilities.* Chicago: Science Research Associates.

Toran-Allerand, C. D. (1991). Organotypic culture of the developing cerebral cortex and hypothalamus: Relevance to sexual differentiation. *Psychoneuroendocrinology, 16,* 7–24.

Tyler, L. E. (1965). *The psychology of human differences.* New York: Appleton-Century-Crofts.

Vom Saal, F. S. (1979). Prenatal exposure to androgen influences morphology and aggressive behavior of male and female mice. *Hormones and Behavior, 12,* 1–11.

Voyer, D., Voyer, S., & Bryden, M. P. (1995). Magnitude of sex differences in spatial abilities: A meta-analysis and consideration of critical variables. *Psychological Bulletin, 117,* 250–270.

Watson, N. V., & Kimura, D. (1991). Nontrivial sex differences in throwing and intercepting: Relation to psychometrically-defined spatial functions. *Personality and Individual Differences, 12,* 375–385.

Wechsler, D. (1974). *Wechsler Intelligence Scale for Children–Revised.* New York: The Psychological Corporation.

Wenzel, U., Schneider, M., Zachmann, M., Knorr-Murset, G., Weber, A., & Prader, A. (1978). Intelligence of patients with congenital adrenal hyperplasia due to 21-hydroxylase deficiency, their parents, and unaffected siblings. *Helvetica Paediatrica Acta, 33,* 11–16.

White, P. C., New, M. I., & DuPont, B. (1987). Congenital adrenal hyperplasia. *New England Journal of Medicine, 316,* 1519–1524.

Williams, C. L., Barnett, A. M., & Meck, W. H. (1990). Organizational effects of early gonadal secretions on sexual differentiation in spatial memory. *Behavioral Neuroscience, 104,* 84–97.

Williams, C. L., & Meck, W. H. (1991). The organizational effects of gonadal steroids on sexually dimorphic spatial ability. *Psychoneuroendocrinology, 16,* 155–176.

Zielinski, W. J., vom Saal, F. S., & Vandenbergh, J. G. (1992). The effect of intrauterine position on the survival, reproduction and home range size of female house mice (Mus musculus). *Behavioral Ecology and Sociobiology, 30,* 185–191.

Zucker, K. J., Bradley, S. J., Oliver, G., Blake, J., Fleming, S., & Hood, J. (1996). Psychosexual development of women with congenital adrenal hyperplasia. *Hormones and Behavior, 30,* 300–318.

Early Androgen Effects on Interest in Infants: Evidence From Children With Congenital Adrenal Hyperplasia

Catherine L. Leveroni
Department of Psychology
Finch University of Health Sciences
The Chicago Medical School

Sheri A. Berenbaum
Department of Behavioral and Social Sciences
School of Medicine and Department of Psychology
Southern Illinois University, Carbondale

Early androgens have been shown to facilitate male-typical behavior in people, but little attention has been paid to androgen effects on female-typical behavior. We studied the effects of early androgen on human interest in infants, attempting to extend studies in rodents and primates that indicate that exposure to high levels of androgen in the prenatal and early postnatal periods reduces the expression of maternal behavior in juvenile and adult animals. Parents completed a questionnaire about the behavior of children with congenital adrenal hyperplasia (CAH) who had been exposed to high levels of androgens early in life, and their unexposed siblings. As hypothesized, girls with CAH were reported to have less interest in infants than their sisters. These results suggest that early androgens may act to suppress some aspects of female-typical behavior in people, as in other species, and that sex differences in maternal behavior result, in part, from early hormones.

In the past few years, convincing evidence has accumulated to show that, in human beings, as in other species, gonadal hormones present early in development play a

---

Requests for reprints should be sent to Sheri A. Berenbaum, Department of Behavioral and Social Sciences, School of Medicine, Southern Illinois University, Carbondale, IL 62901-6517. E-mail: sberenbaum@som.siu.edu

major role in the development of sex differences in a variety of behaviors and probably brain structure and function (e.g., Clark & Galef, this issue; Fitch, Cowell, & Denenberg, this issue; Hampson, Rovet, & Altmann, this issue; McFadden, this issue; Michael & Zumpe, this issue; for reviews, see Becker, Breedlove, & Crews, 1993; Berenbaum, Leveroni, & Korman, 1995; Breedlove, 1994; Collaer & Hines, 1995; Goy & McEwen, 1980). Studies in people have focused primarily on behaviors that are more common or higher in males than in females, generally referred to as *male-typical behavior*. These studies indicate that the presence of high levels of masculinizing hormones, such as androgens or androgenizing progestins, in the prenatal and early postnatal periods facilitate the development of male-typical behavior, such as childhood play with boys' toys, childhood and adult spatial ability, and aggression (e.g., Berenbaum & Hines, 1992; Berenbaum & Resnick, 1997; Berenbaum & Snyder, 1995; Ehrhardt & Baker, 1974; Hampson et al., this issue; Reinisch, 1981; Resnick, Berenbaum, Gottesman, & Bouchard, 1986).

There has been little study of the effects of early hormones on behaviors that are more common or higher in females than in males, perhaps because the sex differences on these behaviors are thought to be small or inconsistent. Female-typical behaviors include emotional perception, verbal memory, perceptual speed and accuracy, and maternal behavior (e.g., Hall, 1984; Hall & Halberstadt, 1981; Halpern, 1992; Kramer, Delis, & Daniel, 1988; Maccoby & Jacklin, 1974).

One of the most important female-typical behaviors relates to readiness to care for infants and young children. The sex difference in infant-directed behavior is not limited to adults. Across cultures, girls are more likely than boys to spontaneously care for younger children, and girls engage in more prosocial behavior toward infants than do boys (Maccoby & Jacklin, 1974). This may be because females are more attracted to and interested in infants than are males. When presented with photographs of babies, adult females spend more time than adult males looking at the photographs and have greater pupillary responses (Feldman & Nash, 1978; Fullard & Reiling, 1976; for review, see Berman, 1980). Young and adolescent girls also show greater responses than boys to pictures of infants (Berman, Goodman, Sloan, & Fernander, 1978; Feldman, Nash, & Cutrona, 1977; Nash & Feldman, 1981).

The sex differences have also been confirmed with observational methods. At home, girls are observed more than boys (by researchers and parents) to interact with infant siblings, and to do so in a nurturant manner (e.g., talking to baby, playing with baby, engaging in direct baby care; Blakemore, 1990; Melson, 1987). In experimental situations where participants are exposed to an unfamiliar infant in a waiting room, females are more likely to interact in positive ways with the infant than are males. This is true for preschool children (Berman, Monda, & Meyerscough, 1977; Berman, Smith, & Goodman, 1983; Blakemore, 1981, 1991b; Fogel, Melson, Toda, & Mistry, 1987; Melson & Fogel, 1982; Reid, Tate, & Berman,

1989), school-aged children (Berman & Goodman, 1984; Feldman et al., 1977; Frodi & Lamb, 1978; Nash & Feldman, 1981), adolescents (Blakemore, 1981; Feldman et al., 1977; Feldman & Nash, 1979a), and adults (Feldman & Nash, 1979b). Across studies and ages, the magnitude of the sex difference is large, at least three quarters of a standard deviation.

It is widely believed that this sex difference results from sex-role socialization, particularly imitation and modeling of same-sex others, reinforcement of sex-appropriate behaviors, discouragement of sex-inappropriate behavior, and gender labeling and identification (Feldman & Nash, 1978, 1979a, 1979b; Kuhn, Nash, & Brucker, 1978; Maccoby & Jacklin, 1974; Nash & Feldman, 1980). Although sex-typed socialization may occur, there is little evidence that parents socialize boys and girls differently with respect to infant-directed or nurturant behavior (for a meta-analytic review, see Lytton & Romney, 1991). For example, mothers have not been observed to encourage girls more than boys to interact with infant siblings (Blakemore, 1990), and men and women evaluate nurturant activity as equally desirable in boys and girls (Blakemore, 1991a; Blakemore, Baumgardner, & Keniston, 1988).

Alternatively, sex differences in interest in infants may result from the differential exposure of males and females to androgen early in development. This hypothesis is supported by studies of responsivity to infants in rodents and primates where pre- and perinatal androgen levels have been manipulated, and by suggestive data from girls and women exposed early in development to atypical levels of sex hormones.

In rodents, maternal behavior including pup retrieval, anogenital licking, nest building, nest defense, and crouching over pups is triggered by the hormonal changes that accompany parturition (Rosenblatt, 1990; Terkel & Rosenblatt, 1972). These behaviors can also be induced in virgin females and males when they are placed for a period of time in a cage with a litter of newborn pups. This sensitization occurs more quickly, more frequently, and lasts longer in female rats than in male rats (Brunelli & Hofer, 1990; Rosenblatt, 1990). Moreover, male rats are more likely than females to attack or kill newborn infants (Jakubowski & Terkel, 1985). Juvenile rats display similar maternal-like behaviors, and respond more readily to young pups than they do to same-age siblings, pup-sized warm objects, or dead pups (Bridges, Zarrow, Goldman, & Denenberg, 1974; Mayer & Rosenblatt, 1979).

Similarly, in most species of nonhuman primates, females of all ages are more responsive to infants than are males (e.g., Chamove, Harlow, & Mitchell, 1967; Devore, 1963; Eaton, Johnson, Glick, & Worlein, 1985; Gibber & Goy, 1985). For example, free-living adult female baboons will interrupt an activity to approach a mother–infant pair and groom and touch the infant, whereas adult males show a more perfunctory interest in infants; juvenile female macaques show more prosocial behavior toward infants (e.g., social play, physical contact, ventral embrace, grooming, communicative gestures, and facial expressions) than juvenile males.

Moreover, hostility toward infants is displayed exclusively by young male macaques (Chamove et al., 1967).

The sex differences in infant-directed behaviors in rodents and primates are mediated in part by the organizational effects of early hormones. Female rats exposed to high levels of androgen showed reduced responsivity, and castrated male rats showed increased responsivity to pups in adulthood, with exposure to testosterone propionate very early in life (Day 1) appearing to be particularly important for this suppression of maternal behavior (Bridges, Zarrow, & Denenberg, 1973; Ichikawa & Fujii, 1982; Kinsley, 1990; Leon, Numan, & Moltz, 1973; McCullough, Quadagno, & Goldman, 1974; Quadagno & Rockwell, 1972; Rosenberg & Herrenkohl, 1976).

Studies in nonhuman primates on the effects of early androgen on maternal behavior illustrate the complexity of hormonal influences on behavior. Female monkeys exposed to dihydrotestosterone (DHT) early in gestation did not differ significantly from unexposed controls in responsivity to infants (e.g., investigation, communicative responses, contact responses), but male monkeys castrated at birth crouched more often and contacted infants more often than intact males (Gibber & Goy, 1985). These results suggest that the critical period for the masculinization of responsivity to infants in rhesus monkeys may be late prenatal or early postnatal, or that masculinization of responsivity to infants may require a longer period of exposure (including both pre- and postnatal periods), or exposure to a different metabolite of testosterone than DHT (Gibber & Goy, 1985; Goy & McEwen, 1980).

These studies in other species suggest that early hormones might affect responsivity to infants in human beings. A unique opportunity to address this issue is provided by individuals with congenital adrenal hyperplasia (CAH) due to 21-hydroxylase deficiency, who, because of a genetic defect are exposed to high levels of adrenal androgens beginning early in gestation and continuing throughout gestation (New, 1985). Once they are diagnosed, usually shortly after birth, patients with CAH are treated with cortisol, which normalizes androgen levels. Thus, individuals with CAH are exposed to high levels of masculinizing hormones in the prenatal and perinatal periods, but relatively normal levels postnatally with good treatment (White, New, & Dupont, 1987).

There is some evidence that girls and women with CAH have reduced interest in activities related to maternal behavior. Compared to controls, CAH females play less with dolls (Berenbaum & Snyder, 1995; Ehrhardt & Baker, 1974; Ehrhardt, Epstein, & Money, 1968), and are reported by themselves and their mothers to be less interested in infants and in motherhood and more interested in pursuing a career (Dittmann et al., 1990; Ehrhardt & Baker, 1974). They also have been found to score lower than controls on personality measures on which females typically score higher than males: a detachment scale, which measures empathy, intimacy, need for social relations, and maternal and nurturant behavior (Helleday, Edman, Ritzen, & Siwers, 1993); and the Succorance scale of the Personality Research Form (PRF), which measures how an individual responds to another's need for help or comfort (Resnick, 1982).

Unfortunately, no study of CAH females has directly tested the hypothesis that CAH females have less interest in infants than controls. Sex-typed play, interest in dolls, interest in motherhood versus career, detachment, and succorance are not synonymous with interest in infants. The limited evidence that CAH females are less interested than controls in attending to or caring for infants is based on responses to a single question in a semistructured interview (Dittmann et al., 1990; Ehrhardt & Baker, 1974; Ehrhardt et al., 1968). Moreover, sibling controls were not always used, samples were small, and interviewers were not blind to whether the participant was a patient or control.

Thus, we studied whether early androgens reduce human interest in infants in a sample of girls and boys with CAH and their unaffected siblings and cousins, using a parent-report questionnaire found to differentiate the sexes (Melson, 1987). If early androgen plays a role in the development of the sex difference in interest in infants, then girls with CAH should show less interest in infants than their sisters. We had no specific hypotheses for boys with CAH because androgen treatment has inconsistent effects in male experimental animals (Baum & Schretlen, 1975; Diamond, Llacuna, & Wong, 1973), and because males with CAH have not been found to differ from controls on aspects of play behavior in childhood (Berenbaum & Hines, 1992; Berenbaum & Snyder, 1995) or on aggression in childhood or adulthood (Berenbaum & Resnick, 1997).

METHOD

Participants

We studied children 3 to 12 years old participating in an ongoing longitudinal investigation of sex-typed social behavior and cognitive abilities. Children with 21-hydroxylase deficient CAH were recruited through university-affiliated pediatric endocrinology clinics. Siblings and first cousins were recruited as comparisons. Because not all patients had a same-sex control, relatives of male and female patients were combined to form control groups. The sex-typed play and aggression of some of these children has been reported elsewhere (Berenbaum & Hines, 1992; Berenbaum & Resnick, 1997; Berenbaum & Snyder, 1995; Hines & Kaufman, 1994).

Data were available for 23 girls with CAH, 16 boys with CAH, 12 control girls (11 sisters and 1 female first cousin), and 22 control boys (20 brothers and 2 male first cousins). These children represent 31 families. Most patients were diagnosed with CAH in early infancy: The median age at diagnosis was 6 days for girls (range = 0 days–5.3 years), and 21 days for boys (range = 11 days–6.0 years). Most children had the salt-losing form of the disease (90% of girls, 93% of boys); this high rate may result from our recruitment strategy (physicians at university-affiliated clinics may be likely to see the most severely ill children or to conduct a very thorough endocrinological examination). All CAH girls had some genital virilization at birth, but all were reared as girls from birth (on the Prader scale, where 0 is normal female and 6 is normal male, scores for CAH girls ranged from 1 to 4, with an average of 3.0). Patients and controls did not differ significantly in birth order or age at testing. CAH girls had a mean age of 96.39 months (range = 39–151), control girls had a mean age of 94.76 months (range = 67–110), CAH boys had a mean age of 86.22 months (range = 32–134), and control boys had a mean age of 89.9 months (range = 36–137).

Measure and Procedure

Melson's (1987) Questionnaire assesses the extent to which children are regularly involved in playing with and caring for younger siblings, infants, pets, and the elderly. The questionnaire was developed from studies showing that there are not sex differences in nurturance per se, but in the target of nurturance: Girls are more nurturing of infants than are boys, but girls and boys are equally nurturing of pets (Fogel, Melson, & Mistry, 1986). Parents completed the questionnaire because children younger than 10 years old do not reliably report this information (Bryant, 1986; cited in Melson, 1987). Parents were asked to indicate on a 5-point scale ranging from 1 (*never*) to 5 (*almost every day*) how often the child engaged in each of 39 behaviors. The first 24 items relate to time engaged in specific activities, including sports, hobbies, homework, and caring for younger children, pets, and the elderly. The next 15 items relate specifically to frequency of interest in babies. This questionnaire was included in a packet of questionnaires distributed to the parents of children participating in the larger study of sex-typed behavior; other questionnaires assessed emotional adjustment, aggression, and sex-typed activities.

Melson (1987) used this questionnaire with parents of 707 children in preschool, second grade, and fifth grade. Parents reported girls to be more likely than boys to play with and care for babies, to ask more questions about parenthood, to pretend to be a parent, and to show an interest in baby pictures or in unfamiliar infants. When there was a younger sibling in the home, girls were reported to spend more time than boys caring for the child. The sex differences were reported to be significant for all age groups and to increase in size as the children got older (specific numbers were not reported). Parents did not report girls and boys to differ on items assessing interest in pets.

Data Analysis Procedures

Composite measures for interest in infants and interest in pets were calculated in order to increase the reliability of measurement, and thus the power to find significant group differences. The main composite measure of interest in infants (Infant) was computed from 11 items related to the care of, play with, or interest in infants. These items are shown in Table 1 (Part A). Because children without younger siblings were unlikely to have valid scores on the item "Takes care of younger siblings," a second composite measure of interest in infants was computed without this item (Infant2). Because control boys and CAH girls play less with girls' toys than do control girls (Berenbaum & Hines, 1992; Berenbaum & Snyder, 1995; Dittmann et al., 1990; Ehrhardt & Baker, 1974), the item assessing interest in dolls was eliminated from a third composite measure of interest in infants (Infant3) to ensure that group differences were not spuriously inflated by differences in doll play. A fourth composite (Infant4) was constructed that excluded items assessing both care of younger siblings and interest in dolls. All four composites had very good internal consistency reliability: Coefficient alpha was .81 for the main composite, .83 for Infant2, .79 for Infant3, and .80 for Infant4. A composite measure of interest in pets was computed from the five items shown in Table 1 (Part B). Because two items on this scale also relate to interest in infants, we computed a second composite excluding the items about baby animals (Pets2). Alpha coefficients for the two composites were .79 and .64.

Group differences on composite scores were examined with t tests. On measures of interest in infants, sex differences and differences between CAH and control girls were conducted with one-tailed tests because the direction of the differences was clearly specified, whereas tests of differences between CAH and control boys were

TABLE 1
Questionnaire Items Measuring Interest in Infants and Interest in Pets

A. Interest in infants
    Takes care of younger siblings
    Plays with babies other than younger siblings
    Takes care of babies other than younger siblings
    Plays with "baby" dolls
    Is interested in babies in books, photo albums, on TV, etc.
    Is interested in unfamiliar babies when encountered on the playground, bus, supermarket, etc.
    Imitates or pretends to be a parent during play
    Asks questions about babies (where they "come from," what they do, how to take care of them)
    Asks questions about pregnancy
    Shows concern or upset after hearing a baby cry
    Talks or asks about a time when he or she will grow up to be a mommy or daddy
B. Interest in pets
    Plays with pets
    Takes care of pets
    Plays with stuffed animals
    Is interested in pictures of baby animals in books, on TV, etc.
    Is interested in unfamiliar baby animals

two-tailed because no difference between these groups was hypothesized. Group comparisons for the measures of interest in pets were two-tailed because no differences were hypothesized. Type I error was set at .10, because there is no other work on hormonal influences on human interest in infants, so it is reasonable to increase the probability of Type I error to minimize the probability of Type II error.

RESULTS

Sex Differences

Control girls were reported to have more interest in infants than were control boys as indicated by scores on the composite measure of interest in infants, Infant, shown in Table 2, columns 1 and 4, $t(32) = -2.62$, $p < .01$. The sex difference was also present on the revised composites: Infant2, which excludes caring for younger siblings, $t(32) = -2.69$, $p < .01$; Infant3, which excludes play with dolls, $t(32) = -1.99$, $p < .05$; and Infant4, which excludes both items, $t(32) = -2.00$, $p < .05$ (see Table 2). Control boys and control girls did not differ in the percentage of

TABLE 2
Sex Differences and CAH Patient–Control Comparisons on Interest in Infants

	Girls			Boys			Sex Difference Controls d^e
	Control[a]	CAH[b]	d	Control[c]	CAH[d]	d	
Interest in infants							
M	30.42	25.91	–0.71**	24.14	24.38	0.04	–0.98***
SD	5.58	7.09		7.19	6.52		
Interest in infants, modified 2[f] (Infant2)							
M	27.50	23.70	–0.63**	21.77	21.69	–0.01	–0.99***
SD	5.44	6.63		6.16	6.13		
Interest in infants, modified 3[g] (Infant3)							
M	27.25	23.83	–0.62*	22.82	22.81	–0.00	–0.77**
SD	4.63	6.42		6.89	5.92		
Interest in infants, modified 4[h] (Infant4)							
M	24.33	21.61	–0.52*	20.46	20.13	–0.06	–0.75**
SD	4.50	5.90		5.84	5.50		

Note. CAH = congenital adrenal hyperplasia.
[a]$n = 12$. [b]$n = 23$. [c]$n = 22$. [d]$n = 16$. [e]d = mean difference expressed in standard deviation units. [f]Composite excludes item "Takes care of younger siblings." [g]Composite excludes item "Plays with dolls." [h]Composite excludes items "Takes care of younger siblings" and "Plays with dolls."
*$p < .10$. **$p < .05$. ***$p < .01$.

participants having younger siblings in the home (57% vs. 73%, respectively; Fisher Exact Test = .21).

Control boys and control girls did not differ in their scores on either composite measure of interest in pets, Pets, $t(32) = .16$, ns, and Pets2, $t(32) = .19$, ns, as shown in Table 3, columns 1 and 4. This occurred despite the fact that control boys were more likely to have pets than were control girls (81% vs. 50%; Fisher Exact Test = .06). When analyses were restricted to children who had pets at home, the same pattern of results was found, for Pets, $t(21) = .81$, ns, and for Pets2, $t(21) = .60$, ns.

Comparisons of CAH Girls and Control Girls

The finding of sex differences on the composite measures of interest in infants indicates that they are valid measures for testing the hypothesis that CAH girls have less interest in infants than do their sisters. As shown in Table 2, columns 1 and 2, CAH girls were reported to be less interested in infants than were control girls, as measured by scores on the composite measure of interest in infants (Infant), $t(33) = -1.91$, $p < .05$, and on the three revised composites: Infant2, which excludes caring for younger siblings, $t(33) = -1.71$, $p < .05$; Infant3, which excludes doll play, $t(33) = -1.63$, $p < .10$; and Infant4, which excludes both items, $t(33) = -1.40$, $p < .10$. CAH girls and control girls did not differ in the percentage of participants having younger siblings in the home (67% vs. 73%, respectively; Fisher Exact Test = .53).

CAH girls were reported to be more interested in pets than were control girls, as indicated by higher scores on both composite measures of interest in pets, Pets, $t(33) = 2.52$, $p < .05$, and Pets2, $t(33) = 2.97$, $p < .01$ (see Table 3, columns 1 and

TABLE 3
Sex Differences and CAH Patient–Control Comparisons on Interest in Pets

	Girls			Boys			Sex Difference Controls d^e
	Control^a	CAH^b	d	Control^c	CAH^d	d	
Interest in pets							
M	12.92	16.74	0.93*	13.18	12.56	−0.13	0.06
SD	3.80	4.46		4.87	4.87		
Interest in pets, modified 2^f (Pets2)							
M	7.33	10.13	1.10**	7.55	7.75	0.06	0.08
SD	2.27	2.82		3.52	3.17		

Note. CAH = congenital adrenal hyperplasia.
$^a n = 12$. $^b n = 23$. $^c n = 22$. $^d n = 16$. $^e d$ = mean difference expressed in standard deviation units. ^{f}Composite excludes items "Is interested in pictures of baby animals in books, on TV, etc." and "Is interested in unfamiliar baby animals."
*$p < .05$. **$p < .01$.

2). These differences occurred despite the fact that CAH girls were not significantly more likely than control girls to have pets at home (65% vs. 50%, respectively; Fisher Exact Test = .30). When analyses were restricted to girls who had pets at home, the same pattern of results was found, for Pets, $t(19) = 2.44$, $p < .05$, and for Pets2, $t(19) = 2.92$, $p < .01$.

For CAH girls, neither interest in infants nor interest in pets was significantly correlated with age at diagnosis ($r = .09$, ns, and $r = .23$, ns, respectively), or Prader score ($r = .16$, ns, $r = -.08$, ns, respectively). Girls with salt-wasting versus simple-virilizing CAH could not be compared because only 2 CAH girls had the simple-virilizing form of the disease.

Comparisons of CAH Boys and Control Boys

There were no differences between CAH boys and control boys on any of the composite measures of interest in infants, as shown in Table 2, columns 4 and 5: Infant, $t(36) = .11$, ns; Infant2, $t(36) = -.04$, ns; Infant3, $t(36) = -.00$, ns; Infant4, $t(36) = -.18$, ns. Control boys and CAH boys did not differ in the percentage of participants having younger siblings in the home (57% vs. 46%, respectively; Fisher Exact Test = .23).

CAH boys and control boys did not differ on either composite measure of interest in pets, Pets, $t(36) = -.39$, ns, and Pets2, $t(36) = .18$, ns (see Table 3, columns 4 and 5). This occurred despite the fact that CAH boys were less likely than control boys to have pets in the home (47% vs. 81%; Fisher Exact Test = .03). When analyses were restricted to boys who had pets at home, the groups were still not significantly different, for Pets, $t(22) = -.19$, ns, and for Pets2, $t(22) = .74$, ns.

For CAH boys, age at diagnosis was not significantly correlated with interest in infants ($r = -.23$, ns) or interest in pets ($r = -.40$, ns). Boys with salt-wasting versus simple-virilizing CAH could not be compared because only 1 CAH boy had the simple-virilizing form of the disease.

Effects of Age

For the entire sample ($n = 73$), age was significantly correlated with interest in infants, $r = -.32$, $p < .01$, but not with interest in pets, $r = -.07$, ns. The groups did not differ significantly in age. Analyses with age as a covariate (conducted to increase statistical power) produced the same patterns of results with respect to all group differences.

DISCUSSION

The results support the hypothesis that early androgen exposure inhibits interest in infants in human beings. CAH girls were reported by parents to have reduced interest in infants compared to their sisters, and the size of the difference is substantial (approximately two thirds of a standard deviation). The differences between CAH girls and their sisters on the composite measures of interest in infants parallel the sex differences observed in this sample and others (Berman & Goodman, 1984; Berman et al., 1977; Blakemore, 1981, 1990; Feldman et al., 1977; Fogel et al., 1987; Frodi & Lamb, 1978; Melson, 1987; Melson & Fogel, 1982; Nash & Feldman, 1981; Reid et al., 1989).

The finding that CAH girls are less interested in infants than are their sisters is consistent with studies in other species showing that androgen exposure inhibits infant-directed behavior. Female rats (Ichikawa & Fujii, 1982; Quadagno & Rockwell, 1972) and rabbits (Anderson, Zarrow, & Denenberg, 1970) treated with androgen in the prenatal and early postnatal periods are less responsive to pups than are untreated females. Moreover, in males, neonatal castration and antiandrogen treatment increase pup responsivity in rats (Leon et al., 1973; McCullough et al., 1974; Quadagno & Rockwell, 1972; Rosenberg & Herrenkohl, 1976) and increases maternal gestures and contact with infants in rhesus monkeys (Gibber & Goy, 1985).

Methodological Considerations

There are two primary methodological issues to consider in interpreting the results of this investigation. First, interest in infants was not measured directly. Parent report may be less reliable and valid than direct observations of children's interactions with babies. This would likely have worked against the hypothesis by reducing power to find differences between CAH girls and control girls. It is also possible that parents would underreport interest in infants in boys because they view it as inconsistent with the male gender role. In the same way, parents may underreport interest in infants in CAH girls because they view the girls as masculine. This is unlikely to account for the observed result for a number of reasons: (a) men and women view infant-directed behavior as equally desirable in boys and girls (Blakemore, 1991a), (b) CAH girls are reared as girls and have female gender identity, (c) there is little evidence that CAH girls are viewed as more masculine than their sisters (Berenbaum & Hines, 1992; Ehrhardt & Meyer-Bahlburg, 1981; Resnick, 1982), and (d) differences between CAH girls and controls in other behavior (sex-typed toy or activity preferences) are seen with both objective and parent report measures, so differences are unlikely to reflect parental responding (Berenbaum & Snyder, 1995). The advantages of parent report measures are reduced reactivity to an observer and increased time sampling. Still, the best test of the hypothesis that CAH girls are less interested in infants than are controls would include observational measures, such as a waiting room situation.

A second methodological concern is that CAH girls do not provide a perfect test of the behavioral effects of early androgen exposure because other factors also differ between CAH girls and their sisters. Children with CAH have abnormalities in other hormones, such as progesterone and corticosteroids, in addition to androgen. It is not likely that these other hormones are responsible for behavioral defeminization because their effects on behavior are smaller and less consistent than those of androgen and are sometimes demasculinizing (Erpino, 1975; Hull, Franz, Snyder, & Nishita, 1980). Moreover, CAH boys also have these same abnormalities, but they do not differ from control boys in interest in infants.

CAH girls have virilized genitalia, which may cause parents to treat them in a more masculine and less feminine fashion, leading the girls to engage in feminine activities less frequently than do their sisters (Quadagno, Briscoe, & Quadagno, 1977). Nevertheless, parents do not report that they treat CAH girls differently than their sisters (Berenbaum & Hines, 1992; Ehrhardt & Baker, 1974), and, in fact, appear to be unconcerned with tomboyish behavior in CAH girls, or to encourage feminine behavior (Ehrhardt & Meyer-Bahlburg, 1981). This is consistent with data from androgenized female rhesus macaques that maternal behavior was unrelated to androgen-influenced offspring behavior (Goy, Bercovitch, & McBrair, 1988). Moreover, degree of genital virilization was not related to interest in infants in this study, and has not been shown to correlate with masculinization of other behaviors in CAH girls (Berenbaum & Hines, 1992; Dittmann et al., 1990; Slijper, 1984) or in androgenized female macaques (Goy et al., 1988).

CAH children have a chronic illness, so parents may be overprotective and restrict the child's amount of responsibility. Thus, the parents might discourage children with CAH from taking care of infants. This might explain CAH girls' reduced interest in infants, but this explanation seems unlikely because CAH boys were not found to be less interested in infants than control boys.

Early Androgen Effects: Facilitation of Male-Typical Behavior

Thus, CAH girls' reduced interest in infants most likely results from early exposure to high levels of androgen. Previous behavioral studies of CAH girls have also revealed behavioral effects of early androgen exposure consistent with those found in other species, specifically by changing behavior in a masculine direction. Compared to control females, CAH females play more with boys' toys (Berenbaum & Hines, 1992; Berenbaum & Snyder, 1995; Ehrhardt & Baker, 1974), are more likely to be considered tomboys (Ehrhardt & Baker, 1974), are more aggressive (Berenbaum & Resnick, 1997), have higher spatial ability (Hampson et al., this issue; Resnick et al., 1986), and are more likely to have homosexual or bisexual fantasies (Dittmann, Kappes, & Kappes, 1992; Zucker et al., 1996). Similarly, girls and women exposed in utero to masculinizing hormones because of maternal ingestion of drugs to prevent miscarriage have been reported to have increased aggression (Reinisch, 1981), increased rates of homosexuality or bisexuality

(Ehrhardt et al., 1985; Meyer-Bahlburg et al., 1995), and male-typical patterns of cerebral lateralization (Hines & Shipley, 1984).

Behavioral masculinization has also been associated with prenatal hormones in normal individuals. As an apparent result of exposure to testosterone in utero, female dizygotic twins with a male cotwin are more masculine than female dizygotic twins with a female cotwin on several traits: They have higher spatial ability (Cole-Harding, Morstad, & Wilson, 1988) and higher sensation seeking (Resnick, Gottesman, & McGue, 1993), and a male-typical pattern on some auditory characteristics (McFadden, 1993, this issue). Girls who had high levels of testosterone in amniotic fluid have faster rates of mental rotation than girls who had low amniotic testosterone (Grimshaw, Sitarenios, & Finegan, 1995).

Early Androgen Effects: Inhibition of Female-Typical Behavior

Thus, a relation between early androgen levels and behavioral masculinization has been established in humans. The finding of reduced interest in infants in girls with CAH is noteworthy because it suggests that androgen may inhibit female-typical behavior, as well as facilitate male-typical behavior. In all species, sexually dimorphic behaviors do not simply represent opposite ends of a continuum; animals may display both female-typical (e.g., lordosis) and male-typical behavior (e.g., mounting). In many species (including guinea pig, rat, mouse, dog, rhesus monkey), the extent to which an animal displays male-typical and female-typical behavior can be altered by early hormonal manipulations, and behavioral masculinization and defeminization are differently affected by different characteristics of hormone exposure, including critical period, duration of exposure, or specific hormone or its metabolite (for reviews, see Becker et al., 1993; Breedlove, 1994; Goy & McEwen, 1980).

Interestingly, studies in other species indicate that the masculinizing and defeminizing effects of early androgen can be decoupled, so that androgen exposure can masculinize but not defeminize a behavior, and vice versa (Davis, Chaptal, & McEwen, 1979; Debold & Whalen, 1975; Goldfoot, Feder, & Goy, 1969). For example, exposing female rats to androgen during different periods of development can induce mounting behavior without decreasing lordosis (Davis et al., 1979). Thus, masculinization and defeminization are related but separate processes, and should be considered separately.

The observation that CAH girls have reduced interest in infants compared to their sisters adds to a small literature showing behavioral defeminization in CAH girls. Interviews with CAH females and their mothers have revealed that, compared to their sisters, girls and women with CAH have less interest in romance, marriage, and motherhood, and less interest in feminine appearance, including jewelry and makeup (Ehrhardt & Baker, 1974; Ehrhardt et al., 1968; Ehrhardt & Meyer-

Bahlburg, 1981). CAH girls also play less with girls' toys than do their sisters (Berenbaum & Hines, 1992). Women with CAH also score lower than controls on three traits that typically show sex differences in favor of females: succorance (Resnick, 1982), indirect aggression (Helleday et al., 1993), and attachment (Helleday et al., 1993). The results of several studies are thus consistent with ours and support the hypothesis that androgen can act to defeminize as well as masculinize human behavior.

It is interesting to consider whether interest in infants reflects a general social responsiveness or need for affiliation, and, thus, whether reduced interest in infants by girls with CAH and typical boys reflects a reduction in a broader social behavior. Although there are sex differences in some aspects of interpersonal social behavior, such as social closeness and desire for intimacy (DiLalla, 1996; Maccoby & Jacklin, 1974; Reisman, 1990), and there is indirect evidence that females with CAH show reductions in some of these characteristics (Helleday et al., 1993), it is unclear how these traits are related to interest in infants. Further, some aspects of interpersonal social behavior, such as sociability, do not show sex differences (Buss & Plomin, 1984; Maccoby & Jacklin, 1974), and early androgens can have a selective effect on maternal behavior in rodents (Bridges et al., 1973; Ichikawa & Fujii, 1982; Kinsley, 1990; Leon et al., 1973; McCullough et al., 1974; Quadagno & Rockwell, 1972; Rosenberg & Herrenkohl, 1976). It will be interesting to study interest in infants in relation to other aspects of social behavior in individuals with CAH and in typical males and females.

It is important to emphasize that sex-typed behavior is also affected by other hormones and that it is not simply the amount of androgen that determines the degree to which behavior is male-or female-typical. This appears to be particularly true for traits that are more common in females than in males. Thus, there is increasing evidence that ovarian estrogens play an active role in the development of female-typical traits (e.g., Fitch et al., this issue; Fitch & Denenberg, in press; Stewart & Cygan, 1980; Toran-Allerand, 1984).

Interest in Pets

An unexpected finding was that CAH girls spent more time playing with and caring for their pets than did control girls. Because a sex difference was not found in interest in pets in this or other studies (Fogel et al., 1986; Melson, 1987), CAH girls' increased interest in pets compared to controls is unlikely to reflect a direct effect of prenatal androgen exposure. It is also unlikely that CAH girls spend more time with pets because they are sick and thus discouraged from other kinds of play, because CAH boys are not reported to be more interested in pets than control boys.

Alternatively, these results might be explained by CAH girls' preference for boys' toys but girl playmates (Berenbaum & Snyder, 1995). Children with sex-atypical interests may interact less with their peers than do children who engage in traditional sex-typed activities (Maccoby, 1988). Because CAH girls do not share common activity interests with their peers, they may spend less time playing with other children, and look to pets for companionship. Moreover, because pets are an outlet for the expression of nurturant behavior (Fogel et al., 1986; Melson, 1987), CAH girls may spend more time with pets because they are less interested in infants, but not less nurturant overall than controls.

Implications for the Development of Maternal Behavior

It is widely assumed that sex differences in interest in infants result from sex-role socialization (e.g., Berman & Goodman, 1984; Berman et al., 1977; Feldman & Nash, 1978, 1979a, 1979b; Reid et al., 1989). The findings from this study provide evidence against a pure social environmental explanation for sex differences. CAH girls are reared as girls and develop a female gender identity. Nonetheless, despite socializing forces that would encourage the expression of interest in infants, they are less interested in infants than are their sisters. This finding is consistent with direct tests of social learning explanations of infant-directed behavior that showed that parents do not encourage girls more than boys to interact with infants: They request help equally from boys and girls in taking care of infant siblings and they reward and punish boys and girls equally for interacting with infant siblings (Blakemore, 1990). In fact, a meta-analytic review of the research on parental socialization has revealed that neither mothers nor fathers encourage nurturant behavior more in girls than boys (Lytton & Romney, 1991).

The results of this study do not suggest that social factors are irrelevant in shaping behavior, but they do indicate that biological factors play a role in aspects of sex-role development. CAH girls' reduced interest in infants compared to their sisters suggests that early hormone exposure might create a behavioral predisposition that is then reinforced by the environment, both imposed and self-selected (Scarr & McCartney, 1983). In this way, individuals who have a predisposition to approach infants will seek out experiences with infants. This experience will foster greater skill and comfort with infants, evoke reinforcement from the environment (e.g., parents), and lead to even more involvement with infants. Evidence for self-selection has been found in another domain of sex-typed behavior. Newcombe and Dubas (1992) reported that girls with high spatial ability at age 11 were more likely than girls with low spatial ability to engage in spatial activities at age 16, whereas activities at age 11 did not predict spatial ability at age 16.

The results of the current investigation suggest that early exposure to androgen is one mechanism predisposing a person to be more or less interested in infants, and thus to be more or less likely to seek involvement in child care. Future investigations might address the interests and activities of CAH girls and their sisters at more than one point in time in order to test the hypothesis that interest in infants leads to increased involvement with infants over time.

In summary, the results of this study show that interest in infants may be reduced by early exposure to high levels of androgen. These data add to a literature indicating that prenatal or perinatal exposure to androgen can defeminize as well as masculinize behavior in people, as in other species. Moreover, the finding that CAH girls are less interested in infants than their sisters provides evidence that social forces are not the sole determinants of this aspect of sex-typed behavior.

ACKNOWLEDGMENTS

This study represents Catherine Leveroni's master's thesis research and was supported by National Institutes of Health Grant HD19644. We thank the following people who contributed to this project: Stephen Duck, Orville Green, David Klein, Ora Pescovitz, Gail Richards, and Julio Santiago generously provided access to their patients and answered medical questions; Kristina Korman, Elizabeth Snyder, Kim Ketterling, Robyn Reed, George Vineyard, and Cindy Tubbs assisted in data collection or processing; Stephen Duck examined medical records and provided ratings on degree of genital virilization; Michael Seidenberg, Susan Resnick, and two reviewers provided thoughtful and helpful comments on the article. We are very grateful to the participants and their parents for their participation in the study.

REFERENCES

Anderson, C. O., Zarrow, M. X., & Denenberg, V. H. (1970). Maternal behavior in the rabbit: Effects of androgen during gestation upon the nest-building behavior of the mother and her offspring. *Hormones and Behavior, 1,* 337–345.

Baum, M. J., & Schretlen, P. (1975). Neuroendocrine effects of perinatal androgenization in the male ferret. *Progress in Brain Research, 42,* 343–355.

Becker, J. B., Breedlove, S. M., & Crews, D. (Eds.). (1993). *Behavioral endocrinology.* Cambridge, MA: MIT Press.

Berenbaum, S. A., & Hines, M. (1992). Early androgens are related to childhood sex-typed toy preferences. *Psychological Science, 3,* 203–206.

Berenbaum, S. A., Leveroni, C., & Korman, K. (1995). Early hormones and sex differences in cognitive abilities. *Learning and Individual Differences, 7,* 303–321.

Berenbaum, S. A., & Resnick, S. M. (1997). Early androgen effects on aggression in children and adults with congenital adrenal hyperplasia. *Psychoneuroendocrinology, 22,* 505–515.

Berenbaum, S. A., & Snyder, E. (1995). Early hormonal influences on childhood sex-typed activity and playmate preferences: Implications for the development of sexual orientation. *Developmental Psychology, 31,* 31–42.

Berman, P. W. (1980). Are women more responsive than men to the young? *Psychological Bulletin, 88,* 668–695.

Berman, P. W., & Goodman, V. (1984). Age and sex differences in children's responsiveness to babies: Effects of adult's caretaking requests and instructions. *Child Development, 55,* 1071–1077.

Berman, P. W., Goodman, V., Sloan, V. L., & Fernander, L. (1978). Preference for infants among black and white children: Sex and age differences. *Child Development, 49,* 917–919.

Berman, P. W., Monda, L. D., & Meyerscough, R. P. (1977). Sex differences in young children's responses to an infant: An observation within a day-care setting. *Child Development, 48,* 711–715.
Berman, P. W., Smith, V. L., & Goodman, V. (1983). Development of sex differences in response to an infant and to the care-taker role. *Journal of Genetic Psychology, 143,* 283–384.
Blakemore, J. E. O. (1981). Age and sex differences in interaction with a human infant. *Child Development, 52,* 386–388.
Blakemore, J. E. O. (1990). Children's nurturant interactions with their infant siblings: An exploration of gender differences and maternal socialization. *Sex Roles, 22,* 43–57.
Blakemore, J. E. O. (1991a). Adults' evaluation of children caring for a baby: The effects of gender and behavior. *Sex Roles, 24,* 541–549.
Blakemore, J. E. O. (1991b). The influence of gender and temperament on children's interaction with a baby. *Sex Roles, 24,* 531–537.
Blakemore, J. E. O., Baumgardner, S. R., & Keniston, A. H. (1988). Male and female nurturing: Perceptions of style and competence. *Sex Roles, 18,* 449–459.
Breedlove, S. M. (1994). Sexual differentiation of the human nervous system. *Annual Review of Psychology, 45,* 389–418.
Bridges, R. S., Zarrow, M. X., & Denenberg, V. H. (1973). The role of neonatal androgen in the expression of hormonally induced maternal responsiveness. *Hormones and Behavior, 4,* 315–322.
Bridges, R. S., Zarrow, M. X., Goldman, B. D., & Denenberg, V. H. (1974). A developmental study of maternal responsiveness in the rat. *Physiology and Behavior, 12,* 149–151.
Brunelli, S. A., & Hofer, M. A. (1990). Parental behavior in juvenile rats: Environmental and biological determinants. In N. A. Krasnegor & R. S. Bridges (Eds.), *Mammalian parenting: Biochemical, neurobiological, and behavioral determinants* (pp. 372–399). New York: Oxford University Press.
Buss, A. H., & Plomin, R. (1984). *Temperament: Early developing personality traits.* Hillsdale, NJ: Lawrence Erlbaum Associates, Inc.
Chamove, A., Harlow, H. F., & Mitchell, G. D. (1967). Sex differences in the infant directed behavior of preadolescent rhesus monkeys. *Child Development, 38,* 329–335.
Clark, M. M., & Galef, B. G., Jr. (1998/this issue). Effects of intrauterine position on the behavior and genital morphology of litter-bearing rodents. *Developmental Neuropyschology, 14,* 197–211.
Cole-Harding, S., Morstad, A. L., & Wilson, J. R. (1988). Spatial ability in members of opposite-sex twin pairs [Abstract]. *Behavior Genetics, 18,* 710.
Collaer, M. L., & Hines, M. (1995). Human behavioral sex differences: A role for gonadal hormones during early development? *Psychological Bulletin, 118,* 55–107.
Davis, P. G., Chaptal, C. V., & McEwen, B. S. (1979). Independence of the differentiation of masculine and feminine behavior in rats. *Hormones and Behavior, 12,* 12–19.
Debold, J. F., & Whalen, R. E. (1975). Differential sensitivity of mounting and lordosis control systems to early androgen treatment in male and female hamsters. *Hormones and Behavior, 6,* 196–209.
Devore, I. (1963). Mother–infant relations in free ranging baboons. In H. L. Reingold (Ed.), *Maternal behavior in mammals* (pp. 305–335). New York: Wiley.
Diamond, M., Llacuna, A., & Wong, C. L. (1973). Sex behavior after neonatal progesterone, testosterone, estrogen, or antiandrogens. *Hormones and Behavior, 4,* 73–88.
DiLalla, D. L. (1996). Computerized administration of the Multidimensional Personality Questionnaire. *Assessment, 3,* 365–374.
Dittmann, R. W., Kappes, M. E., & Kappes, M. H. (1992). Sexual behavior in adolescent and adult females with congenital adrenal hyperplasia. *Psychoneuroendocrinology, 17,* 153–170.
Dittmann, R. W., Kappes, M. H., Kappes, M. E., Borger, D., Stegner, H., Willig, R. H., & Wallis, H. (1990). Congenital adrenal hyperplasia I: Gender-related behaviors and attitudes in female patients and their sisters. *Psychoneuroendocrinology, 15,* 401–420.
Eaton, G. G., Johnson, D. F., Glick, B. B., & Worlein, J. M. (1985). Development in Japanese macaques (Macaca fuscata): Sexually dimorphic behavior during the first year of life. *Primates, 26,* 238–248.

Ehrhardt, A. A., & Baker, S. W. (1974). Fetal androgens, human central nervous system differentiation, and behavior sex differences. In R. C. Friedman, R. R. Richart, & R. L. Vande Weile (Eds.), *Sex differences in behavior* (pp. 33–51). New York: Wiley.
Ehrhardt, A. A., Epstein, R., & Money, J. (1968). Fetal androgens and female gender identity in the early treated adrenogenital syndrome. *Johns Hopkins Medical Journal, 122,* 160–167.
Ehrhardt, A. A., & Meyer-Bahlburg, H. F. L. (1981). Effect of prenatal sex hormones on gender-related behavior. *Science, 211,* 1312–1318.
Ehrhardt, A. A., Meyer-Bahlburg, H. F. L., Rosen, L. R., Feldman, J. F., Veridiano, N. P., Zimmerman, I., & McEwen, B. S. (1985). Sexual orientation after prenatal exposure to exogenous estrogens. *Archives of Sexual Behavior, 14,* 57–77.
Erpino, M. J. (1975). Androgen-induced aggression in neonatally androgenized female mice: Inhibition by progesterone. *Hormones and Behavior, 6,* 149–157.
Feldman, S. S., & Nash, S. C. (1978). Interest in babies during young adulthood. *Child Development, 49,* 617–622.
Feldman, S. S., & Nash, S. C. (1979a). Changes in responsiveness to babies during adolescence. *Child Development, 50,* 942–949.
Feldman, S. S., & Nash, S. C. (1979b). Sex differences in responsiveness to babies among mature adults. *Developmental Psychology, 15,* 430–436.
Feldman, S. S., Nash, S. C., & Cutrona, C. (1977). The influence of age and sex on responsiveness to babies. *Developmental Psychology, 13,* 675–676.
Fitch, R. H., Cowell, P. E., & Denenberg, V. H. (1998/this issue). The female phenotype: Nature's default? *Developmental Neuropsychology, 14,* 213–231.
Fitch, R. H., & Denenberg, V. H. (in press). A role for ovarian hormones in sexual differentiation of the brain. *Behavioral and Brain Sciences.*
Fogel, A., Melson, G. F., & Mistry, J. (1986). Conceptualizing the determinants of nurturance: A reassessment of sex differences. In A. Fogel & G. F. Melson (Eds.), *Origins of nurturance: Developmental, biological, and cultural perspectives on caregiving* (pp. 53–67). Hillsdale, NJ: Lawrence Erlbaum Associates, Inc.
Fogel, A., Melson, G. F., Toda, S., & Mistry, J. (1987). Young children's responses to unfamiliar infants: The effect of adult involvement. *International Journal of Behavioral Development, 10,* 37–50.
Frodi, A. M., & Lamb, M. E. (1978). Sex difference in responsiveness to infants: A developmental study of psychological and behavioral responses. *Child Development, 49,* 1182–1188.
Fullard, W., & Reiling, A. M. (1976). An investigation of Lorenz's "babyness." *Child Development, 47,* 1191–1193.
Gibber, J. R., & Goy, R. W. (1985). Infant directed behavior in young rhesus monkeys: Sex difference and effects of prenatal androgen. *American Journal of Primatology, 8,* 235–237.
Goldfoot, D. A., Feder, H. H., & Goy, R. W. (1969). Development of bisexuality in the male rat treated neonatally with androstenedione. *Journal of Comparative and Physiological Psychology, 67,* 41–45.
Goy, R. W., Bercovitch, F. B., & McBrair, M. C. (1988). Behavioral masculinization is independent of genital masculinization in prenatally androgenized female rhesus macaques. *Hormones and Behavior, 22,* 552–571.
Goy, R. W., & McEwen, B. S. (1980). *Sexual differentiation of the brain.* London: Oxford University Press.
Grimshaw, G. M., Sitarenios, G., & Finegan, J. K. (1995). Mental rotation at 7 years: Relations with prenatal testosterone levels and spatial play experience. *Brain and Cognition, 29,* 85–100.
Hall, J. A. (1984). *Nonverbal sex differences: Communication accuracy and expressive style.* Baltimore: Johns Hopkins University Press.
Hall, J. A., & Halberstadt, A. G. (1981). Sex roles and nonverbal communication skills. *Sex Roles, 7,* 273–287.
Halpern, D. F. (1992). *Sex differences in cognitive abilities* (2nd ed.). Hillsdale, NJ: Lawrence Erlbaum Associates, Inc.

Hampson, E., Rovet, J. F., & Altmann, D. (1998/this issue). Spatial reasoning in children with congenital adrenal hyperplasia due to 21-hydroxylase deficiency. *Developmental Neuropsychology, 14*, 299–320.

Helleday, J., Edman, G., Ritzen, M., & Siwers, B. (1993). Personality characteristics and platelet MAO activity in women with congenital adrenal hyperplasia (CAH). *Psychoneuroendocrinology, 18*, 343–354.

Hines, M., & Kaufman, F. (1994). Androgen and the development of human sex-typical behavior: Rough-and-tumble play and sex of preferred playmates in children with congenital adrenal hyperplasia (CAH). *Child Development, 65*, 1042–1053.

Hines, M., & Shipley, C. (1984). Prenatal exposure to diethylstilbestrol (DES) and the development of sexually dimorphic cognitive abilities and cerebral lateralization. *Developmental Psychology, 20*, 81–94.

Hull, E. M., Franz, J. R., Snyder, A. M., & Nishita, J. K. (1980). Perinatal progesterone and learning, social, and reproductive behavior in rats. *Physiology and Behavior, 24*, 251–256.

Ichikawa, S., & Fujii, Y. (1982). Effect of prenatal androgen treatment on maternal behavior in the female rat. *Hormones and Behavior, 16*, 224–233.

Jakubowski, M., & Terkel, J. (1985). Incidence of pup killing and parental behavior in virgin females and male rats (rattus norvegicus): Differences between Wistar and Sprague-Dawley stocks. *Journal of Comparative Psychology, 99*, 93–97.

Kinsley, C. H. (1990). Prenatal and postnatal influences on parental behavior in rodents. In N. A. Krasnegor & R. S. Bridges (Eds.), *Mammalian parenting: Biochemical, neurobiological, and behavioral determinants* (pp. 347–372). New York: Oxford University Press.

Kramer, J. H., Delis, D. C., & Daniel, M. (1988). Sex differences in verbal learning. *Journal of Clinical Psychology, 44*, 907–915.

Kuhn, D., Nash, S. C., & Brucker, L. (1978). Sex role concepts of two- and three-year-olds. *Child Development, 49*, 445–451.

Leon, M., Numan, M., & Moltz, H. (1973). Maternal behavior in the rat: Facilitation through gonadectomy. *Science, 179*, 1018–1019.

Lytton, H., & Romney, D. M. (1991). Parents' differential socialization of boys and girls: A meta-analysis. *Psychological Bulletin, 109*, 267–296.

Maccoby, E. (1988). Gender as a social category. *Developmental Psychology, 24*, 755–765.

Maccoby, E. E., & Jacklin, C. N. (1974). *The psychology of sex differences*. Palo Alto, CA: Stanford University Press.

Mayer, A. D., & Rosenblatt, J. S. (1979). Ontogeny of maternal behavior in the laboratory rat: Early origins in 18- to 27-day-old young. *Developmental Psychobiology, 12*, 407–442.

McCullough, J., Quadagno, D. M., & Goldman, B. D. (1974). Neonatal gonadal hormones: Effect on maternal and sexual behavior in the male rat. *Physiology and Behavior, 12*, 183–188.

McFadden, D. M. (1993). A masculinizing effect on the auditory systems of human females having male co-twins. *Proceedings of the National Academy of Science, 90*, 11900–11904.

McFadden, D. M. (1998/this issue). Sex differences in the auditory system. *Developmental Neuropsychology, 14*, 261–298.

Melson, G. F. (1987, October). *The role of pets in the development of children's nurturance*. Paper presented at the Delta Society Conference, Vancouver, Canada.

Melson, G. F., & Fogel, A. (1982). Young children's interest in unfamiliar infants. *Child Development, 53*, 693–700.

Meyer-Bahlburg, H. F. L., Ehrhardt, A. A., Rosen, L. R., Gruen, R. S., Veridiano, N. P., Vann, F. H., & Neuwalder, H. F. (1995). Prenatal estrogens and the development of homosexual orientation. *Developmental Psychology, 31*, 12–21.

Michael, R. P., & Zumpe, D. (1998/this issue). Developmental changes in behavior and in steroid uptake by the male and female macaque brain. *Developmental Neuropsychology, 14*, 233–260.

Nash, S. C., & Feldman, S. S. (1980). Responsiveness to babies: Life-situation specific sex differences in adulthood. *Sex Roles, 6,* 751–758.

Nash, S. C., & Feldman, S. S. (1981). Sex-related differences in the relationship between sibling status and responsivity to babies. *Sex Roles, 7,* 1035–1042.

New, M. I. (Ed.). (1985). Congenital adrenal hyperplasia. *Annals of the New York Academy of Sciences, 458.*

Newcombe, N., & Dubas, J. S. (1992). A longitudinal study of predictors of spatial ability in adolescent females. *Child Development, 63,* 37–46.

Quadagno, D. M., Briscoe, R., & Quadagno, J. S. (1977). Effects of perinatal gonadal hormones on selected nonsexual behavior patterns: A critical assessment of the nonhuman and human literature. *Psychological Bulletin, 84,* 62–80.

Quadagno, D. M., & Rockwell, J. (1972). The effect of gonadal hormones in infancy on maternal behavior in the adult rat. *Hormones and Behavior, 3,* 55–62.

Reid, P. T., Tate, C. S., & Berman, P. W. (1989). Preschool children's self-presentation in situations with infants: Effects of sex and race. *Child Development, 60,* 710–714.

Reinisch, J. M. (1981). Prenatal exposure to synthetic progestins increases potential for aggression in humans. *Science, 211,* 1171–1173.

Reisman, J. M. (1990). Intimacy in same-sex friendships. *Sex Roles, 23,* 65–82.

Resnick, S. M. (1982). *Psychological functioning in individuals with congenital adrenal hyperplasia: Early hormonal influences on cognition and personality.* Unpublished doctoral dissertation, University of Minnesota, Minneapolis.

Resnick, S. M., Berenbaum, S. A., Gottesman, I. I., & Bouchard, T. J. (1986). Early hormonal influences on cognitive functioning in congenital adrenal hyperplasia. *Developmental Psychology, 22,* 191–198.

Resnick, S. M., Gottesman, I. I., & McGue, M. (1993). Sensation seeking in opposite-sex twins: An effect of prenatal hormones? *Behavior Genetics, 23,* 323–329.

Rosenberg, D. A., & Herrenkohl, L. R. (1976). Maternal behavior in male rats: Critical times for the suppressive action of androgens. *Physiology and Behavior, 16,* 293–297.

Rosenblatt, J. S. (1990). Landmarks in the physiological study of maternal behavior with specific reference to the rat. In N. A. Krasnegor & R. S. Bridges (Eds.), *Mammalian parenting: Biochemical, neurobiological, and behavioral determinants* (pp. 40–60). New York: Oxford University Press.

Scarr, S., & McCartney, K. (1983). How people make their own environments: A theory of genotype → environment effects. *Child Development, 54,* 424–435.

Slijper, F. M. E. (1984). Androgens and gender role behavior in girls with congenital adrenal hyperplasia (CAH). In G. J. DeVries, J. P. C. DeBruin, H. B. M. Uylings, & M. A. Corner (Eds.), *Progress in brain research* (Vol. 61, pp. 417–422). Amsterdam: Elsevier.

Stewart, J., & Cygan, D. (1980). Ovarian hormones act early in development to feminize adult open-field behavior in the rat. *Hormones and Behavior, 14,* 20–32.

Terkel, J., & Rosenblatt, J. S. (1972). Humoral factors underlying maternal behavior at parturition: Cross transfusion between freely moving rats. *Journal of Comparative and Physiological Psychology, 80,* 365–371.

Toran-Allerand, C. D. (1984). Gonadal hormones and brain development: Implications for the genesis of sexual differentiation. *Annals of the New York Academy of Sciences, 435,* 101–110.

White, P. C., New, M. I., & Dupont, B. (1987). Congenital adrenal hyperplasia. *New England Journal of Medicine, 316,* 1519–1524.

Zucker, K. J., Bradley, S. J., Oliver, G., Blake, J., Fleming, S., & Hood, J. (1996). Psychosexual development of women with congenital adrenal hyperplasia. *Hormones and Behavior, 30,* 300–318.

A Reexamination of the Visuospatial Deficit in Turner Syndrome: Contributions of Working Memory

Lori Buchanan
Department of Psychology
The University of Alberta
Edmonton, Canada

Jelena Pavlovic
Department of Psychology
The University of Waterloo
Waterloo, Canada

Joanne Rovet
Department of Pediatrics
The University of Toronto
Toronto, Canada

Studies describing deficits in children with Turner Syndrome (TS) typically report that visual and spatial processing are impaired relative to verbal processing (Rovet & Netley, 1982). The exact nature of this deficit is not entirely clear, however, because the tasks that have been used to date (e.g., mental rotation, part–whole and left–right decisions, etc.) do not distinguish between what Kosslyn (1980) described as the two components of visual processing: locating an object in space (where?) and determining the identity of an object (what?). We report findings from an experiment designed to examine visual processing and working memory in children with TS and normal control children. However, unlike previous examinations of visuospatial processing in TS, the reported experiments tease apart what and where aspects of the visual

---

Requests for reprints should be sent to Lori Buchanan, Department of Psychology, The University of Alberta, Edmonton, Alberta, Canada T6G 2E9. E-mail: lori@psych.ualberta.ca

system. Moreover, they examine separately the contributions of both visual and verbal working memory to visuospatial processing. Differences between children with TS and normal controls indicate that the core deficit is in visuospatial working memory. Correlations with karyotype information from the girls with TS provide some preliminary support for a gene-dosage hypothesis.

Sex differences in cognitive ability have long been recognized (Maccoby & Jacklin, 1974) to the extent that males generally perform better on visuospatial tasks, whereas females show an advantage on verbal tasks (e.g., Halpern, 1986; Johnson & Meade, 1987; Linn & Petersen, 1985). This sexual dimorphism has traditionally been attributed to the gonadal hormones that differentiate the two sexes, although factors such as growth rate (Waber, 1979) and genetic differences (Money, 1963) have also been considered. The latter has been studied primarily in individuals with abnormal sex chromosome complements and is based on the observation of verbal deficits (Rovet, Netley, Bailey, Keenan, & Stewart, 1995) in individuals with a supernumerary X chromosome (Klinefelter syndrome in males and trisomy X syndrome in females) and of visuospatial deficits (Rovet, 1995) in those missing an X chromosome (Turner syndrome).

Turner syndrome (TS) affects 1 in 3,000 to 5,000 females (Hook & Warburton, 1983; Lippe, 1982). Caused by the loss of some material from the X chromosome, usually an entire X chromosome, its physical manifestations include short stature, a defect in lymphatic clearance, mild skeletal abnormalities, and gonadal dysgenesis (Lippe, 1991; Money & Granoff, 1965; Wilson & Foster, 1985). Gonadal dysgenesis results in the lack of estrogen production and abnormal development of secondary sex characteristics. Consequently, adolescents and women with TS require estrogen replacement therapy in order to mature sexually (Hier, Atkins, & Perlo, 1980; Rosenfeld & Grumbach, 1990; Ross, 1996). Although all individuals with TS are short, and most are infertile, there exists considerable variability as to severity and type of stigmata. Recent molecular genetics studies indicate there may be as many as five genes located in different regions of the X chromosome that contribute to these abnormalities (Page, 1995) and possibly to the phenotypic variability. Different genetic karyotypes and, in particular, the presence or absence of different combinations of these genes, is thought to be associated with variations in the TS physical stigmata.

In addition to an unusual physical phenotype, females with TS also demonstrate an uneven profile of cognitive strengths and weaknesses suggestive of a nonverbal learning disability (Rovet, 1995). Impairments in tasks of visuospatial processing, arithmetic, and selective aspects of social processing are typically reported in individuals with TS whereas verbal abilities are generally unaffected (e.g., Garron, 1977; McCauley, Kay, Ho, & Treder, 1987; Money & Alexander, 1966; Murphy et al., 1994; Ross, Roeltgen, & Cutler, 1995; Rovet, 1993; Temple & Carney, 1993; Waber, 1979). TS has also been associated with difficulties in working memory, attention, and executive processing (e.g., Ross et al., 1995; Silbert, Wolff, & Lilienthal, 1977; Waber, 1979; Williams, Richman, & Yarbrough, 1991). Neuroanatomical studies reveal structural and functional abnormalities in brain regions linked to the cognitive profile of TS (e.g., Elliot, Watkins, Messa, Lippe, & Chugani, 1996; Johnson, Rohrbaugh, & Ross, 1993; Johnson & Ross, 1994; Kolb & Heaton, 1975; Molland & Purcell, 1974; Portellano-Perez, Bouthelier, & Monge, 1996; Reske-Nielsen, Christensen, & Nielson, 1982; Shucard, Shucard, Clopper, & Schacter, 1992; Tsuboi & Nielsen, 1976).

Because endogenous estrogen production is entirely absent in most cases and estrogen therapy is often delayed until mid- to late adolescence, individuals with TS provide a unique population to study hormonal influences on cognitive abilities and to separate chromosomal from hormonal effects (Collaer & Hines, 1995). Although no study has, as yet, systematically investigated both factors in tandem, Ross and her colleagues are making important strides in this direction (see Ross & Zinn, in press). It may be that hormones and chromosomes independently contribute to different kinds of processing deficits: impaired perceptual detection reflecting a congenital abnormality and impaired selective attention and orientation reflecting an acquired abnormality. This hypothesis was proposed by Johnson and Ross (1994), to explain why, in their small sample, perceptual impairments were evident across ages but attentional and organizational deficits were found only in older adolescents.

TS is considered a prototype for understanding the biological bases of brain–behavior relations (Reiss, Mazzoco, Greenlaw, Freund, & Ross, 1995). However, a major difficulty with the extant TS literature is the lack of adequate empirical methods for assessing specific deficits, as almost all studies have employed only psychometric tests. Although these measures are useful for detecting clinically important global impairments, they are not effective in isolating a defective processing component, especially one that may be coincident with the neuroanatomical abnormalities described in this population. The field of cognitive neuroscience offers a model with the potential to identify deficient processes and their neuroanatomical loci. This model of visuospatial processing assumes two distinct pathways for processing visual identity and spatial location information: the what and where pathways (Kosslyn, 1980). Findings from a retrospective study, based on clinical test data, suggest that these pathways may be differentially affected in TS (Rovet & Buchanan, in press).

This article describes preliminary data from our first attempt to explore systematically the manner by which children and adolescents with TS process visuospatial information. Our approach involves the use of an experimental paradigm that dissociates *what* from *where* cognitive processes. In addition, because the cognitive descriptions that existed in this population do conform to a pattern expected in working memory impairments (Berch, 1996), the procedure also explores the involvement of the visual and verbal working memory systems (cf. Baddeley,

1986). A further goal of this study is to determine whether specific deficits can be mapped to a locus on the X chromosome. This is accomplished by comparing different subgroups of individuals with TS who differ in presence or absence of specific chromosomal segments.

CHROMOSOMAL ABNORMALITIES IN TS

Approximately 50% of all affected individuals have the classic TS karyotype in which there is only a single X chromosome (45,X). Some remaining individuals have a variety of chromosomal abnormalities that differ as to portion of the second chromosome (typically an X but occasionally a Y) that is missing. These karyotypes include: a deletion of a short arm (Xp) or long arm (Xq); a rearrangement or translocation of part of a chromosome to or from the X; a ring chromosome; and an isochromosome, in which the chromosome consists of two long arms and is missing the short arm. In addition, a significant number of individuals have mosaicism that reflects the presence of two or more cell lines: Simple mosaicism is characterized by a 45,X/46,XX constitution, and more complex mosaicisms involve two or more abnormal cell lines. Both physical and cognitive characteristics in TS appear to vary with karyotype: A ring chromosome, for example, is associated with more marked physical stigmata and mental retardation (Migeon, Luo, Jani, & Jeppesen, 1994). Among the other karyotypes, short stature appears to be associated with the loss of short arm material, whereas infertility is associated with loss of either arm, thus suggesting that input from genes in both locations is required.

Because TS is a genetic disorder, direct genetic influences have often been proposed to account for neurocognitive defects. These mechanisms include imprinting, X-linked mental retardation, and reduced dosage of an essential gene product for brain development. Imprinting effects result from a genetic process whereby there are vastly different consequences, including different age of onset, different levels of severity, and even totally different diseases, if the expressed gene is maternal or paternal in origin (Deal, 1995). Ross and Zinn (in press) examined imprinting effects in 20 children with a monosomy X karyotype and found essentially identical IQ profiles, regardless of the parental origin of the child's X chromosome. This suggests that imprinting is an unlikely explanation for the cognitive deficit found in TS.

A second explanation concerns the possibility that TS reflects an X-linked recessive condition, as has been linked to neurodevelopmental abnormalities in other conditions. Thus, problems should be more frequent in TS than in the general female population because only the recessive gene is expressed. Although this may account for the increased incidence of mental retardation that occurs in a small percentage of this population (Rovet, 1990), it cannot explain the pervasiveness of the selective cognitive disabilities.

A more likely hypothesis is that the neurocognitive phenotype in TS arises from a reduced dosage of an as yet unidentified gene or set of genes on the X chromosome. Originally, it was thought that there could be no direct effects of the loss of an X chromosome because one of the two X chromosomes normally becomes inactivated during early development (Lyon, 1962). However, recent evidence from molecular genetics indicates that although this holds for the majority of X-chromosome genes, there are potentially five sites that do not "lyonize," and it is these genes and the lack of their associated protein products that contribute to the TS phenotype (Page, 1995). A dosage effect reflects the number of copies of relevant genes that guide specific aspects of development (Zinn, Page, & Fisher, 1993). Because most individuals with TS have only a single copy of each of these five (vs. two copies for normal females), the group with TS will have a reduced expression of the proteins associated with these genes. Individuals with monosomy X will have a dosage of 1; individuals with mosaicism will have a dosage effect between 1 and 2; individuals with an isochromosome or deletion will have a dosage of 1 for genes on one arm only and a normal dosage (or greater in the case of the long arm in isochromosomes) for the other arm. By comparing individuals with monosomy and mosaic constitutions, one can test the dosage hypothesis. Also, by comparing individuals with loss to one region only with others for whom this region is present, one is in the position to map the genetic locus of a specific deficit.

Recently, Ross and Zinn (in press) tested the dosage hypothesis by contrasting neurocognitive profiles of children with a 45,X karyotype and children with simple mosaicism. Differences between the groups, favoring mosaics, were observed in global IQ and in tasks that placed demands on auditory attention and visual memory. However, the groups did not differ in their visuospatial or visual-motor skills. Similar findings have been reported by a number of other groups of investigators (Murphy et al., 1993; Pennington et al., 1985; Temple & Carney, 1993). The lack of effect of chromosome complement on visuospatial processing in TS suggests a hormonal influence in addition to the genetic contribution. However, Murphy et al. (1993) showed that among individuals with mosaicism, those with a higher percentage of normal 46,XX cells produced the best performance on tasks of visuospatial processing. Although the neurocognitive deficit has not yet been mapped to a specific locus on the X chromosome, a previous study from this lab (Rovet et al., 1995) showed that individuals with a translocation, rearrangement, or ring chromosome had the highest incidence of behavioral problems, whereas individuals with mosaicism and an isochromosome of the long arm had the lowest incidence of impairment. Grouping participants according to number of copies of each chromosomal arm offers an attractive initial approach for studying the relations between genes and neurocognitive abilities. However, one must control for confounding effects of trisomy in the duplicated arm of an isochromosome, as trisomy X has also been associated with a distinct pattern of abilities and disabilities (Rovet et al., 1995).

HORMONAL ABNORMALITIES IN TS

In TS, premature ovarian failure arises from a massive loss of oocytes in utero and shortly after birth, leading to streak or dysgenic ovaries. This is caused by an atretic process, which is typical for all females and culminates in menopause. For some unknown reason, this process is highly accelerated in individuals with TS (Singh & Carr, 1966). For the vast majority of persons with TS, ovarian dysgenesis results in a lack of secondary sexual development and infertility, although about 10% may have spontaneous menses, usually for a brief time. A few individuals with TS have even given birth to normal, healthy offspring.

Sex steroid hormones may modulate certain abilities. The animal literature demonstrates effects of sex hormone manipulation on sexually dimorphic behaviors in several species (Collaer & Hines, 1995). Of particular interest is the finding that visuospatial processes and working memory are influenced by sex hormones during critical periods of development (Williams & Meck, 1991). Other articles in this special issue discuss the contributions of sex hormones to cognitive processes in more detail. Our interest is focused primarily on gaining an understanding of this one population within which hormonal abnormalities are a central symptom.

In TS, neurocognitive deficits may arise from a lack of estrogen during the first year of life when there is normally a period of increased ovarian estrogen production (Ross & Zinn, in press). Other deficits may be associated with lack of estrogen during early puberty prior to receiving estrogen replacement therapy. Still others may reflect abnormal levels of circulating hormone. Nyborg (1990) theorized that there is a curvilinear relation between spatial ability and serum estrogen levels. He found a marked improvement on selective spatial tasks following a short-term trial of estrogen replacement therapy. Ross is currently investigating the effects of low-dose estrogen therapy in a placebo-controlled study of 8- to 12-year-old TS patients to assess both positive and negative effects, but results from these studies are still pending (Ross & Zinn, in press). Previously, Johnson and Ross (1994) reported a normal behavioral profile and normal event-related potentials (ERPs) from a single case study of a TS female with normal endogenous estrogen production. In contrast, they showed that patients without endogenous production, who received estrogen therapy later in adolescence, demonstrated abnormalities on both behavioral and electrophysiological measures.

NEUROANATOMICAL ABNORMALITIES IN TS

TS has been associated with a number of neuroanatomical defects through a variety of methodologies and, although a great deal of variability exists, there are also commonalities across studies. Studies using cerebral lateralization techniques have reported atypical hemispheric organization for processing verbal and spatial information: In individuals with TS, the left hemisphere appears to be less involved than normal in processing verbal information and more involved in processing nonverbal information (Gordon & Galatzer, 1980; Lewandowski, Costenbader, & Richman, 1985, McGlone, 1985; Netley, 1977; Rovet, 1990; Rovet & Netley, 1982; Waber, 1979). Examinations of brain activation patterns in TS support a view of right-hemisphere dysfunction to the extent that individuals with TS produce electroencephalogram maps that show greater right-hemisphere activation for reading and greater left parietal activation for arithmetic than controls (Portellano-Perez et al., 1996). Shucard et al. (1992) similarly found that the right hemisphere of individuals with TS was less efficient than normal in handling irrelevant or competing information.

More definitive neuropathological and neuroimaging studies have allowed investigators to localize potential sites of the TS neuroanatomic defect. Neuropathologies in cerebral cortical organization and developmental deviation of structures in the posterior fossa were evident in most, but not all, of the handful of cases examined on autopsy (Kolb & Heaton, 1975; Molland & Purcell, 1974; Reske-Nielsen et al., 1982). In awake women with TS, a bilateral reduction of glucose uptake in parietal and occipital lobes has been reported in positron emission tomography (PET) studies (Clark, Klonoff, & Hayden, 1990). Studies using magnetic resonance imaging (MRI) have reported reductions in gray and white matter in right temporal and parietal and in left parietal perisylvian regions (Reiss et al., 1995); cerebellum and pons (Reiss et al., 1993); and hippocampus, lenticular nucleus, and thalamus (Murphy et al., 1993). However, major hemispheric differences have not been found with MRI (Reiss et al., 1995), and anomalies in frontal regions have not been consistently observed. The discrepancy between the reported involvement of subcortical structures in Murphy's (1993) study of mature women and the lack of involvement in Reiss et al.'s (1995) study of children may reflect the influence of hormonal factors on brain maturation during puberty (Ross & Zinn, in press). There also appears to be genetic involvement in the neuroanatomical abnormalities associated with TS: Murphy et al. (1993) reported that the level of neuroanatomical abnormalities in TS women with a mosaic karyotype is intermediary between controls and women with a 45,X karyotype. Moreover, Elliot et al. (1996) reported a unique pattern of glucose uptake in one girl with a small ring karyotype that included overall reductions in uptake and an unusual reduction specific to the temporal lobe.

The view that both hormonal and genetic influences may be involved in TS brain abnormalities gains support from a study conducted by Johnson and Ross (1994). These researchers compared ERP profiles of girls and adolescents with TS during two different cognitive paradigms, a discrimination task of line drawings of hands shown in different rotations, and an auditory oddball task. Two distinct abnormalities were found: The first abnormality was observed in the N2 wave component during the visual discrimination task. This abnormality was thought to represent a congenitally produced difficulty in stimulus detection, as it was observed in all participants regardless of age. The second abnormality, thought to be acquired during adolescence, occurred in the O wave component during the auditory oddball task, which older participants with TS performed like the younger controls. The TS group failed to show the developmental changes in the ability to contextualize information, overrating the impacts of events instead of putting them in the proper context, a difficulty that normally resolves during midpuberty. Although the mechanisms that contribute to these abnormalities are not clear, Johnson et al. (1993) suggested there may be a critical period of neuroanatomical development during which estrogen is required and, if it is missing, normal adolescent maturation of selective brain systems fails to occur. The additional deficits in hippocampus, caudate, and other subcortical structures observed by Murphy et al. (1993) in adult women, which were not observed by Reiss et al. (1995) with children, may reflect this maturational deficiency.

Summary

Across methods, the findings suggest that the development of parietal and occipital structures tends to be atypical in TS. Because abnormal development of these structures is associated with deficits in visuospatial processing (Kosslyn, 1980), it is not surprising that both behavioral and neuroanatomical abnormalities coexist in TS. Also observed are abnormalities in other structures such as the hippocampus and caudate, which are associated with memory and attention. As these abnormalities were more frequently reported in older participants with TS, there is a suggestion that impairments in these domains may be more evident during midadolescence and adulthood and may reflect the influences of abnormal hormonal levels in early puberty. Abnormalities in frontal structures have seldom been observed, with the exception of a single case study of twins discordant for TS (Reiss et al., 1993), who also differed in their executive processing skills.

COGNITIVE ABNORMALITIES

Shaffer (1962) first reported a selective impairment in cognitive processing in TS shortly after the original physical descriptions of the syndrome. Since that time, numerous studies have revealed a significant impairment for processing visuospatial information although verbal skills are normal (e.g., Money & Alexander, 1966; Garron, 1977; Murphy et al., 1994; Temple & Carney, 1993). In a synthesis of the findings from 19 studies involving 226 women and children with TS, Rovet (1990) found a 12-point IQ advantage for verbal over performance scales with the discrepancy ranging from 4 to 29 points. On more specific indices from intelligence tests, individuals with TS were found to score significantly below controls on factors of perceptual organization and freedom from distractibility but not verbal comprehension (Rovet, 1996). Although the majority of studies concur that their performance is below normal on all nonverbal subtests, several studies have reported that block design, the presumed most spatial of all performance subtests, is least affected in TS (McGlone, 1985; Ross & Zinn, in press; Silbert et al., 1977; Waber, 1979). Use of verbal strategies, small sample sizes, and atypical controls have all been offered to account for these differences.

On more specific tasks of visuospatial processing, individuals with TS do poorly on construction (Murphy et al., 1994), design copying (Waber, 1979), directional sense (Alexander, Walker, & Money, 1964), extrapersonal space perception (Alexander & Money, 1966), mazes (Nielsen, Nyborg, & Dahl, 1977), mental rotation (Berch & Kirkendall, 1986; Rovet & Netley, 1982), part–whole perception (Silbert et al., 1977), the rod and frame task (Nyborg, 1990), spatial and visual reasoning (Money & Alexander, 1966; Murphy et al., 1994), visual discrimination (Silbert et al., 1977), visual imagery (Downey et al., 1991), visual memory (Murphy et al., 1994; Ross et al., 1995), visual sequencing (Robinson et al., 1986), and visual-motor integration (Lewandowski et al., 1985). In comparing visuospatial skills from several domains, Ross (1996) reported greater difficulty on tasks assessing *how things go together* and *spatial location and orientation* than tasks of *object identity*, although all are significantly impaired. A retrospective analysis of how participants with TS performed on multiple tasks of spatial processing in our lab similarly revealed less difficulty with tasks that were primarily visual than tasks that were spatial or constructional, although all were affected (Rovet & Buchanan, in press).

Most examinations of the cognitive deficits in TS have used clinical psychometric tests, which do not adequately measure component mental processes. In one of the few exceptions, Rovet and Netley (1982) gave participants with TS and matched controls two laboratory-based cognitive processing tasks: a mental rotation task of abstract cubic stimuli (Sheppard & Metzler, 1971) and a sentence verification task (Just & Carpenter, 1976). Decomposition of reaction revealed a disruption only on the mental transformation component of the visual, but not the verbal, task. Visual discrimination abilities were unaffected. Furthermore, TS reaction times were consistently slower across tasks. In contrast, Murphy et al. (1994) recently gave women with TS an alternate version of the mental rotation task involving letter stimuli and found no deficit in the TS group relative to the controls. The discrepancy between studies may be indicative of a specific working memory deficit rather than a visuospatial processing impairment because the alphanumeric characters placed fewer demands on working memory than the complex figures used by Rovet and Netley. Indeed, Berch (1996) posited that problems in memory may be the core cognitive deficit in TS. Similarly, Murphy et al. (1994) reported that participants with TS did not differ from controls on tasks of face matching during the immediate presentation condition but were significantly worse during delayed presentation; they were also outperformed by controls in memory for line drawings and stories.

In addition to visuospatial and memory problems, individuals with TS demonstrate difficulty on tasks of attention (Ross et al., 1995; Williams et al., 1991); auditory sequencing (Silbert et al., 1977); executive functioning in the areas of verbal fluency, planning, organization, and flexibility (Temple, Carney, & Mullarkey, 1996; Waber, 1979); facial identity and face affect processing (McCauley et al., 1987; Ross et al., 1995; Waber, 1979); numerical computation (Rovet, 1993, 1996; Rovet, Szekely, & Hockenberry, 1994); and social competency (Rovet & Ireland, 1994).

Summary

These studies indicate that difficulties in visuospatial processing and memory are commonplace among most females with TS and extend across a wide range of tasks. Tasks involving a "where" or "how things go together" judgment or that involve a memory component seem to provide the greatest degree of difficulty. Although neuroanatomical differences have also been consistently observed in this population, correlations between these effects and cognitive deficits are surprisingly weak (Reiss et al., 1995). This may reflect the fact that the majority of tasks in these correlational studies assessed a mixture of processing components with tasks that are limited to commonly used neuropsychological assessments (e.g., the Stroop task) that are not well understood in terms of component processes. This lack of theoretical and experimental sophistication remains a major impediment in the study of a specific cognitive phenotype in TS. In order to specify brain–behavior relations and their biological determinants in this population, it is necessary to assess specific cognitive processes using tasks that are well grounded in principled cognitive theory.

A COGNITIVE NEUROSCIENCE APPROACH TO STUDY VISUOSPATIAL DEFICITS

We conceive the visuospatial processing system as a combination of three distinct parts. Each of these three subsystems can be thought of as a potential site for a specific deficit in TS. These are the parvocellular and magnocellular pathways from the retina to the thalamus, followed by the dorsal/ventral (or "what/where") streams, and, at the higher end of the cognitive ladder, working memory. Each of these potential sites of damage is investigated in this study.

The visual system diverges very early, prior to the lateral geniculate nucleus (LGN) of the thalamus. The parvocellular (P) cells are capable of processing information that is conveyed by color changes, whereas the magnocellular (M) cells are virtually color-blind (Merigan & Maunsell, 1993). Tasks in which stimuli are conveyed by changes in color (i.e., when background and stimuli are equiluminant) should force processing through the P pathway. It is therefore expected that if the

TS visuospatial deficit reflects an abnormality early in the M system, differences from controls should be greater when stimuli are defined by changes in luminance (black background–white stimuli) than by changes in color (red background–green stimuli). A contrast of these conditions may provide information about possible deficits early in the system.

Ames (1955) described an object as being represented in two dimensions: identity and location. Kosslyn (1980) repeated this description with a more formalized view of the two visual processes. Since then, advances in neuroscience have identified the existence of two parallel neuroanatomical pathways in the visual system (Mishkin & Ungerleider, 1982; Mishkin, Ungerleider, & Macko, 1983) that reflect Ames's and Kosslyn's distinction. The pathway that projects to the inferotemporal cortex is assumed to subserve object identification and is known as the "what" pathway. The pathway that projects to the occipital cortex to the posterior parietal cortex is assumed to subserve object location and is known as the "where" pathway. The where or dorsal stream seems to have evolved earlier than the what or ventral stream (Merigan & Maunsell, 1993). Because developmental trajectories often mimic evolutionary trajectories, it may be that the two pathways develop at different stages and could be disrupted by different factors such as genetic and hormonal abnormalities.

This pathway distinction was originally discovered in primates for which ablations to temporal and parietal regions disrupted abilities in discriminating objects and spatial locations, respectively (Mishkin et al., 1983). The dichotomy has also been observed in human patients with localized brain damage (Bauer & Rubens, 1985; De Renzi, 1982; Levine, Warach, & Farah, 1985) and in normals using PET (Haxby, Grady, Ungerleider, & Horowitz, 1991; Kosslyn et al., 1993; McIntosh et al., 1994; Sergent, Ohta, & MacDonald, 1992; Sergent, Zuck, Levesque, & MacDonald, 1992). Neuropsychological studies show that patients with lesions in the inferotemporal region lose the ability to identify common objects or recognize faces but they can orient themselves in their environment and know how objects are constructed and located. In contrast, patients with lesions in the posterior parietal region can recognize objects and faces but have difficulty locating and mentally transforming them and are poor at interpreting emotional expression. This dissociation is similar to that found in TS, in which object identification appears less affected than constructional and spatial processes (e.g., Ross, 1996; Rovet & Buchanan, in press).

Tresch, Sinnamon, and Seamon (1993) showed that it was possible, experimentally, to dissociate visual and spatial processing in college students. In their study, participants made shape versus location decisions about stimuli during trials in which secondary interference tasks were presented. The use of what versus where interference tasks produced dissociations in performance between the shape and location decisions. As their tasks generated dissociable information about where and what processing, we proposed that the use of a modified version of this paradigm in TS could provide a more finely grained approach for the analysis of their visuospatial processing abilities. If the TS deficit were uniquely spatial, performance of individuals with TS would be more affected on the location decision task than the shape decision task, whereas if it were primarily visual, the reverse would be true. If both pathways were defective, their performance would be poorer than controls on both tasks.

The difficulties in visuospatial processing associated with TS may be due to deficits in higher order processing, such as attention or memory. If so, no dissociation and no difference from controls would be observed on these simple what and where tasks. Because it is possible to tap memory effects in visuospatial processing by introducing secondary interference tasks that vary as to type and modality of demand on short-term or working memory, we propose that these manipulations can identify these higher order deficits. Our view of working memory follows the basic model proposed by Baddeley and colleagues (Baddeley, 1986; Baddeley & Hitch, 1994) in which there is a verbal (phonological loop) and a nonverbal (visuospatial sketchpad) subsystem in short-term or working memory. In the experiments reported here, we test the integrity of both subsystems by introducing secondary tasks that draw on either the visual or the verbal components of working memory.

This article describes our preliminary efforts to disentangle visuospatial processes using data from an experiment that was conducted on children and adolescents with TS. It involves an experimental paradigm that distinguishes between visual and spatial processes. This paradigm also allows for the identification of deficits that occur lower (background manipulation) or higher (delay manipulations) in the system. It was anticipated that participants with TS would show a deficit on location relative to shape tasks and that they would be impaired in visual working memory, akin to Baddeley's (1986) visuospatial sketchpad, but not in verbal working memory.

In order to assess the contribution of gene dosage and location to specific deficits, we compared performance of different karyotype groups. It was hypothesized that because the three groups differ in number and type of critical genes that are missing, if any one group is more affected than the others on a specific aspect of cognitive processing, this will provide critical information about the specific genes that affect distinct processing pathways, for which the neuroanatomic underpinnings are known. This approach will serve to describe the role of genetic factors in the specialization of brain structure.

METHOD

Participants

The study participants included nine 12- to 18-year-old adolescents with TS and eight female controls matched for age[1] and verbal IQ. The TS group was recruited

---

[1]Time constraints for this special issue made it impossible for us to obtain a full sample of controls. We were unable to obtain an age-matched control for one 15-year-old girl in the TS group.

with the assistance of staff endocrinologists at the Hospital for Sick Children in Toronto, Canada, and from the clinical files of one of the authors. Participants with TS included 3 with a 45,X karyotype, 2 with mosaicism (both of whom had one normal and one abnormal cell line), and 2 with an isochromosome for the long arm (i.e., duplication of long arm material and the absence of short arm material). All had short stature and were currently or previously on growth hormone replacement therapy. Five of the eight were receiving estrogen replacement therapy at the time of testing, and most displayed the classic phenotypic characteristics of TS.[2] Controls were sisters of the girls in the TS group ($n = 3$) and local teenage volunteers ($n = 5$). The controls and the TS came from roughly similar socioeconomic status groups (the children were all from middle-class professional families in southern Ontario, Canada).

Procedure

Each participant received, by mail, a letter of introduction describing the purpose and requirements of the study. Two weeks after receipt of the letter, a phone call was made and an appointment scheduled for testing in either the psychology department at the Hospital for Sick Children or the home of one of the investigators. After informed consent or assent was obtained, each participant was tested in a quiet, dimly lit room. Testing duration was approximately 3.5 hr. Approximately half of this time was spent on the study described here and the remainder to psychometric testing procedures described elsewhere (Buchanan, Pavlovic, & Rovet, in press).

Tests

Verbal intelligence. This was estimated with the Similarities and Vocabulary subtests of the Wechsler Intelligence Scale for Children–III (WISC–III; Wechsler, 1991). A prorated verbal IQ was determined by calculating the mean percentiles for the Similarities and Vocabulary subtests. This score was used to ensure that the TS group and the controls did not differ in terms of verbal intelligence. These groups did not differ: The mean for the TS group was 100.3 and the mean for the control group was 101.25, $t(16) < 1$.

Visuospatial processing tasks. Testing consisted of a series of six task blocks. All trials were presented via a personal computer with a 14-in. color display

---

[2]There were no effects of estrogen therapy for any of our studies, but these effects may be evident when larger samples are tested.

monitor (see Figure 1 for trial examples). All tasks required a participant to make a same–different judgment about two visual displays that varied in shape (circle, square, or rectangle) and display location (one of three points on an equilateral triangle that subtended approximately 7° of visual angle). Participants were required to judge whether the two stimuli had the same shape or same location as specified by the examiner. For example, if a triangle appeared in both displays, the correct answer for a shape judgment was "yes," whereas if these triangles appeared in different locations, the correct answer for a location judgment was "no." Responses for both shape and location items were mapped onto the ? and z keys of a standard keyboard, representing yes and no responses, respectively.

For each phase, the tasks varied as to background color, simultaneous versus successive, with an intervening lag condition, and type of secondary task manipulation during the intervening lag condition. The basic task (immediate black) consisted of a fixation cross shown in the center of the screen for 50 msec, followed by the experimental display, which remained on the screen until a response was made. The display contained two stimuli drawn in white and shown simultaneously

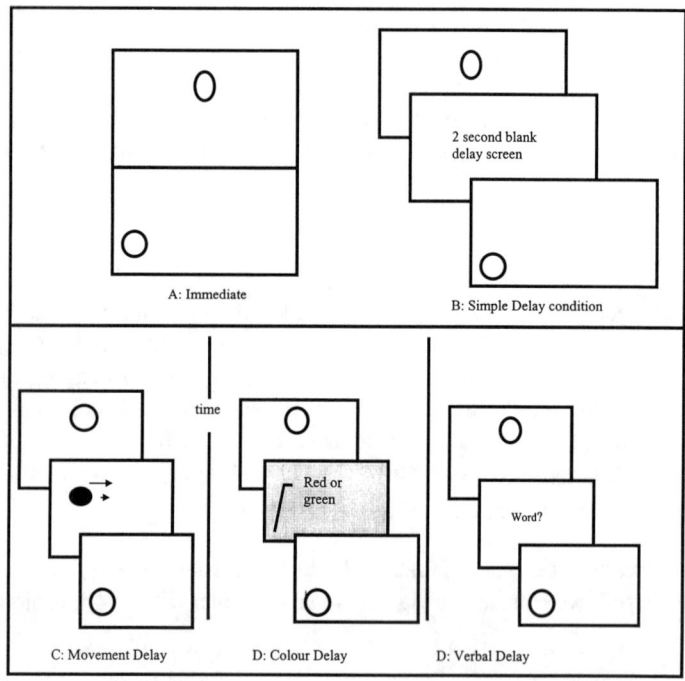

FIGURE 1 Examples of trials from the experimental procedure.

on a black computer screen. The displays were presented one on the top and one on the bottom half of the screen. The task was to determine whether the bottom display matched the top display on the relevant (identity or location) dimension. The immediate red condition was identical except the background was red and stimuli were roughly equiluminant green.

In the four delay conditions, the top display appeared for 250 msec. It was replaced first for 50 msec by random-length white lines, and for 2,000 msec either by a blank screen or by screens that differed in color or showed either moving or stationary dots or letter strings. This was followed by the bottom display. For the intervening tasks, participants were to decide whether the screen was red (color delay), the dot was moving (movement delay), or the letter string was a real English word (lexical delay). Participants were instructed to complete as many secondary tasks as possible within the 2,000-msec interval (this worked out to be approximately four decisions per trial and at least one of these secondary tasks had to be completed prior to the onset of the second display of the primary task) and then decide whether the bottom display matched the top display on the criterion dimension. All responses were made via the ? and z keys (for yes and no responses, respectively).

The tasks were presented such that half the participants from each group carried out the six location-decision blocks first and the other half did the six identity-decision blocks first. Within each decision condition, half of the participants performed the immediate black followed by immediate red blocks first and half did them in the reverse order. The third block consisted of simple delay for all participants, and the fourth to sixth blocks consisted of the three secondary tasks, the order of which were counterbalanced across participants. Following completion of the first six blocks of either identity- or location-decision conditions, participants received the psychometric tests. Then, the remaining six blocks requiring the other decision were provided in the same order as in the first six blocks. For ease of presentation, we now report each phase of this study individually and describe the hypotheses tested and the outcome. Table 1 provides mean reaction times (RTs) and error rates for all of the phases in the experiment; however, each analysis of interest has its own figure depicting relevant mean RTs for reasons of clarity.

CONTRASTS OF WHAT AND WHERE DECISIONS

The major question of interest was whether the TS group and controls differed in terms of their ability to process what and where information. By using stimulus location and stimulus identity as the two varying dimensions in this paradigm, we had hoped to answer this question. Specifically, a comparison of shape and location decisions was expected to supply information about the relative functioning of what and where processes in girls with TS versus controls.

TABLE 1
Mean Reaction Times and Error Rates for Turner Syndrome (TS) and Control Groups for All Experimental Conditions

	Reaction Times (msec)					Errors				
	TS		Control			TS		Control		
	M	SD	M	SD	Difference	MD	SD	M	SD	Difference
Shape decisions										
Black immediate	1,072	284	889	289	183*	1.33	1.5	.375	.74	.955
Red immediate	1,004	290	795	307	209*	.88	.92	.87	.64	.01
Simple delay	1,294	390	963	339	331*	1.77	.97	1.12	1.24	.65
Color delay	2,304	569	1,380	456	924*	4.22	2.94	3	1.85	1.22*
Movement delay	2,349	538	1,356	407	993*	4.22	3.15	2.5	2.26	1.72*
Lexical delay	1,829	338	1,260	340	569*	3.6	1.87	2.5	2.92	1.1
Grand means	1,652		1,107		545*	2.67		1.72		.95
Location decisions										
Black immediate	1,180	168	781	176	399*	1.88	1.26	1.6	1.18	.28
Red immediate	946	291	741	180	205*	1.55	1.23	1	1.19	.55
Simple delay	1,464	349	992	362	472*	1.44	.88	.625	.91	.81
Color delay	2,319	591	1,335	442	984*	5.55	1.87	2.5	1.30	3.05*
Movement delay	2,575	492	1,269	433	1,306*	5.33	1.65	1.75	.88	3.58*
Lexical delay	1,773	567	1,181	354	592*	3.55	2.24	1.375	1.06	2.18*
Grand means	1,709		1,049		659*	2.97		1.37		1.6*

*$p < .05$.

Results

We expected that the TS group would differ from controls on the experimental tasks. This expectation was confirmed with a significant main effect of group for RTs, $F(1, 15) = 7.49$, $p < .01$, and for errors, $F(1, 15) = 8.01$, $p < .01$. Inspection of the means indicates that the TS group was slower and made more errors than the controls on all tasks. We predicted that the group with TS would be more impaired on the location decision than the identity decision. This was assessed by comparing the groups' performance on the two decision conditions. As illustrated by Figure 2, the decision manipulation resulted in neither a main effect for RTs, $F(1, 15) = 1.08, p < .1$, nor for error data, $F(1, 15) < 1$. Also, the Group × Decision interaction was not significant, $F(1, 15) < 1$, for both RT and errors.

These results, therefore, do not support the hypothesis that where processes are differentially impaired in TS. Although this failure to find a significant difference may be a function of our limited sample size, the fact that there does not appear to be any trend toward a deficit in the location decision in the RT data suggests it most likely does not exist. The error data do suggest that a where deficit may be found

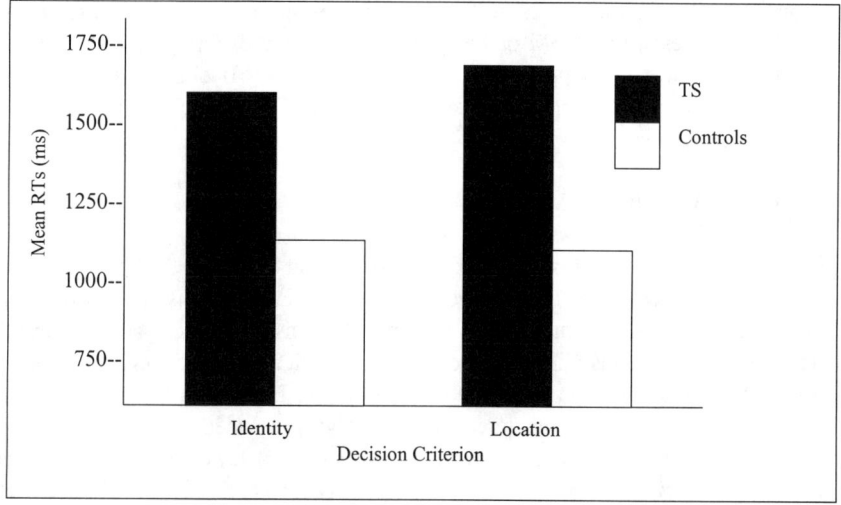

FIGURE 2 Reaction times for Turner syndrome (TS) group and control group as a function of what versus where decisions. There is a significant main effect of group but no interaction.

given a larger sample size; however, we are reluctant to endorse this view given the speed–accuracy trade-off present in the data from the control group.

Red Versus Black Background Manipulation

The manipulation in this phase took advantage of the color processing abilities of the P and M pathways to determine if the deficit was early in the visuospatial system (perhaps at the detection stage, as suggested by Johnson & Ross, 1994). Because color is processed by only the P pathway, the presentation of stimuli at equiluminance should favor the P pathway, thus equating TS and control groups, if the deficit in TS is limited to the magnocells. In one condition, stimuli were presented in white on a black background and in the second condition they were presented in green on a (roughly equiluminant[3]) red background.

A Group × Background manipulation (i.e., red vs. black background conditions) repeated measures mixed analysis of variance revealed that the black background had significantly shorter RTs than the red background, $F(1, 15) = 4.32, p < .05$ (see

---

[3]Due to our concern for overtaxing participants, we did not require them to individualize the luminance using psychophysical measures. We based our luminance decision on mean red–green–blue values generated during minimum motion detection tests of 6 University of Waterloo graduate students. Consequently, equiluminance is only approximate.

Figure 3), but there was not a significant effect present in the error data, $F(1, 15) < 1$. Our hypothesis that the M pathway of the TS group differed from that of the normal group was not supported, as neither the Group × Background interaction nor the Group × Background × Decision interaction, $F(1, 15) < 1$, for both RT and errors, was significant.

Immediate Versus Delayed Conditions

Our next question of interest was whether visuospatial deficits in the TS population could be explained on the basis of working memory impairments. To answer this, we included a time lag manipulation in which decisions were made to stimuli presented simultaneously in one condition and with a 2-sec delay between presentation of the two stimuli in the second condition (see Figures 1a and 1b).

The three conditions considered in this analysis included the two immediate conditions (red and black backgrounds) and the simple delay condition. There was a significant main effect of condition for RTs, $F(2, 30) = 17.43, p < .001$, but not for errors, $F(2, 30) < 1$. Neither the main effect of group, $F(1, 15) < 1$, nor the Group × Condition interaction, $F(1, 15) < 1$, was significant. As Figure 4 shows, the main effect of condition in the RT data resulted from the simple delay producing longer

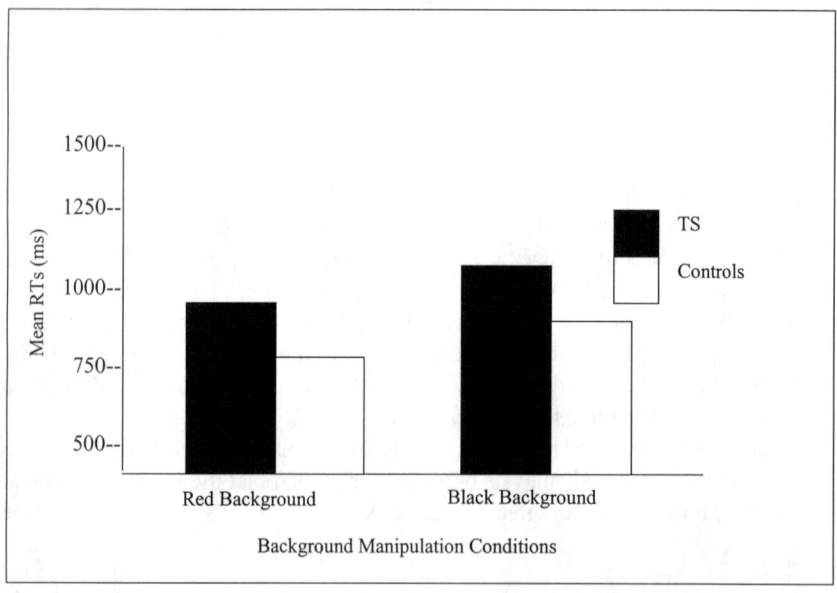

FIGURE 3 Reaction times for Turner syndrome (TS) group and control group as a function of red versus black background manipulation. There is a significant main effect for both group and background but no interaction.

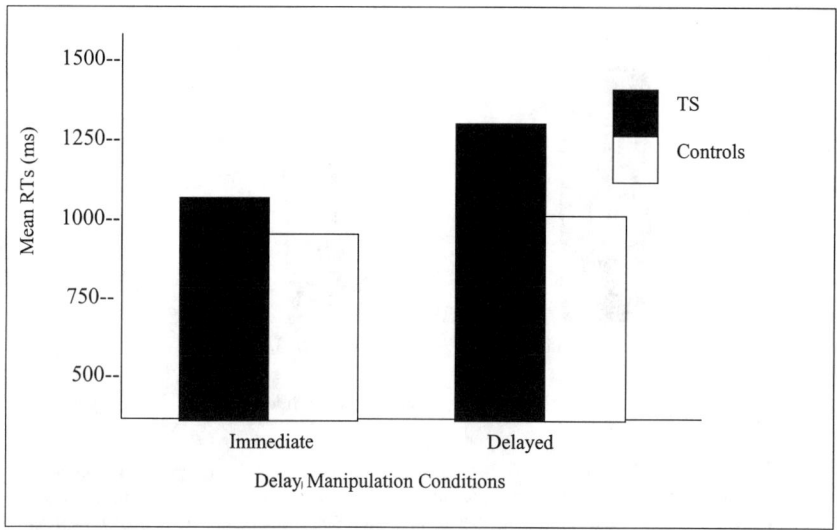

FIGURE 4 Reaction times for Turner syndrome (TS) group and control group as a function of immediate versus delayed presentation (red and black background are combined conditions for the immediate condition). There is a significant main effect of presentation but no interaction, despite a trend favoring the immediate condition over the delayed for the TS group.

responses than the immediate conditions; $t(17) = 3.84$, $p < .01$, delay versus immediate black background, and $t(17) = 4.31$, $p < .01$, delay versus immediate red background. Although the Group × Delay interaction was not significant, Figure 4 indicates that the TS group appeared to have more difficulty than the controls when the task placed demands on working. The following phase extended the examination of this impairment by placing even greater demands on working memory.

Secondary Interference Tasks

Working memory was studied by introducing a secondary interference task manipulation during the 2-sec delay between the presentation of the first and the second shapes (Figures 1c, 1d, and 1e depict these conditions). In these conditions, children had to maintain information about the target shapes in memory while making supplementary decisions on either visual (detecting either color or movement in a display) or verbal information (deciding whether a letter string was a real word).

The conditions considered for this analysis included the three secondary task delay conditions (i.e., screen color, moving dot, and lexical decision). As Figure 5 shows, there was a significant main effect of group for RTs, $F(1, 15) = 8.04$, $p = .01$, and errors, $F(1, 15) = 59.01$, $p < .01$. There was also a significant main effect of condition for RTs, $F(2, 30) = 27.16$, $p < .01$, and for errors, $F(2, 30) = 4.76$, $p <$

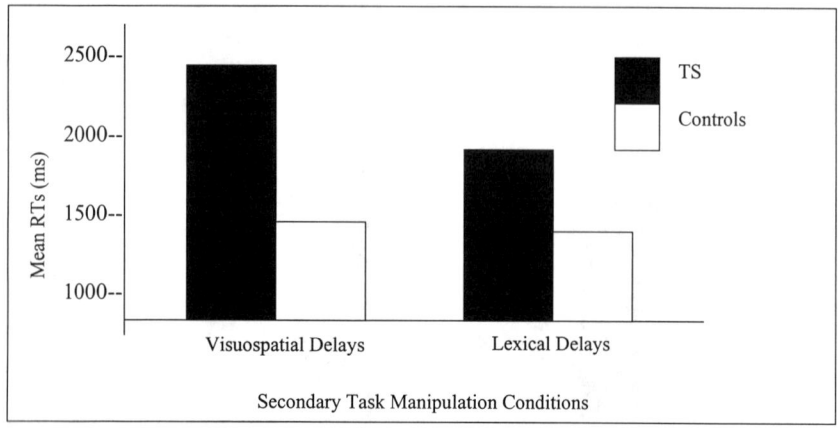

FIGURE 5 Reaction times for Turner syndrome (TS) group and control group as a function of visual versus lexical secondary task manipulation (color and movement conditions are combined for the visual condition). There is a significant interaction with the TS group performing relatively poorly in the visual condition.

.05, and a significant Group × Condition interaction for RTs, $F(2, 30) = 3.71, p < .01$, but not for errors, $F(2, 30) < 1$. Further analysis of this interaction revealed that the control group ($n = 8$) did not produce significant differences when the three secondary task conditions were contrasted in separate t tests, $t(7) = 1.57, p > .55$ for color versus movement; $t(7) = 1.42, p > .20$ for color versus lexical, and $t(7) = 1.23, p > .25$ for movement versus lexical. In contrast, the TS group ($n = 9$) did show selective disadvantages when these secondary conditions were contrasted, $t(8) = .96, p > .35$ for color versus movement; $t(8) = 1.93, p < .10$, for color versus lexical; and $t(8) = 4.86, p < .01$ for movement versus lexical. This advantage for verbal over nonverbal interference conditions can be seen in Figure 5, which presents the mean RTs for the two visual tasks combined, versus the mean RT for the verbal task.

Investigation of Genetic Contributions

As a supplementary goal, we sought to determine whether performance on the experimental task could be predicted by the karyotype of the girls with TS. To do this, we calculated a measure of visuospatial memory interference. Comparing the difference between reaction times for the verbal and the visuospatial interference tasks and dividing that difference by overall reaction time for each individual determined this visuospatial interference score. Although our numbers were limited, a trend suggests that the various TS karyotype groups may differ with respect to this visuospatial interference score (see Figure 6). The same was not true for

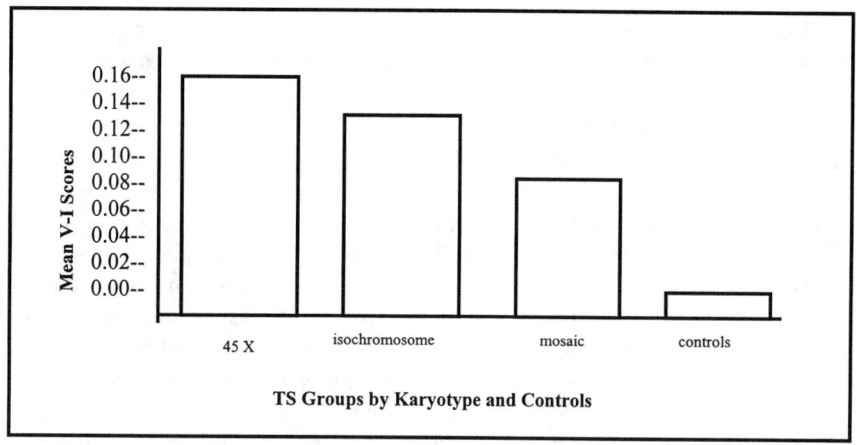

FIGURE 6 Visual interference scores for Turner syndrome (TS) group (by karyotype) and controls.

general processing speed because grouping by karyotype did not reveal any trends in overall RT data, despite the fact that the TS group was consistently slower in every condition.

DISCUSSION

Overall, our findings indicate a global impairment in visuospatial processing in TS: The TS group was slower and less accurate than the control group in all experimental conditions. Contrary to expectations, the findings of this study suggest that females with TS do not show a specific deficit on one of the two pathways that characterize the visuospatial system. Rather, these results show that if there are specific visuospatial deficits in TS, they reflect a higher order cognitive impairment. This was supported by the lack of difference on the basic task between location-decision and shape-decision conditions and the lack of an effect for the background manipulation condition, and the fact that an introduction of tasks that placed demands on the visual working memory system showed deficits in the TS group (color delay and movement delay). These results, therefore, support Berch's (1996) claim that a deficiency in working memory may represent the primary deficit in TS. Furthermore, the lack of effect on participants' ability to make identity and location judgments when demands were placed on verbal working memory (lexical delay) indicates that the working memory deficit is confined to visuospatial memory. It also suggests that the use of verbal strategies did not differ between the girls with TS and the control group.

Visual working memory is a component process in most of the psychometric tests of spatial ability in which TS groups have shown deficits. For example, visual working memory is required in delayed copying tasks, computing mental rotations, solving mazes and puzzles, and reading maps—all of which have been reported to be impaired in previous studies of individuals with TS (see the introduction of this article for the complete list). These findings are, therefore, in agreement with our experimental findings and with neurophysiological studies that point in a similar direction. For example, Shucard et al. (1992) reported that the right hemisphere of individuals with TS was less efficient in handling irrelevant or competing information than normal. The competing information from the visuospatial secondary tasks appeared to affect performance for the TS group more than did competing, presumably left-hemisphere-linked verbal information. Furthermore, the neuroanatomical substrates of visuospatial working memory (Jonides et al., 1993) are those in which TS have reduced volume relative to controls (i.e., the right parietal, occipital, and prefrontal cortices). Thus, although the results are based on a limited sample size and are subject to question in that regard, they fit well with existing information about cognitive and neuroanatomical abnormalities in TS.

Although these findings do not show a specific deficit in either visual or spatial processing per se, the use of a very simple spatial task in which locations could be coded verbally may have restricted our ability to observe this deficit. Similarly, the type of stimuli, which also can be verbally coded quite readily, may have allowed for alternate modes of processing. Moreover, this study had a very limited number of participants, so the power to find effects was somewhat limited. However, the complex within-subject design of the experiment, to some extent, ameliorated this limitation. We are presently conducting a follow-up study that is expected to overcome these limitations.

Because the stimuli were easily named it could be argued that the TS group used a different, more verbal strategy than the control group. However, it seems from the data that the TS group did not have a preference for verbal encoding over the control group. If the TS group was using a verbal strategy to remember the shapes and locations, then the introduction of a secondary verbal task would have a had a greater impact on their ability to remember the stimuli. This was not the case, as both groups were equally affected by the introduction of a verbal task. Consequently, although we do recognize the limitation of the stimulus set, we do not believe that this limitation compromises our claims that a specific visuospatial working memory deficit is at the heart of the cognitive difficulties associated with TS.

The preliminary analysis of genetic influences might be viewed as somewhat premature because of our small sample size. However, the results, based only on descriptive comparisons, did indicate that the TS subgroup that was missing the entire X chromosome was more affected than the TS subgroups with some material from a second X chromosome. This finding suggests that the dosage hypothesis may well provide at least a partial answer to questions about the cause of cognitive deficits in TS. Increasing the size of our sample to include other chromosomal variants in TS will undoubtedly allow us to pinpoint the genetic locus of the cognitive deficits. This step is one that is critical to developing an understanding of the contribution of genes to cognitive deficits in TS.

In conclusion, this preliminary report suggests that our method of examination offers a powerful approach for identifying deficient mental processes in TS. Because these processes have their roots in well-defined neuroanatomical systems, the methods used here have the potential for identifying unique brain–behavior relations and their biological determinants. Future studies involving larger samples, additional karyotypic subgroups, improved test stimuli, and hormonal data will serve to describe more precisely the processing deficits and contributing genetic and hormonal factors.

This issue on hormonal determinants of cognitive functions illustrates the variety of ways researchers attempt to understand the biological basis of behavior. This understanding has both theoretical and practical importance and has become an increasingly more attainable goal with technology advances. TS provides a unique model for disentangling genetic and hormonal contributions to a cognitive deficit. Although the means of mapping these contributions are not yet available, we are confident that genetic and endocrinological advances in the near future will allow us to do so. In the meantime, our projects are aimed at gaining a clearer understanding of the nature of the deficits in TS. We believe that the findings reported in this article are a first step in this direction.

ACKNOWLEDGMENTS

Lori Buchanan was supported by a RESTRACOM postdoctoral Fellowship awarded by the Research Institute at the Hospital for Sick Children, Toronto, Canada. Financial support for some of this research came from Eli Lilly, Toronto, Canada. We thank all the participants in this study as well as the staff of the Endocrinology Department at the Hospital for Sick Children, Toronto, Canada, and Masashi Yanagisawa for their helpful comments.

REFERENCES

Alexander, D., & Money, J. (1966). Turner's syndrome and Gerstmann's syndrome: Neuropsychologic comparisons. *Neuropsychologia, 4,* 265–273.

Alexander, D., Walker, H., & Money, J. (1964). Studies in direction sense. *Archives of General Psychiatry, 10,* 337–339.

Ames, A. (1955). *The nature of our perception, apprehension and behavior.* Princeton, NJ: Princeton University Press.

Baddeley, A. D. (1986). *Working memory.* New York: Oxford University Press.

Baddeley, A. D. & Hitch, G. J. (1994). Developments in the concept of working memory. *Neuropsychology, 8,* 485–493.

Bauer, R. M., & Rubens, A. B. (1985). Agnosia. In K. M. Heilman & E. Valenstein (Eds.), *Clinical neuropsychology* (2nd ed., pp. 187–241). New York: Oxford University Press.

Berch, D. B. (1996). Memory. In J. Rovet (Ed.), *Turner syndrome across the lifespan* (pp. 140–145). Toronto: Klein Graphics.

Berch, D. B. & Kirkendall, K. L. (1986). Spatial information processing in 45,X children. In A. Robinson (Chair), *Cognitive and psychosocial dysfunctions associated with sex chromosome abnormalities*. Symposium presented at the meeting of the American Association for the Advancement of Science, Philadelphia.

Buchanan, L., Pavlovic, J., & Rovet, J. (in press). The contribution of visuospatial working memory to impairments in facial processing and arithmetic in Turner syndrome. *Brain and Cognition*.

Clark, C., Klonoff, H., & Hayden, M. (1990). Regional cerebral glucose metabolism in Turner syndrome. *Canadian Journal of Neurological Sciences, 17,* 140–144.

Collaer, M., & Hines, M. (1995). Human behavioral sex differences: A role for gonadal hormones during early development? *Psychological Bulletin, 118,* 55–107.

Deal, C. L. (1995). Parental genomic imprinting. *Current Opinions in Pediatrics, 7,* 445–448.

De Renzi, E. (1982). Memory disorders following focal neocortical damage. *Philosophical Transactions of the Royal Society of London—Series B: Biological Sciences, 298*(1089), 73–83.

Downey, J., Elkin, E., Ehrhardt, E., Meyer-Bahlburg, A., Bell, H., & Akira, J. (1991). Cognitive ability and everyday functioning in women with Turner syndrome. *Journal of Learning Disabilities, 24,* 32–39.

Elliott, T. K., Watkins, J. M., Messa, C., Lippe, B., & Chugani, H. (1996). Positron emission tomography and neuropsychological correlations in children with Turner's syndrome. *Developmental Neuropsychology, 12,* 365–386.

Garron, D. (1977). Intelligence among persons with Turner's syndrome. *Behavior Genetics, 7,* 105–127.

Gordon, H. W., & Galatzer, A. (1980). Cerebral organization in patients with gonadal dysgenesis. *Psychoneuroendocrinology, 5,* 235–244.

Halpern, D. F. (1986). *Sex differences in cognitive abilities.* Hillsdale, NJ: Lawrence Erlbaum Associates, Inc.

Haxby, J., Grady, C., Ungerleider, L., & Horowitz, B. (1991). Mapping the functional neuroanatomy of the intact human brain with brain work imaging. *Neuropsychologia, 29,* 539–555.

Hier, D. B., Atkins, L., & Perlo, V. P. (1980). Learning disorders and sex chromosome aberrations. *Journal of Mental Deficiency Research, 24,* 17–26.

Hook, E. B., & Warburton, D. (1983). The distribution of chromosomal genotypes associated with Turner's syndrome: Livebirth prevalence rates and evidence for diminished fetal mortality and severity in genotypes associated with structural abnormalities or mosaicism. *Human Genetics, 64,* 24–27.

Johnson, E. S., & Meade, A. C. (1987). Developmental patterns of spatial ability: An early sex difference. *Child Development, 58,* 725–740.

Johnson, R., Rohrbaugh, J., & Ross, J. (1993). Altered brain development in Turner's syndrome. *Neurology, 43,* 801–808.

Johnson, R., & Ross, J. (1994). Event-related potential indications of altered brain development in Turner syndrome. In S. Broman & J. Grafman (Eds.), *Atypical cognitive deficits in developmental disorders: Implications for brain function* (pp. 217–242). Hillsdale, NJ: Lawrence Erlbaum Associates, Inc.

Jonides, J., Smith, E. E., Koeppe, R. A., Awh, E., Minoshima, S., & Mintun, M. A. (1993). Spatial working memory in humans as revealed by PET. *Nature, 363,* 623–625.

Just, M. A., & Carpenter, P. A. (1976). Eye fixations and cognitive processes. *Cognitive Psychology, 8,* 441–480.

Kolb, J., & Heaton, R. (1975). Lateralized neurologic deficits and psychopathology in a Turner syndrome patient. *Archives of General Psychiatry, 32,* 1198–1200.

Kosslyn, S. E. (1980). *Image and mind.* Cambridge, MA: Harvard University Press.
Kosslyn, S. E., Alpert, N. M., Thompson, W. L., Chabris, C. F., Rauch, S. L., & Anderson, A. K. (1993). *Components of object identification: PET investigations.* Unpublished manuscript, Harvard University, Cambridge, MA.
Levine, D. N., Warach, J., & Farah, M. J. (1985). Two visual systems in mental imagery: Dissociations of "what" and "where" in imagery disorders due to bilateral posterior cerebral lesions. *Neurology, 35,* 1010–1018.
Lewandowski, L., Costenbader, V., & Richman, R. (1985). Neuropsychological aspects of Turner syndrome. *International Journal of Neuropsychology, 1,* 144–147.
Linn, M. C., & Petersen, A. C. (1985). Emergence and characterization of sex differences in spatial abilities: A meta analysis. *Child Development, 56,* 1479–1498.
Lippe, B. M. (1982). Primary ovarian failure. In S. A. Kaplan (Ed.), *Clinical pediatric and adolescent endocrinology* (pp. 325–366). Philadelphia: Saunders.
Lippe, B. M. (1991). Turner syndrome. *Endocrinology and Metabolism Clinics of North America, 20,* 121–152.
Lyon, M. F. (1962). Sex chromatin and gene action in the mammalian X-chromosome. *American Journal of Human Genetics, 14,* 135–148.
Maccoby, E. E., & Jacklin, C. N. (1974). *The psychology of sex differences.* Stanford, CA: Stanford University Press.
McIntosh, A. R., Grady, C. L., Ungerleider, L. G., Haxby, J. V., Rapoport, S. I., & Horwitz, B. (1994). Network analysis of cortical visual pathways mapped with PET. *The Journal of Neuroscience, 14,* 655–666.
McCauley, E., Kay, T., Ito, J., & Treder, R. (1987). The Turner's syndrome: Cognitive deficits, affective discrimination and behavior problems. *Child Development, 58,* 464–473.
McGlone, J. (1985). Can spatial deficits in Turner's syndrome be explained by focal CNS dysfunction or atypical speech lateralization? *Journal of Clinical and Experimental Neuropsychology, 7,* 375–394.
Merigan, W. H., & Maunsell, J. H. (1993). How parallel are the primate visual pathways? *Annual Review of Neuroscience, 16,* 369–402.
Migeon, B. R., Luo, S., Jani, M., & Jeppesen, P. (1994). The severe phenotype of females with tiny ring X chromosomes is associated with inability of these chromosomes to undergo X inactivation. *American Journal of Human Genetics, 55,* 497–504.
Mishkin, M., & Ungerleider, L. G. (1982). Contribution of striate inputs to the visuospatial functions of parieto–preoccipital cortex in monkeys. *Behavioral Brain Research, 6,* 57–77.
Mishkin, M., Ungerleider, L. G., & Macko, K. A. (1983). Object vision and spatial vision: Two cortical pathways. *Trends in Neuroscience, 6,* 414–417.
Molland, E. A., & Purcell, M. (1974). Biliary atresia and the Dandy-Walker anomaly in a neonate with 45,X Turner's Syndrome. *Journal of Pathology, 115,* 227–231.
Money, J. (1963). Cytogenetic and psychosexual incongruities with a note on space-form blindness. *American Journal of Psychiatry, 119,* 820–827.
Money, J., & Alexander, D. (1966). Turner's syndrome: Further demonstration of the presence of specific cognitional deficiencies. *Journal of Medical Genetics, 3,* 47–48.
Money, J., & Granoff, D. (1965). IQ and the somatic stigmata of Turner's syndrome. *American Journal of Mental Deficiency, 70,* 69–77.
Murphy, D., Allen, G., Haxby, J., Largay, K., Daly, E., White, B., Powell, C., & Schapiro, M. (1994). The effects of sex steroids, and the X chromosome, on female brain function: A study of the neuropsychology of adult Turner syndrome. *Neuropsychologia, 32,* 1309–1323.
Murphy, D., DeCarli, C., Daly, E., Haxby, J., Allen, G., White, B., McIntosh, A., Powell, C., Horwitz, B., Rapoport, S., & Schapiro, M. (1993). X–chromosome effects on female brain: A magnetic resonance imaging study of Turner's syndrome. *Lancet, 342,* 1197–1200.

Netley, C. (1977). Dichotic listening of callosal agenesis and Turner's syndrome patients. In C. Netley (Ed.), *Language and development and neurological theory* (pp. 133–143). New York: Academic.

Nielsen, J., Nyborg, H., & Dahl, G. (1977). Turner's syndrome: A psychiatric-psychological study of 45 women with Turner's syndrome, compared with their sisters and women with normal karyotypes, growth retardation, and primary amenorrhea. *Acta Jutlandica, 45*(Medicine Series 21), 190.

Nyborg, H. (1990). Sex hormones, brain development, and spatio–perceptual strategies in Turner syndrome. In D. Berch & B. Bender (Eds.), *Sex chromosomes abnormalities and human behavior: Psychological studies* (pp. 100–129). Boulder, CO: Westview.

Page, D. C. (1995). Mapping and targeting Turner genes. In K. A. Albertsson-Wikland & M. B. Ranke (Eds.), *Turner syndrome in a life span perspective: Research and clinical aspects* (pp. 11). Amsterdam: Elsevier.

Pennington, B. F., Heaton, R. K., Karzmark, P., Pendelton, R., Lehman, R., & Shucard, D. W. (1985). The neuropsychological phenotype in Turner's syndrome. *Cortex, 21,* 391–404.

Portellano-Perez, J. J. A., Bouthelier, R. G., & Monge, I. A. (1996). New neurophysiological and neuropsychological contributions on Turner syndrome. In J. Rovet (Ed.), *Turner syndrome across the lifespan* (pp. 52–57). Toronto: Klein Graphics.

Reiss, A. L., Freund, L., Plotnick, L., Baumgartner, T., Green, K., Sozer, A. C., Reader, M., Boehm, C., & Denkla, M. B. (1993). The effects of X monosomy on brain development: Monozygotic twins discordant for Turner's syndrome. *Annals of Neurology, 34,* 97–105.

Reiss, A. L., Mazzocco, M. M., Greenlaw, R., Freund, L., & Ross, J. L. (1995). Neurodevelopmental effects of X monosomy: A volumetric imaging study. *Annals of Neurology, 38,* 731–738.

Reske-Nielsen, E., Christensen, A., & Nielsen, J. (1982). A neuropathological and neuropsychological study of Turner's syndrome. *Cortex, 18,* 181–191.

Robinson, A., Bender, B., Borelli, J., Puck, M., Salbenglatt, J., & Winter, J. (1986). Sex chromosomal aneuploidy: Prospective and longitudinal studies. In S. Ratcliffe & N. Paul (Ed.), *Prospective studies on children with sex chromosome aneuploidy* (pp. 23–73). New York: Liss.

Rosenfeld, R. G., & Grumbach, M. M. (Eds.). (1990). *Turner syndrome.* New York: Marcel Dekker.

Ross, J. L. (1996). Estrogen therapy in the treatment of Turner syndrome. In J. Rovet (Ed.), *Turner syndrome across the lifespan* (pp. 93–96). Toronto: Klein Graphics.

Ross, J. L., Roeltgen, D., & Cutler, G. B. (1995). The neurodevelopmental transition between childhood and adolescence in girls with Turner syndrome. In K. A. Albertsson-Wikland & M. B. Ranke (Eds.), *Turner syndrome in a life span perspective: Research and clinical aspects* (pp. 297–308). Amsterdam: Elsevier.

Ross, J. L., & Zinn, A. (in press). Turner syndrome: Potential hormonal and genetic influences on the neurocognitive profile. In H. Tager-Flusberg (Ed.), *Neurodevelopmental disorders: Contributions to a new framework from the cognitive neurosciences.* Cambridge, MA: MIT Press.

Rovet, J. (1990). The cognitive and neuropsychological characteristics of children with Turner syndrome. In D. Berch & B. Bender (Ed.), *Sex chromosome abnormalities and human behavior: Psychological studies* (pp. 38–77). Boulder, CO: Westview.

Rovet, J. (1993). The psychoeducational characteristics of children with Turner syndrome. *Journal of Learning Disabilities, 26,* 333–341.

Rovet, J. (1995). Behavioral manifestations of Turner syndrome in children: A unique phenotype. In K. A. Albertsson-Wikland & M. B. Ranke (Eds.), *Turner syndrome in a life span perspective: Research and clinical aspects* (pp. 285–295). Amsterdam: Elsevier.

Rovet, J. (1996). Arithmetic processing in Turner syndrome. In J. Rovet (Ed.), *Turner syndrome across the lifespan* (pp. 44–51). Toronto: Klein Graphics.

Rovet, J., & Buchanan, L. (in press). Turner syndrome: A cognitive neuroscience approach. In H. Tager-Flausberg (Ed.), *Neurodevelopmental disorders: Contributions to a new framework from the cognitive neurosciences.* Cambridge, MA: MIT Press.

Rovet, J., & Ireland, L. (1994). The behavioral phenotype of children with Turner syndrome. *Journal of Pediatric Psychology, 19,* 779–790.

Rovet, J., & Netley, C. (1982). Processing deficits in Turner's syndrome. *Developmental Psychology, 18,* 77–94.

Rovet, J., Netley, C., Bailey, J., Keenan, M., & Stewart, D. (1995). Intelligence and achievement in children with extra X aneuploidy: A longitudinal perspective. *American Journal of Medical Genetics (Neuropsychiatric Genetics), 60,* 356–363.

Rovet, J., Szekely, C., & Hockenberry, M. (1994). Specific arithmetic deficits in children with Turner syndrome. *Journal of Clinical and Experimental Neuropsychology, 16,* 820–839.

Sergent, J., Ohta, S., & MacDonald, B. (1992). Functional neuroanatomy and object processing. A positron emission tomography study. *Brain, 1,* 15–36.

Sergent, J., Zuck, E., Levesque, M., & MacDonald, B. (1992). Positron emission tomography study of letter and object processing: Empirical findings and methodological considerations. *Cerebral Cortex, 2,* 68–80.

Shaffer, J. W. (1962). A specific cognitive deficit observed in gonadal aplasia (Turner syndrome). *Journal of Clinical Psychology, 18,* 403–406.

Sheppard, R. N., & Metzler, J. (1971). Mental rotation of three-dimensional objects. *Science, 171,* 701–703.

Shucard, D. W., Shucard, J. L., Clopper, R. J., & Schacter, M. (1992). Electrophysiological and neuropsychological indices of cognitive processing deficits in Turner syndrome. *Developmental Neuropsychology, 8,* 299–323.

Silbert, A., Wolff, P., & Lilienthal, J. (1977). Spatial and temporal processing in patients with Turner's syndrome. *Behavior Genetics, 7,* 11–21.

Singh, R., & Carr, H. (1966). The anatomy and histology of human embryos and fetuses. *Anatomy Research, 155,* 369–384.

Temple, C., & Carney, R. (1993). Intellectual functioning of children with Turner syndrome: A comparison of behavioural phenotypes. *Developmental Medicine and Child Neurology, 35,* 691–698.

Temple, C., Carney, R., & Mullarkey, S. (1996). Frontal lobe function and executive skills in children with Turner's syndrome. *Developmental Neuropsychology, 12,* 343–363.

Tresch, M. C., Sinnamon, H. M., & Seamon, J. G. (1993). Double dissociation of spatial and object visual memory: Evidence from selective interference in intact human subjects. *Neuropsychologia, 31,* 211–219.

Tsuboi, T., & Nielsen, J. (1976). Electroencephalographic examination of 50 women with Turner's syndrome. *Acta Neurologica Scandinavica, 54,* 359–365.

Waber, D. (1979). Neuropsychological aspects of Turner syndrome. *Developmental Medicine and Child Neurology, 21,* 58–70.

Wechsler, D. (1991). *Wechsler Intelligence Scale for Children* (3rd ed.). New York: Psychological Corporation.

Williams, C. L., & Meck, W. H. (1991). The organizational effects of gonadal hormones on sexually dimorphic spatial ability. *Psychoneuroendocrinology, 16,* 155–176.

Williams, J., Richman, L., & Yarbrough, D. (1991). A comparison of memory and attention in Turner syndrome and learning disability. *Journal of Pediatric Psychology, 16,* 585–593.

Wilson, J. D., & Foster, D. W. (Eds.). (1985). *Williams textbook of endocrinology* (7th ed.). Philadelphia: Saunders.

Zinn, A., Page, D., & Fisher, E. (1993). Turner syndrome: The case of the missing sex chromosome. *Trends in Genetics, 9,* 90–93.

Female Sexual Orientation and Pubertal Onset

Wendy N. Tenhula and J. Michael Bailey
Department of Psychology
Northwestern University

Both sexual orientation and pubertal onset are sexually dimorphic. Biologic theories of sexual orientation emphasize the role of early androgens in sexual differentiation of partner preference. If homosexual individuals have been subject to atypical androgenizing influences, such influences may also affect other sexually dimorphic traits, such as pubertal timing. Based on this rationale as well as promising evidence from a prior twin study, we examined the onset of puberty in lesbians. We hypothesized that lesbians would have a later (i.e., more masculine) age of pubertal onset compared to heterosexual women. We investigated this hypothesis in a sample of community volunteers and a second sample of discordant twins. Contrary to our hypothesis, we found no significant differences in pubertal onset between homosexual and heterosexual women.

Human sexual orientation is highly sexually dimorphic, with the vast majority of men preferring female partners, and women preferring male partners (Diamond, 1993). Pubertal timing is also sexually dimorphic, with girls experiencing puberty on average 2 years earlier than boys (Kulin & Müller, 1996; Wheeler, 1991). The sexual differentiation of neither sexual orientation nor pubertal timing in humans is well understood. However, indirect evidence suggests that both may be influenced by the organizational effects of prenatal androgens (e.g., Herbosa & Foster, 1996; LeVay, 1991). If so, then individuals who have been subject to atypical prenatal androgenization may be atypical both in their sexual orientation and in their pubertal onset. For example, lesbians may have masculine (i.e., relatively late)

Requests for reprints should be sent to J. Michael Bailey, Department of Psychology, Northwestern University, Evanston, IL 60208. E-mail: jm-bailey@nwu.edu

pubertal onset compared with other women; gay men may have feminine (i.e., relatively early) pubertal onset compared with other men.

In the study reported herein, we examined pubertal onset in lesbians and heterosexual women. Before we report our study, we review some research concerning the role of prenatal androgens in sexual differentiation of both sexual orientation and pubertal timing, as well as evidence that homosexual people have sex-atypical pubertal onset.

NEUROHORMONAL ASPECTS OF SEXUAL ORIENTATION

Much recent attention has focused on the possibility that sexual orientation is influenced by innate processes (Gladue, 1994; Hamer & Copeland, 1994; LeVay, 1993). The most prominent biological theory of sexual orientation (which we refer to as the *neuroendocrine theory*) specifies that sexual orientation toward females occurs if androgens masculinize relevant brain structures, and orientation toward males develops if those structures are not androgenized (Ellis & Ames, 1987; Meyer-Bahlburg, 1979, 1984). Androgenizing processes are hypothesized to account for both between-sex and within-sex differences in sexual orientation. Like observable sex differences in gross morphology, such as genitalia, sex differences in sexual orientation are hypothesized to result from differences in the amount of androgens present during early, probably prenatal, developmental periods. Within-sex differences in sexual orientation might result either from differences in circulating prenatal androgens during the relevant critical period or from insensitivity of relevant tissue to the effects of androgens.

Several lines of research have been pursued in an attempt to delineate the neurohormonal processes that may be related to homosexuality. For example, studies have investigated behavioral outcomes resulting from hormonal manipulations in nonhuman animals, sexual behaviors in humans exposed to unusual hormonal environments, neuroanatomic correlates of sexual orientation, and sexually dimorphic characteristics in humans. This study is an example of the latter approach, in which we studied a sexually dimorphic characteristic believed to be influenced by hormonal factors, and that theory and prior evidence suggest may be related to sexual orientation. Specifically, we investigated the relation between sexual orientation and the timing of the onset of puberty in women. Before reporting our findings, we briefly summarize the research relevant to the neuroendocrine theory of sexual orientation.

One source of support for the neuroendocrine theory of sexual orientation has been research on the effects of hormones on sexual behavior in nonhuman animals. This work, which has primarily focused on rodents, has shown clearly that sex-typical behavior patterns depend on the organizing effects of early androgens. Depriving a genetic male rat of androgens during the first 2 to 3 days of postnatal life will lead to a substantial increase in female-typical sexual behavior (lordosis) and a decrease in male-typical sexual behavior (mounting) in adulthood (Gorski, 1987). Similarly, giving a neonatal genetic female rat high levels of androgens will lead, with appropriate hormonal priming, to high levels of mounting in adulthood (Gorski, 1987). There are, however, limits to the analogy between human sexual orientation and sex-typicality of rat mating behavior. Most important, differences in human sexual orientation are not directly analogous to the mounting–lordosis dimension in rodents, which limits the utility of the latter findings as support for a neuroendocrine model of human sexual orientation (Adkins-Regan, 1988; Byne & Parsons, 1993; Meyer-Bahlburg, 1984). On the other hand, researchers examining behavior more akin to sexual orientation (e.g., whether an adult elects to spend more of its time with a same-sex or opposite-sex conspecific) have also found that organizational hormonal effects are important (e.g., Baum, Kornberg, Erskine, & Weaver, 1990).

Another line of evidence for the neuroendocrine hypothesis includes studies of women who have been exposed to unusual patterns of hormones in utero. The most extensively studied condition has been congenital adrenal hyperplasia (CAH). Females with CAH are exposed to high levels of androgens in utero, and thus are often born with varying degrees of masculinized genitalia. The large majority of these women now have their genitalia surgically feminized in infancy and are treated with ongoing hormonal therapy. The neuroendocrine theory of sexual orientation should predict an increase in homosexuality among CAH women due to the effects of prenatal exposure to androgens on the developing brain. Most studies have found elevated rates of bisexual feelings among such women (Dittmann et al., 1992; Ehrhardt, Evers, & Money, 1968; Money, Schwartz, & Lewis, 1984; Zucker et al., 1996), although two studies did not (Lev-Ran, 1974; Mulaikal, Migeon, & Rock, 1987). In the most recent and most detailed report, for example, Zucker et al. (1996) found elevated rates of (infrequent) bisexual feelings compared with controls. In all studies, however, the majority of CAH women reported exclusively heterosexual feelings and behavior (Berenbaum, 1990).

Other support for the neuroendocrine theory has come from the study of women prenatally exposed to diethylstilbestrol (DES), which has been shown to have masculinizing effects in female mammals. One study found elevated rates of bisexual and homosexual feelings compared with controls (Meyer-Bahlburg et al., 1995). Similar to studies of CAH, however, the majority of participants were strictly heterosexual.

Less direct evidence for a neuroendocrine hypothesis includes findings that gay men's brains are similar to women's in certain respects (Allen & Gorski, 1992; LeVay, 1991). LeVay (1991) found that the third interstitial nucleus of the anterior hypothalamus was less than half as large in heterosexual women and homosexual men as in heterosexual men. Allen and Gorski (1992) found a sex and sexual orientation difference in the anterior commissure of the corpus callosum. Although the anterior commissure is not thought to be directly related to sexual behavior, it may reflect generalized effects of neurohormonal influences that do affect the areas of the brain directly related to sexual orientation.

If homosexual people have been subject to atypical patterns of brain androgenization, it is likely that those influences affected other sexually dimorphic traits as well. That is, gay men should be more feminine, and lesbians more masculine, in respects other than sexual orientation. Studies of childhood sex-typed behavior have uniformly confirmed this general prediction. On average, gay men and lesbians were sex-atypical as children in their play patterns, interests, and in some cases, gender identity (Bailey & Zucker, 1995; Green, 1987). On the other hand, not all sexually dimorphic characteristics covary with sexual orientation. For instance, homosexual individuals of both sexes have sex-typical genitalia. Sexually dimorphic characteristics will covary with sexual orientation if their development is affected by overlapping processes. This could happen if a particular characteristic had the same critical period of development as sexual orientation, or if its development depended on the same tissue. Traits investigated using this rationale have included spatial ability (e.g., Gladue & Bailey, 1995b), aggression (e.g., Gladue & Bailey, 1995a), occupational interests (e.g., Bailey, Finkel, & Bailey, 1996), dermatoglyphic asymmetry (e.g., Hall & Kimura, 1994), and biodemographic variables such as pubertal timing (e.g., Blanchard & Bogaert, 1996). At this point, theories of neither sexual orientation nor most other sexually dimorphic characteristics are sufficiently well specified to make strong predictions about which particular sexually dimorphic characteristics will be associated with sexual orientation.

PUBERTAL ONSET

Physical changes that occur at puberty are preceded by changes in hormone levels. The hormonal modulation system that controls timing of the onset of pubertal events differentiates prenatally and then is suppressed until puberty (Petersen & Brooks-Gunn, 1988; Thomas & Rebar, 1989), but little is known about the mechanism that regulates this process in humans. Studies of nonhuman primates suggest that female pubertal onset depends on the maturation of the neuroendocrine control system directing the pulsatile secretion of gonadotropin-releasing hormone from the hypothalamus (Wildt, Knobil, & Marshall, 1980).

Studies of nonhuman species have also suggested that sex differences in pubertal timing are influenced by organizational androgens. For example, the timing of puberty onset in sheep (and many other seasonal breeders) is dependent on day length (photoperiod) in females but not in males. Early androgens defeminize the female reproductive response to photoperiod (Herbosa & Foster, 1996). On the other hand, we know of no evidence that early-treated CAH is associated with later puberty in females, and a study of DES-exposed women found such women to have similar ages of menarche compared with unexposed women (Hines & Shipley, 1984).

SEXUAL ORIENTATION AND PUBERTAL TIMING

Because pubertal timing appears to depend on neural structures that differentiate prenatally, it is reasonable to study whether homosexual people have sex-atypical pubertal onsets. That is, according to the neuroendocrine theory, homosexual men would be expected to have earlier puberties and homosexual women later puberties. One difficulty with studying the timing of pubertal development is that puberty is an ongoing process rather than a discrete event that can easily be measured or recalled precisely. This is particularly problematic with respect to men, for whom no signal event, such as menarche, is correlated strongly with pubertal developmental rate. Moreover, it is often necessary to rely on retrospective reporting of events that occurred years earlier. Nevertheless, there is some evidence that homosexual men undergo sexual development earlier than heterosexual men and recall experiencing the milestones of puberty (e.g., first ejaculation, voice change, sexual feelings) earlier than heterosexual men (e.g., Blanchard & Bogaert, 1996; Manosevitz, 1970, 1972; Saghir & Robins, 1973; Stephan, 1973; Tripp, 1982).

In women, these issues are less problematic, because the markers of pubertal development are more distinctive and are believed to be more salient for girls than for boys (Brooks-Gunn & Petersen, 1984). However, the association between sexual orientation and pubertal onset has been studied less systematically for females than for males. There is some evidence consistent with a neuroendocrine prediction. In a report on four monozygotic (MZ) twin pairs separated at birth and discordant for sexual orientation (i.e., one is homosexual and one is heterosexual), the lesbian twins began menstruating 2 years later than their heterosexual twins, on average, and were later in all four cases (Eckert, Bouchard, Bohlen, & Heston, 1986). Even adjusted for small sample size, the estimated effect size was large (1.4). This is a remarkable difference because identical twins reared together typically reach menarche within a few months of each other (Fischbein, 1977). Less direct evidence includes findings that both lesbians (Bailey & Zucker, 1995) and late-maturing girls (Jones & Mussen, 1958) are less stereotypically sex-typed than early maturers. For example, many lesbians recall being tomboys, preferring to play with boys, and disliking sex-stereotypic activities and clothing.

An alternative theory relating homosexuality to pubertal timing was proposed by Storms (1981). He suggested that early maturers of either sex are more likely to develop a homosexual "erotic orientation" because their sexual interest develops at a time in their lives when most friendships are with members of the same sex (homosocial groups). Like the neuroendocrine theory, Storms's theory predicts earlier pubertal onset in gay men. However, in contrast to the neuroendocrine theory, Storms's theory should predict that homosexual women would have experienced pubertal events earlier than a heterosexual control group. Some existing evidence suggests that Storms's theory is unlikely to hold for females. Early-maturing girls have a tendency to date earlier and show more interest in heterosexual relationships than on-time or late-maturing girls (Simmons & Blyth, 1987).

The studies reported here were designed to investigate the timing of puberty in homosexual and heterosexual women. In accordance with the neuroendocrine theory, we predicted that homosexual women would report having experienced their first menstrual period and other pubertal events later in life than heterosexual women. In Study 1, we examined the association of sexual orientation and the timing of the onset of puberty in a relatively large sample of community volunteers. In Study 2, we compared the pubertal timing of twins discordant for sexual orientation.

STUDY 1

Method

Participants. Heterosexual and homosexual women were recruited using advertisements in a free alternative newspaper. Additional homosexual participants were recruited through advertisements in gay and lesbian publications. Separate advertisements were placed for each sexual orientation group. Aside from the sexual orientation specified in each ad, the advertisements were identical, requesting individuals 20 to 40 years of age to participate in a study of personality, cognitive abilities, interests, and sexual behavior. This restricted age range was used due to constraints regarding other hypotheses being tested in the study. Participants were paid $20 each for their participation.

Participants were assigned to either the homosexual or heterosexual groups according to self-identification. Those who considered themselves to be homosexual/lesbian or bisexual were assigned to the homosexual group. These self-reports were confirmed by more detailed assessments (see Bailey, Gaulin, Agyei, & Gladue, 1994, for additional information). The final sample included 91 homosexual women and 74 heterosexual women.

The homosexual participants ($M = 28.9$, $SD = 5.9$) were older than the heterosexual participants ($M = 25.1$, $SD = 4.6$), $t(162) = 4.56$, $p < .01$, but age was uncorrelated with any of the variables of interest. The sample was 72% White, 15% African American, 3% Hispanic, 3% Asian, and 7% of unspecified ethnicity. Ethnicity did not differ significantly between homosexual and heterosexual groups. The educational levels of the two groups were comparable, $t(162) = 1.64$, $p = .09$.

Procedures. Timing of the onset of puberty was assessed using a 15-item questionnaire that included questions about the age and school grade when significant pubertal events (e.g., menarche, breast development, and body hair growth) occurred. Participants also rated their perception of the relative timing of these events and of their overall pubertal development compared with their peers. For these ratings, a 5-point rating scale was used: 1 (*much earlier;* more than 2 years), 2 (*somewhat earlier;* between 6 months and 2 years), 3 (*same time;* within 6 months), 4 (*somewhat later;* between 6 months and 2 years), and 5 (*much later;* more than 2 years).

Retrospective reports of age at menarche are reliable and valid over long periods of time. Damon and Bajema (1974) found a correlation of .60 between actual and recalled time of menarche after 39 years. Other studies have found higher correlations for briefer periods of recall (Damon, Damon, Reed, & Valadian, 1969; Livson & McNeil, 1962). Dubas, Graber, and Petersen (1991) found that individuals' memories of pubertal timing were more accurate by 12th grade than they had been several years earlier. We know of no studies of the accuracy of recall of other pubertal events such as breast development, growth of underarm and pubic hair, or wearing a bra. These items were included to increase the reliability (by aggregation) of retrospective reports of pubertal timing.

Results

A principal factor analysis was performed on the responses to the puberty questionnaire. A scree test indicated that there was one general puberty factor, and this factor accounted for 43.9% of the items' variance. Items with factor loadings of at least .7 were standardized and combined into a single scale. These items included age of menarche, school grade at the time of menarche, age at the beginning of breast development, school grade at the time breast development began, age and school grade when the participant began wearing a bra, and overall rating of pubertal timing relative to peers. In addition, the two individual items concerning menarche were analyzed separately, because it is plausible that memories are much more accurate for menarche than for other milestones.

The mean age of menarche for the participants in Study 1 was 12.7 years (SD = 1.5). There was a trend for lesbians to recall earlier menarche (by 0.4 years) than heterosexual women, $t(160) = 1.79$, $p = .08$. Scores on the general puberty scale for homosexual and heterosexual women did not differ significantly, $t(160) = -0.63$, ns. None of the other items (either those included in the scale or those, such as pubic hair development, that were not included) yielded a significant difference (Table 1).

TABLE 1
Age of Onset for Pubertal Events

	Heterosexual		Homosexual		
Variable	M	SD	M	SD	t^a
Age at first period	12.9	1.3	12.5	1.7	−1.79
Grade at first period	7.4	1.5	7.1	1.6	−1.43
Age at first breast development	11.7	1.8	11.6	1.8	−0.13
Grade at first breast development	6.4	1.8	7.2	2.4	0.76
Age began wearing bra	12.0	1.3	11.9	1.6	−0.51
Grade began wearing bra	6.7	1.5	6.7	1.6	0.10
Overall development compared to peers[b]	3.0	0.9	3.0	0.9	−0.10

[a] all $p > .05$, two-tailed test. [b] 1 (*much earlier*; more than 2 years), 2 (*somewhat earlier*; between 6 months and 2 years), 3 (*same time*; within 6 months), 4 (*somewhat later*; between 6 months and 2 years), 5 (*much later*; more than 2 years).

STUDY 2

Method

Participants. In order to recruit participants for Study 2, we recontacted female twins who had participated in a previous study in our laboratory on the heritability of female sexual orientation (Bailey, Pillard, Neale, & Agyei, 1993). For the previous study, we advertised for lesbians with twin sisters, ensuring that at least one member of each twin pair was a lesbian (the proband). Each proband was then asked for permission to contact her twin.

Zygosity of the twin pairs was determined using the questionnaire developed by Nichols and Bilbro (1966). Sexual orientation of the probands was determined on the basis of their sexual identities, which must have been either lesbian or bisexual to meet initial criteria, and was confirmed by their combined Kinsey fantasy and behavior ratings (Kinsey, Pomeroy, & Martin, 1948; Kinsey, Pomeroy, Martin, & Gebhard, 1953), which must have been at least a score of 2 (indicating strong bisexual feelings). Sexual orientation of the cotwins was assessed in two ways. First, probands were asked what they believed their twin's sexual orientation to be and how certain they were of their assessment. Second, the cotwins who were contacted were asked to rate themselves as homosexual/lesbian, heterosexual, or bisexual and to give their combined Kinsey fantasy and behavior ratings. There was a very close correspondence between probands' reports of twins' sexual orientations and the twins' self-reports. Thus, even when probands' twins did not participate, we still had good estimates of their sexual orientations. This allowed us to use some of the data provided by probands about their twins, even in cases when the twin did not respond.

Procedures. Probands and cooperating cotwins from the previous twin study were sent pubertal timing questionnaires. This questionnaire was identical to the one used in Study 1 except that the participants in Study 2 were also asked to compare the relative timing of their own pubertal events to their twin sisters'. Each of these items was rated on a 5-point Likert-type scale with the following assigned values: 1 (*much earlier;* more than 1 year), 2 (*somewhat earlier;* between 3 months and 1 year, 3 (*same time;* within 3 months), 4 (*somewhat later;* between 3 months and 1 year), and 5 (*much later;* more than 1 year).

Results

Recruitment results. Fifty-one (44.7%) probands and 45 twins (48.4%) returned their questionnaires. Thirty-seven pairs of twins both returned questionnaires, so we had at least some data from 57 twin pairs. The primary data of interest were from those twin pairs who were discordant for sexual orientation (i.e., twin pairs in which the cotwin was heterosexual). Fifty-four percent (19 of 35) of the MZ cotwins were heterosexual and 86% (19 of 22) of the dizygotic (DZ) cotwins were heterosexual. We had at least partial data (i.e., at least one twin's data) from 19 discordant MZ pairs and 19 discordant DZ pairs, and complete data from 12 discordant MZ pairs and 9 discordant DZ pairs.

Correlational findings. Among all the MZ twin pairs from whom we had complete data, the correlation between the reported age of the proband's first period and the reported age of the cotwin's first period was .69 (95% confidence interval, .20–.91). Among the DZ twin pairs who both returned their questionnaires, menarcheal age correlated .71 (95% confidence interval, .09–.93). For both MZ and DZ twin pairs there also were significant correlations between probands' scores and cotwins' scores on the general puberty factor (MZ: $r = .79, p < .01$; DZ: $r = .75, p < .05$). Although in our sample, MZ pairs were not more similar than DZ pairs, confidence intervals on our twin correlations were sufficiently wide to be consistent with substantial heritability.

Because the twins also provided estimates of their pubertal onset relative to their twin sisters, this gave us the opportunity to investigate the validity of those memories. Sisters' responses to the comparison items were negatively correlated. That is, proband reports that they experienced milestones earlier than their twin sisters tended to be accompanied by sisters' reports that they experienced such milestones later than the probands: for menarche, $r = -.57, p < .01$; for age at which the participants began to wear bras to school, $r = -.47, p < .01$; for age at which the participants first began to notice body hair, $r = -.53, p < .01$; and for rate of general pubertal development, $r = -.47, p < .01$. These correlations supported the validity of the comparison ratings made by one twin about the relative timing of her sister's pubertal development relative to her own development.

Comparison of pubertal timing among discordant twin pairs. In considering the pubertal timing of the twin pairs, we first present the findings for MZ pairs who were discordant for sexual orientation followed by the findings for discordant DZ pairs. Any differences between homosexual and heterosexual MZ twins on measures of pubertal timing reflect environmental differences because MZ twins are genetically identical. Differences between homosexual and heterosexual DZ twins can be indicative of either genetic or environmental differences. Finally, we also consider together the data for both MZ and DZ twins who were discordant for sexual orientation. If a difference between homosexual and heterosexual twins reflects difference in prenatal hormonal factors, it should exist whether the twin pairs are MZ or DZ.

The 12 MZ twin pairs who were discordant for homosexuality and who both returned their questionnaires showed a nonsignificant trend for the lesbian member of the pair to report an older menarche (by .44 years) than their sisters, paired $t(11) = 1.8$, *ns*. This is opposite to the trend seen in the nontwin participants. There were no differences between the discordant MZ twins on any of the other puberty variables.

For the DZ probands who had heterosexual twins, the mean age of menarche was 12.5 years ($SD = 1.5$). The respective figure for their twins was 12.6 years ($SD = 1.4$). For the nine pairs of discordant DZ twins who both returned their questionnaires, this mean difference of 0.1 years was not significant, paired $t(8) = -.27$, *ns*. There was also not a difference between the probands and cotwins on the general puberty factor, paired $t(8) = 0.21$, *ns*. Among the discordant DZ pairs there was a significant difference such that the heterosexual cotwins reported that they began wearing a bra to school earlier than the probands reported—for age, paired $t(8) = 3.0$, $p < .01$; for grade, paired $t(8) = 4.74$, $p < .01$—but there were no other differences between the probands and their heterosexual DZ twins on any of the other pubertal timing variables. Thus, the discordant DZ twins reported experiencing the developmental milestones of puberty at about the same time as each other with the exception of the age and grade at which they began wearing a bra.

When the data from MZ and DZ pairs discordant for sexual orientation were combined, the mean reported age of menarche for the lesbian probands was 12.9 years ($SD = 1.4$). For the heterosexual twins the mean reported age of menarche was 12.7 years ($SD = 1.2$). This difference of 0.2 years was not significant, paired $t(20) = 0.66$, *ns*. There was no significant difference on the general puberty factor or on any of the items contributing to it (see Table 2).

In a final set of analyses, we examined the items that explicitly asked participants to compare their pubertal timing with that of their twin sisters. We rescaled probands' responses so that for both lesbian probands and their heterosexual sisters, higher scores indicated that the proband was later. For each discordant pair, we averaged twins' ratings when both were available. When only one twin's ratings were available, we used hers because sisters showed reasonable interrater reliability

TABLE 2
Timing of Puberty in 21 Discordant Twin Pairs

Variable	Proband		Twin		Paired t^a
	M	SD	M	SD	
Age at first period	12.9	1.4	12.7	1.2	1.00
Grade at first period	7.1	1.4	7.3	1.3	−0.40
Age at breast development	11.9	2.0	11.5	1.7	0.96
Grade at breast development	6.6	1.9	6.2	1.7	0.55
Age began wearing bra	12.3	1.5	12.0	1.3	1.71
Grade began wearing bra	6.9	1.6	6.7	1.4	1.70
Overall development compared to peers[b]	3.3	1.0	3.0	0.8	1.55

[a]all $p > .05$, two-tailed test. [b]1 (*much earlier*; more than 2 years), 2 (*somewhat earlier*; between 6 months and 2 years), 3 (*same time*; within 6 months), 4 (*somewhat later*; between 6 months and 2 years), 5 (*much later*; more than 2 years).

on these items. Scores of 3 indicated that sisters experienced relevant events simultaneously. Thus, we tested the difference between the average ratings from 3, across the discordant pairs. We did this for both the rate of general pubertal development and menarche, for discordant MZ twins, DZ twins, and combined MZ and DZ twins. Although consistent with our hypothesis all average ratings exceeded 3, none did so significantly. For general pubertal development, MZ, DZ, and combined groups' means were, respectively, 3.2, $t(15) = 1.2$, *ns;* 3.4, $t(17) = 1.5$, *ns;* and 3.3, $t(33) = 1.8$, *ns*. For menarche, they were 3.2, $t(17) = 1.3$, *ns;* 3.1, $t(18) = 0.4$, *ns;* and 3.2, $t(36) = 1.0$, *ns*.

GENERAL DISCUSSION

The purpose of this study was to investigate hypotheses about hormonal influence on both sexual orientation and pubertal onset by examining their covariation in women. We hypothesized, based on the neuroendocrine theory of sexual orientation and previous empirical evidence, that homosexual women would report delayed onset of puberty relative to heterosexual women. Study 1 examined a large sample of self-identified lesbian women and compared their retrospective reports of pubertal timing to women who identified themselves as heterosexual. Study 2 investigated reports of pubertal timing in a sample of lesbian probands who have twin sisters who are heterosexual.

Contrary to our prediction, there was no significant difference in the overall timing of puberty between lesbians and heterosexual women in either discordant twin pairs or in nontwin participants. Homosexual twins reported having started their periods slightly, but not significantly, later than their heterosexual identical twin sisters. On the other hand, the nontwin lesbians in our sample showed a nonsignificant trend to have started their periods earlier than the heterosexual controls. This difference was a nonsignificant trend and was opposite to our prediction.

One methodological concern regarding our results is the retrospective reporting of pubertal events. The timing of puberty may be difficult to measure because pubertal development is an ongoing process rather than a discrete event (Blanchard & Bogaert, 1996; Bogaert & Blanchard, 1996). However, we attempted to avoid this potential problem by asking about specific discrete events that should be easier to recall. This is especially true for menarche. Longitudinal studies have shown a correlation of 0.60 between reported and actual age of first period up to 39 years after menarche.

The average age of menarche in developed countries has gradually declined during the 20th century. This trend seems to have leveled off in the past 2 decades (Gerver, DeBruin, & Drayer, 1994). Even if this were the case, however, one would expect older participants to report having experienced puberty at later ages than younger participants. Because the lesbian participants in our large nontwin sample were on average 3.7 years older than the female heterosexual participants, the trend for lesbians in that sample to start their periods at younger ages cannot be attributed to such a cohort effect. Also, age was not significantly correlated with any of the other puberty variables (all correlations .10 or less), which suggests that any cohort effect on the age of menarche is small within the age ranges of our sample.

Another potential concern is ascertainment bias. Neither the probands for the twin study nor the participants for the nontwin study were obtained through systematic sampling. However, because pubertal timing was not mentioned in the advertisements or on the phone at the time of scheduling, it is unlikely that this aspect of the study would have affected the pattern of participation of one group of individuals differently from the other or that the data would be systematically biased due to sampling fluctuations.

Another methodological concern is statistical power. The sample size of the twin study, especially, was not large. However, the nontwin sample was large enough to detect a moderate effect, and furthermore, our twin sample was substantially larger than that of Eckert et al. (1986), who were able to detect a significant difference in pubertal timing between MZ twins discordant for sexual orientation. Even restricting our sample to discordant MZ twins, we had statistical power of greater than .80 to detect an effect size as large as that implied by the earlier twin study (Eckert et al., 1986).

Our results do not support any theory, either biological or psychological, that links sexual differentiation of puberty timing and sexual orientation. For example, they do not support a neuroendocrine theory in which both sexual orientation and pubertal timing are influenced by the same prenatal events. Nor do they support Storms's (1981) theory of erotic orientation development.

The failure to find a difference between heterosexual and homosexual women on the timing of the onset of puberty does not necessarily mean that sexual orientation in women is unaffected by hormonal processes. It is possible that the neurohormonal processes that affect sexual orientation are different from those that affect the timing of the onset of puberty. For instance, hormonal differences associated with pubertal development and sexual orientation may occur during developmentally distinct phases of fetal development. If this is the case, sexual orientation would not be expected to be associated with pubertal timing.

Thus, although the findings of the studies reported here do not provide additional support for the current formulation of the neuroendocrine theory of sexual orientation, they also do not provide strong evidence against it. It is quite possible that lesbianism is caused by an androgenizing process that may also affect other sexually dimorphic characteristics, but leaves pubertal timing intact. It is clear that lesbians are not masculinized on all sexually dimorphic traits, as they have sex-typical genitalia, which is the most obvious sexually dimorphic characteristic. Future research should examine other sexually dimorphic physical and psychological traits to see if they are associated with either sexual orientation or pubertal timing. Such research can contribute to a better understanding of sexual differentiation, and specifically, overlap and independence in sexual differentiating processes.

REFERENCES

Adkins-Regan, E. (1988). Sex hormones and sexual orientation in animals. *Psychobiology, 16,* 335–347.

Allen, L. S., & Gorski, R. A. (1992). Sexual orientation and the size of the anterior commissure of the human brain. *Proceedings of the National Academy of Sciences, 89,* 7199–7202.

Bailey, J. M., Finkel, E., & Bailey, T. (1996). *Masculinity, femininity, and sexual orientation.* Manuscript submitted for publication.

Bailey, J. M., Gaulin, S., Agyei, Y., & Gladue, B. A. (1994). Effects of gender and sexual orientation on evolutionarily relevant aspects of human mating psychology. *Journal of Personality and Social Psychology, 66,* 1081–1093.

Bailey, J. M., Pillard, R. C., Neale, M. C., & Agyei, Y. (1993). Heritable factors influence sexual orientation in women. *Archives of General Psychiatry, 50,* 217–223.

Bailey, J. M., & Zucker, K. J. (1995). Childhood sex-typed behavior and sexual orientation: A conceptual analysis and quantitative review. *Developmental Psychology, 31,* 43–55.

Baum, J. M., Kornberg, E., Erskine, M. S., & Weaver, C. E. (1990). Prenatal and neonatal testosterone exposure interact to affect differentiation of sexual behavior and partner preference in female ferrets. *Behavioral Neuroscience, 104,* 183–198.

Berenbaum, S. A. (1990). Congenital adrenal hyperplasia: Intellectual and psychosexual functioning. In C. Holmes (Ed.), *Psychoneuroendocrinology: Brain, behavior, and hormonal interactions* (pp. 227–260). New York: Springer-Verlag.

Blanchard, R., & Bogaert, A. F. (1996). Biodemographic comparisons of homosexual and heterosexual men in the Kinsey interview data. *Archives of Sexual Behavior, 25,* 551–579.

Blanchard, R., & Bogaert, A. F. (in press). Biodemographic comparisons of homosexual and heterosexual men in the Kinsey interview data. *Archives of Sexual Behavior.*

Bogaert, A. F., & Blanchard, R. (1996). Physical development and sexual orientation in men: Height, weight, and age of puberty differences. *Personality and Individual Differences, 21,* 77–84.
Brooks-Gunn, J., & Petersen, A. C. (1984). Problems in studying and defining pubertal events. *Journal of Youth and Adolescence, 13,* 181–196.
Byne, W., & Parsons, B. (1993). Human sexual orientation: The biologic theories reappraised. *Archives of General Psychiatry, 50,* 228–239.
Damon, A., & Bajema, C. J. (1974). Age at menarche: Accuracy of recall after thirty nine years. *Human Biology, 46,* 381–384.
Damon, A., Damon, S. T., Reed, R. B., & Valadian, I. (1969). Age at menarche of mothers and daughters, with a note on accuracy of recall. *Human Biology, 41,* 161–185.
Diamond, M. (1993). Homosexuality and bisexuality in different populations. *Archives of Sexual Behavior, 22,* 291–310.
Dittman, R. W., Kappes, M. E., & Kappes, M. H. (1992). Sexual behavior in adolescent and adult females with congenital adrenal hyperplasia. *Psychoneuroendocrinology, 17,* 153–170.
Dubas, J. S., Graber, J. A., & Petersen, A. C. (1991). A longitudinal investigation of adolescents' changing perceptions of pubertal timing. *Developmental Psychology, 27,* 580–586.
Eckert, E. D., Bouchard, T. J., Bohlen, J., & Heston, L. L. (1986). Homosexuality in monozygotic twins reared apart. *British Journal of Psychiatry, 148,* 421–425.
Ehrhardt, A. A., Evers, L., & Money, J. (1968). Influence of androgen and some aspects of sexually dimorphic behavior in women with the late-treated androgenital syndrome. *Johns Hopkins Medical Journal, 123,* 115–122.
Ellis, L., & Ames, M. A. (1987). Neurohormonal functioning and sexual orientation: A theory of homosexuality-heterosexuality. *Psychological Bulletin, 101,* 233–258.
Fischbein, S. (1977). Onset of puberty in MZ and DZ twins. *Acta Geneticae et Gemallogiae, 24,* 15–30.
Gerver, W. J., DeBruin, R., & Drayer, N. M. (1994). A persisting secular trend for body measurements in Dutch children. The Oosterwolde II Study. *Acta Pediatrica, 83,* 812–814.
Gladue, B. A. (1994). The biopsychology of sexual orientation. *Current Directions in Psychological Science, 3,* 150–154.
Gladue, B. A., & Bailey, J. M. (1995a). Aggressiveness, competitiveness, and human sexual orientation. *Psychoneuroendocrinology, 20,* 475–485.
Gladue, B. A., & Bailey, J. M. (1995b). Spatial ability, handedness, and human sexual orientation. *Psychoneuroendocrinology, 20,* 487–497.
Gorski, R. A. (1987). Sex differences in the rodent brain. In J. M. Reinisch, L. A. Rosenblum, & S. A. Sanders (Eds.), *Masculinity/femininity: Basic perspectives* (pp. 37–67). New York: Oxford University Press.
Green, R. (1987). *The "sissy boy syndrome" and the development of homosexuality.* New Haven, CT: Yale University Press.
Hall, J. A., & Kimura, D. (1994). Dermatoglyphic asymmetry and sexual orientation in men. *Behavioral Neuroscience, 108,* 1203–1206.
Hamer, D. H., & Copeland, P. (1994). *The science of desire: The search for the gay gene and the biology of behavior.* New York: Simon & Schuster.
Herbosa, C. G., & Foster, D. L. (1996). Defeminization of the reproductive response to photoperiod occurs early in prenatal development in the sheep. *Biology of Reproduction, 54,* 420–428.
Hines, M., & Shipley, C. (1984). Prenatal exposure to diethylstilbestrol (DES) and the development of sexually dimorphic cognitive abilities and cerebral lateralization. *Developmental Psychology, 20,* 81–94.
Jones, M. C., & Mussen, P. H. (1958). Self-conceptions, motivations, and interpersonal attitudes of early- and late-maturing girls. *Child Development, 29,* 491–501.
Kinsey, A. C., Pomeroy, W. B., & Martin, C. E. (1948). *Sexual behavior in the human male.* Philadelphia: Saunders.

Kinsey, A. C., Pomeroy, W. B., Martin, C. E., & Gebhard, P. H. (1953). *Sexual behavior in the human female*. Philadelphia: Saunders.
Kulin, H. E., & Müller, J. (1996). The biological aspects of puberty. *Pediatrics in Review, 17,* 75–86.
LeVay, S. (1991). A difference in hypothalamic structure between heterosexual and homosexual men. *Science, 253,* 1034–1037.
LeVay, S. (1993). *The sexual brain*. Cambridge, MA: MIT Press.
Lev-Ran, A. (1974). Gender role differentiation in hermaphrodites. *Archives of Sexual Behavior, 3,* 391.
Livson, N., & McNeil, D. (1962). The accuracy of recalled age of menarche. *Human Biology, 34,* 218–221.
Manosevitz, M. (1970). Early sexual behaviors in adult homosexual and heterosexual males. *Journal of Abnormal Psychology, 76,* 396–402.
Manosevitz, M. (1972). The development of male homosexuality. *Journal of Sex Research, 8,* 31–40.
Meyer-Bahlburg, H. F. L. (1979). Sex hormones and female homosexuality: A critical examination. *Archives of Sexual Behavior, 8,* 101–119.
Meyer-Bahlburg, H. F. L. (1984). Psychoendocrine research on sexual orientation. Current status and future options. In G. J. DeVries, J. P. C. De Bruin, H. M. B. Uylings, & M. A. Corner (Eds.), *Progress in brain research* (Vol. 61, pp. 375–398). Amsterdam: Elsevier.
Meyer-Bahlburg, H. F. L., Ehrhardt, A. A., Rosen, L. R., Gruen, R. S., Veridiano, N. P., Vann, F. H., & Neuwalder, H. F. (1995). Prenatal estrogens and the development of homosexual orientation. *Developmental Psychology, 31,* 12–21.
Money, J., Schwartz, M., & Lewis, V. G. (1984). Adult erotosexual status and fetal hormonal masculinization and demasculinization. *Psychoneuroendocrinology, 9,* 405–414.
Mulaikal, R. M., Migeon, C. J., & Rock, J. A. (1987). Fertility rates in female patients with congenital adrenal hyperplasia due to 21-hydroxylase deficiency. *The New England Journal of Medicine, 316,* 178–182.
Nichols, R. C., & Bilbro, W. C. (1966). The diagnosis of twin zygosity. *Acta Genetica Statistica, 16,* 265–275.
Petersen, A. C., & Brooks-Gunn, J. (1988). Puberty and adolescence. In E. A. Blechman & K. D. Brownell (Eds.), *Handbook of behavioral medicine for women* (pp. 12–27). New York: Pergamon.
Saghir, M. T., & Robins, E. (1973). *Male and female homosexuality*. Baltimore: Williams & Wilkins.
Simmons, R. G., Burgeson, R., Carlton-Ford, S., & Blyth, D. A. (1987). The impact of cumulative change in early adolescence. *Child Development, 58,* 1220–1234.
Stephan, W. G. (1973). Parental relationships and early social experiences of activist male homosexuals and male heterosexuals. *Journal of Abnormal Psychology, 82,* 506–513.
Storms, M. D. (1981). A theory of erotic orientation development. *Psychological Review, 88,* 340–353.
Thomas, M. A., & Rebar, R. W. (1989). The endocrinology of normal and abnormal female puberty. *Current Opinion in Obstetrics & Gynecology, 1,* 259–265.
Tripp, C. A. (1982). Tripp's answer to Bell, Weinberg & Hammersmith's objections to his review of their *Sexual preference: Its development in men and women. Journal of Sex Research, 18,* 366–368.
Wheeler, M. D. (1991). Physical changes of puberty. *Endocrinology and Metabolism Clinics of North America, 20,* 1–14.
Wildt, L., Marshall, G., & Knobil, E. (1980). Experimental induction of puberty in the infantile female rhesus monkey. *Science, 207,* 1373–1375.
Zucker, K. J., Bradley, S. J., Oliver, G., Blake, J., Fleming, S., & Hood, J. (1996). Psychosexual development of women with congenital adrenal hyperplasia. *Hormones and Behavior, 30,* 300–318.

Intrapersonal Motor but Not Extrapersonal Targeting Skill Is Enhanced During the Midluteal Phase of the Menstrual Cycle

Deborah M. Saucier and Doreen Kimura

Department of Psychology
University of Western Ontario
London, Canada

Verbal articulatory speed and small-amplitude manual skills within personal space are usually enhanced during the high-estrogen phases (midluteal and preovulatory) of the menstrual cycle, whereas spatial ability is better in the low-estrogen phase (menstrual). Thirty-three women performed an intrapersonal motor task (the Manual Sequence Box) in both the midluteal and menstrual phases, as well as a spatio-motor task (Targeting) directed at extrapersonal space. The Targeting task reliably yields a large male advantage. Saliva samples were assayed for estrogen and progesterone to confirm the appropriate menstrual phase for each test session.

Performance on the Manual Sequence Box was faster during the high-estrogen midluteal phase relative to the menstrual phase, which confirms previous reports. In contrast, there was no effect of phase on overall targeting accuracy. Although for targeting accuracy, the right hand was more accurate than the left throughout, it was even more accurate than the left in the midluteal phase, consistent with earlier suggestions that high estrogen concentration may facilitate left-hemisphere function relative to the right hemisphere.

Performance on many cognitive tasks is sexually dimorphic. For instance, men outperform women on most tasks of spatial ability and mathematical reasoning, whereas women typically outperform men on verbal fluency tasks and perceptual speed (for a review, see Halpern, 1992; Kimura, 1996). Tasks of small-amplitude

---

Requests for reprints should be sent to Doreen Kimura, Department of Psychology, University of Western Ontario, London, Ontario, Canada N6A 5C2. E-mail: kimura@uwo.ca

motor skill are also typically performed better by women and include such activities as placing pegs into holes (Hall & Kimura, 1995; Tiffin, 1968) and sequencing motor movements, including verbal articulation (Nicholson & Kimura, 1996). All of these tasks are performed within arm's reach of the body; that is, within intrapersonal space. In contrast, certain tasks of large-amplitude motor skill, such as throwing a missile at an external target, are typically performed better by men (Hall & Kimura, 1995; Jardine & Martin, 1983; Peters, 1990; Watson & Kimura, 1989, 1991), as is intercepting a projectile (Watson & Kimura, 1989, 1991). This difference in throwing accuracy is present very early (Gesell, 1940; Lunn, 1987). These tasks require that movements be directed toward extrapersonal space.

Some of these sexually dimorphic tasks are known to be affected by the natural variations in sex hormone levels across the menstrual cycle. Performance on tasks that tend to show a female advantage (articulatory ability and certain manual skills) improved during high-estrogen (E) phases (midluteal or preovulatory) relative to the low-E menstrual phase (Hampson 1990a, 1990b; Hampson & Kimura, 1988). Conversely, performance on spatial tasks that typically show a male advantage was better during the low-E phase relative to the high-E phases (Hampson 1990a, 1990b; Silverman & Phillips, 1993). Furthermore, evidence for variation in functional brain asymmetry has been observed across the menstrual cycle (Hampson, 1990a) and may be a factor in some of the skill differences.

Thus, there is a demonstrated relation between intrapersonal motor skills and naturally occurring changes in hormone levels that occur during the menstrual cycle. However, it is not known how the pattern of performance on an extrapersonal motor skill on which males excel might differ from a motor skill on which females excel. This study compares the performance of intrapersonal (Motor Sequence Box) and extrapersonal (targeting) motor tasks across the menstrual cycle. In addition, we investigated effects on a nonmotor spatial task, as well as a math reasoning task, both of which favor males, and administered a neutral task (vocabulary) as a general IQ measure.

METHOD

Participants

Participants were female students at the University of Western Ontario who were solicited by ads placed in two campus newspapers offering payment for participation. Individuals were prescreened, and those who were left-handed as determined by a questionnaire (Kimura, 1973), had irregular menstrual cycles, or had used oral contraceptives in the 4 months prior to testing were excluded. All participants were screened to ensure that English was their first language. Seventy-seven participants were enrolled in the study, but 12 did not return for the second session, leaving 65 individuals who participated in both phases of the study. However, inclusion in the final sample was based on E concentrations determined by radioimmunoassay (for procedure, see Mead & Hampson, 1996), resulting in the exclusion of an additional 24 participants. In addition, 8 participants had one or more saliva samples that could not be used for the radioimmunoassay and were therefore also excluded from the study. This left 33 participants who ranged in age from 19 to 33 years, with a mean of 22.3 years. These 33 women had an average cycle length of 28.4 days, with a standard deviation of 3.21 days.

One participant had a sliver in her right index finger during the menstrual phase and she did not perform the Manual Sequence Box during that session. Her data were thus excluded from the analyses of all motor tasks.

Procedure

Participants were tested twice approximately 6 weeks apart. Timing of the test sessions was arranged to occur once during the low-E, low-progesterone (P) menstrual phase (3 to 5 days following the onset of menstruation with participants calling us to arrange testing), and once during the high-E, high-P midluteal phase (10 to 5 days prior to predicted menstruation). For test sessions that occurred during the midluteal phase, actual date of menstruation was confirmed by a subsequent telephone message. The dates of testing were thus based on predicted and self-reported occurrence of menstruation. The phase (midluteal or menstrual) that the participants were first tested in was counterbalanced across participants. In addition, testing was performed by an assistant who was unfamiliar with this area of research and who was blind as to the phase of the participant until testing was completed.

Saliva samples. Two saliva samples were collected to be used for later radioimmunoassay to confirm both E and P concentrations. Samples were collected approximately 1 hr apart, one at the beginning and the other at the end of the test session. Samples were collected in polystyrene tubes that were pretreated with sodium azide (an antibacterial agent). Saliva production was aided by chewing sugarless gum, which was inert for radioimmunoassay purposes. *Criterion for inclusion in the final sample was that the E concentrations for both midluteal samples were absolutely greater than the E concentrations for both menstrual samples.*

Tests

Intrapersonal motor (Manual Sequence Box; Kimura, 1977). Participants learned a series of three unique unimanual movements directed at a wooden box with a button, a handle, and a bar on it (Kimura, 1977; Figure 1). They were shown how to press the top button with the index finger, pull the vertical handle with four fingers, and press down on the bottom bar with the side of the thumb. For the

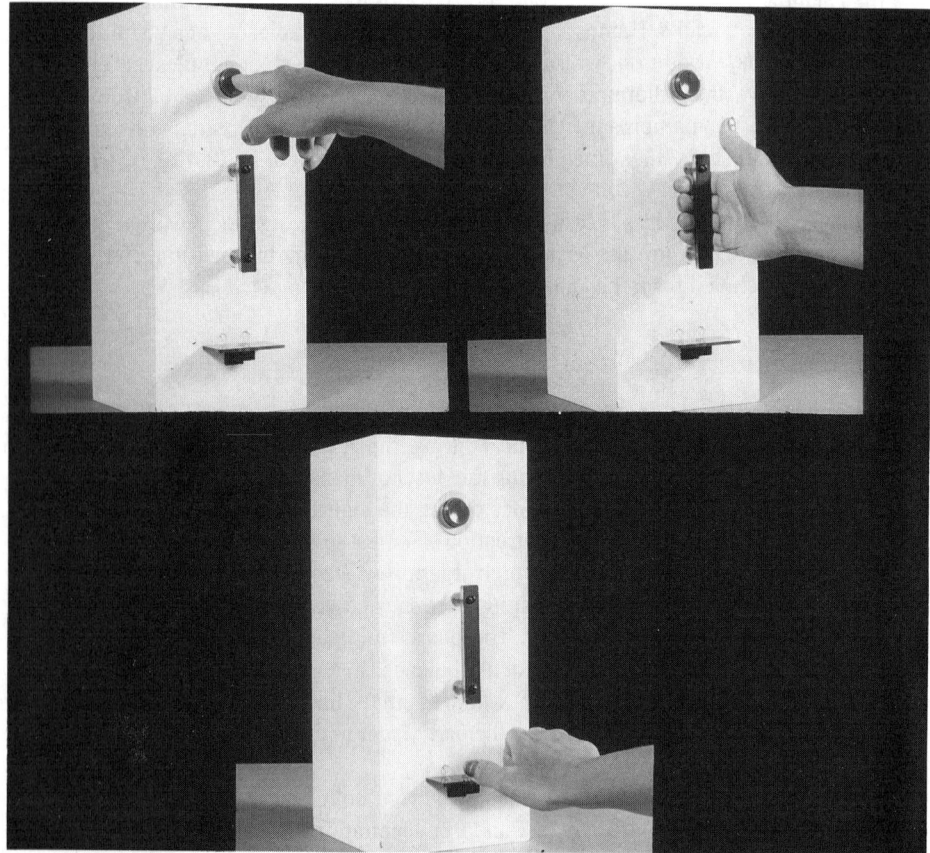

FIGURE 1 The Manual Sequence Box task (Kimura, 1977).

acquisition phase, participants had to perform five consecutive correct sequences. Once this criterion was achieved, participants then performed the sequence as quickly as possible until an additional 10 consecutive correct sequences were performed (performance phase). For both phases of the Manual Sequence Box task, the time required to achieve the criterion was recorded with a digital stopwatch. The hand used first to perform this task was counterbalanced between participants and between test sessions.

Extrapersonal motor (Targeting). Participants threw, underhand, a Velcro-covered ball to a square, carpet-covered frame (1.45 m × 1.45 m) hung on the wall. The center of the square was marked with a 6.5 cm × 6.5 cm red square, which participants were instructed to aim at. Participants stood 2.85 m from the target and the center of the target was 1.5 m from the ground (Hall & Kimura, 1995). Five practice trials were performed with each hand, followed by 10 test trials with the same hand. The order of the throwing hand was counterbalanced between participants and between test sessions. For each test trial, the deviation from the central target was calculated as the distance (in centimeters) from the closest edge of the center square to the actual position of the ball on the target. For each hand, an error measure was computed consisting of the average deviation from the center square for the 10 test trials.

Cognitive tests. Participants were also given three cognitive tests: (a) Mental Rotations (Vandenberg & Kuse, 1978), (b) Math Aptitude (Ekstrom, French, Harman, & Dermen, 1976), and (c) Advanced Vocabulary (Ekstrom et al., 1976). For the two sessions, alternate forms of the tests were given, counterbalanced between participants.

Both Mental Rotations and Math Aptitude tests typically show a male advantage (Benbow, 1988; Hyde, Fennema, & Lamon, 1990; Linn & Petersen, 1985) and scores on the Mental Rotations test have been reported to be higher in the menstrual phase (Silverman & Phillips, 1993). It was therefore anticipated that performance on these tasks might be better at the menstrual phase relative to the midluteal phase. The Advanced Vocabulary test was administered as a measure of general intellectual ability (Vernon, 1971; Wechsler, 1958, pp. 122, 132). It was not anticipated that performance on this test would vary with the phase of the menstrual cycle.

RESULTS

Hormone Levels[1]

Recall that to be included in the study, the participant's E concentration for both midluteal saliva samples had to be absolutely greater than both of the menstrual saliva samples. The final sample of 33 participants had salivary E concentration of 11.15 pg/mL ($SEM = 0.64$) at the midluteal phase, and 6.14 pg/mL ($SEM = 0.57$) at the menstrual phase. These values represent the average of the E concentrations, as determined by radioimmunoassay (for procedure, see Mead & Hampson, 1996), for the two saliva samples produced during each session. For these same participants, the salivary P concentration was 51.24 pg/ml ($SEM = 6.23$) at the midluteal phase, and 26.88 pg/ml ($SEM = 3.41$) at the menstrual phase. The intra-assay coefficient of reliability averaged 4.25% for E and 14% for P.

---

[1]Hormone assays were conducted by a radioimmunoassay technician under the supervision of Professor E. Hampson, who had no participation in, or knowledge of, other test results. We are grateful to Dr. Hampson for assistance with the assays.

The performance of these 33 participants is summarized in Table 1.

Manual Sequence Box

Acquisition. A 2 × 2 repeated measures analysis of variance (ANOVA) with the phase of the menstrual cycle and the hand used to perform the sequence as within-subjects measures was performed on the amount of time taken to perform the acquisition phase of the Manual Sequence Box task (five consecutive correct trials). There were no significant main effects for phase or hand, $F(1, 31) = 0.07$, ns, and $F(1, 31) = 1.90$, ns, respectively; or for interactions, $F(1, 31) = 0.001$, ns, consistent with Hampson and Kimura (1988).

Performance (Figure 2). A 2 × 2 repeated measures ANOVA with phase and hand as within-subjects measures was also performed on the amount of time taken to complete the performance phase of the Manual Sequence Box task (10 consecutive correct trials). There was a significant main effect of phase, $F(1, 31) = 4.24$, $p < .05$, indicating faster performance at the midluteal phase. There was no main effect of hand, $F(1, 31) = 0.01$, ns, and there was no interaction between hand and phase, $F(1, 31) = 1.48$, ns.

TABLE 1
A Summary of the Participants' Performance on the Tests

	Phase			
	Midluteal		Menstrual	
Test	M	SD	M	SD
Targeting (deviation from center in cm)				
Right hand	13.60	5.29	15.20	5.55
Left hand	21.29	7.38	19.40	5.58
Box Task: Acquisition (time to perform 5 trials in sec)				
Right hand	11.22	5.15	11.59	5.99
Left hand	12.54	7.00	12.79	7.05
Box Task: Performance (time to perform 10 trials in sec)				
Right hand	15.24	3.60	19.38	10.80
Left hand	16.63	3.40	18.18	5.49
Cognitive tasks (number correct adjusted for errors)				
Mental Rotations	7.25	4.17	8.59	4.87
Math Aptitude	5.73	2.95	5.52	3.08
Advanced Vocabulary	7.96	4.01	8.06	3.48

Note. $n = 33$.

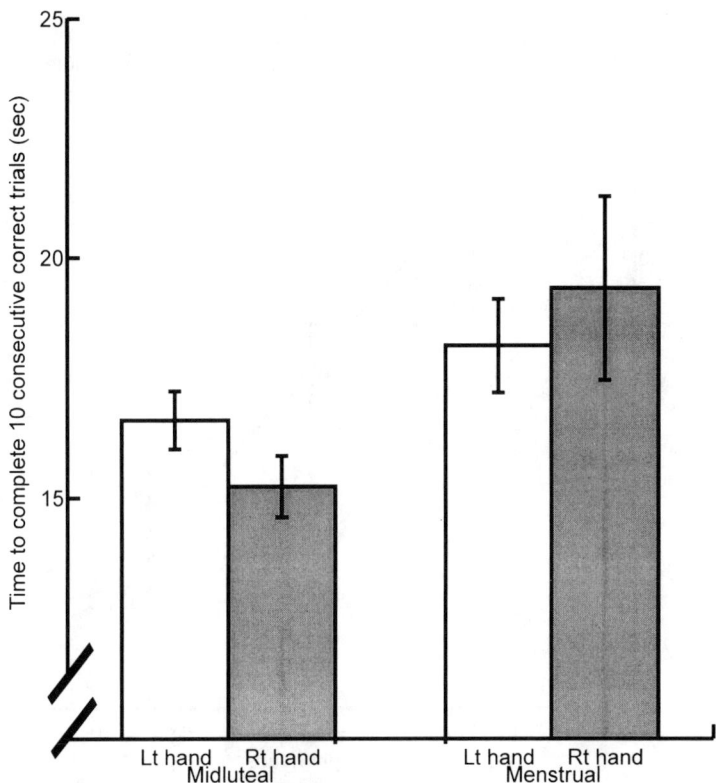

FIGURE 2 Performance of the Box Task for 10 consecutive correct trials after acquisition ($n = 32$). The error bars represent the standard error of measurement.

Targeting (Figure 3)

A 2 × 2 repeated measures ANOVA with the phase of the menstrual cycle and the throwing hand as within-subjects measures was performed on the error measure for the targeting data. There was no main effect of phase, $F(1, 31) = 0.21$, ns, indicating that performance did not differ between the menstrual and midluteal phases.

There was an expected main effect of hand, $F(1, 31) = 44.62, p < .0001$. Post hoc tests (Tukey's) indicated that the left hand was significantly less accurate than the right hand at both the menstrual and midluteal phases.

There was a significant interaction between phase and throwing hand, $F(1, 31) = 7.10, p < .05$, indicating a relatively greater accuracy with the right hand at the midluteal phase than the menstrual phase. Post hoc tests (Tukey's) revealed that

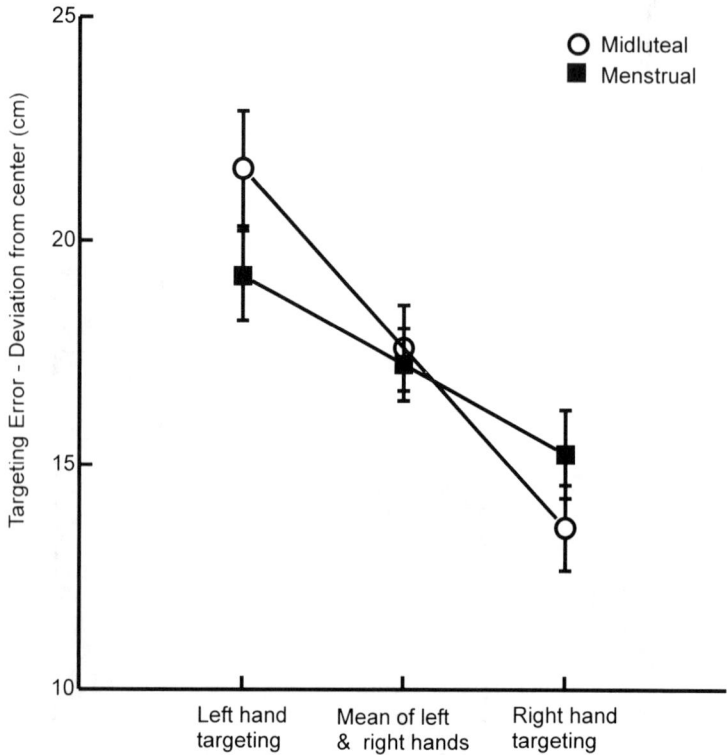

FIGURE 3 Performance on the Targeting task ($n = 32$). The error bars represent the standard error of measurement.

the left hand was significantly more accurate during the menstrual phase than it was during the midluteal phase.

An asymmetry measure comparing the accuracy of the right and the left hands for the two phases was also computed (Harshman, 1988):

$$\frac{\text{left hand error} - \text{right hand error}}{\text{left hand error} + \text{right hand error}}.$$

A paired-difference t test comparing asymmetry across the phases indicated that the right-hand advantage was significantly greater in the midluteal phase ($M = 0.23$, $SD = 0.20$) than in the menstrual phase ($M = 0.12$, $SD = 0.19$), $t(31) = 2.14$, $p < .05$.

Cognitive Tasks (Figure 4)

As expected, performance on the Advanced Vocabulary task did not differ significantly between the midluteal ($M = 8.00$, $SD = 4.01$) and menstrual ($M = 8.06$, $SD = 3.48$) phase, $t(32) = -0.21$, ns. Neither did performance on the Math Aptitude task differ between the midluteal ($M = 5.73$, $SD = 2.95$) and menstrual ($M = 5.52$, $SD = 3.08$) phase, $t(32) = 0.41$, ns. The anticipated advantage for Mental Rotations in the

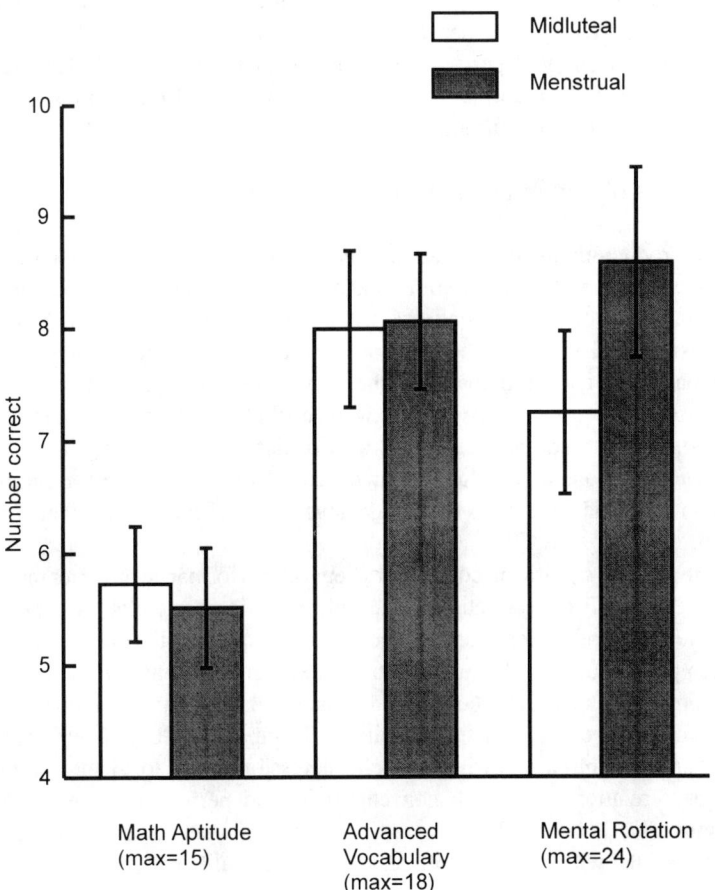

FIGURE 4 Scores on the cognitive tasks ($n = 33$). The error bars represent the standard error of measurement.

menstrual phase (Silverman & Phillips, 1993), although in the expected direction, did not reach statistical significance, $t(32) = -1.41, p = .08$, one-tailed.

Because the Targeting task has a spatial component, a Pearson product–moment correlation was computed, comparing performance on the Targeting task with Mental Rotations scores. For this correlation, scores for the Targeting task were multiplied by –1 so that a more positive score indicated better performance. There were no significant correlations between performance on Mental Rotations and performance on Targeting (overall, collapsed across hands and phase), $r(31) = .01$, ns. Examining the performance by hand and phase, there were no significant correlations for either the midluteal phase (right hand), $r(31) = .01$, ns, and (left hand), $r(31) = .11$, ns, or the menstrual phase (right hand), $r(31) = .18$, ns, and (left hand), $r(31) = .01$, ns, with performance on the Mental Rotations task. This confirms the findings of Watson and Kimura (1991), who also failed to find a significant relation between targeting accuracy and performance on spatial tasks.

Correlations of Performance With Hormone Levels

Pearson product–moment correlations were calculated to examine potential relations between E and P concentrations and performance on the cognitive and motor tasks. For these correlations, only the performance on the first occasion of testing was considered. To increase the range of E and P values, the performance of all 77 individuals who had participated in the first session were considered for these correlations. However, 4 participants were excluded because they had salivary samples that could not be assayed. As well, 1 participant with pregnancy-level E and P concentrations was excluded from the correlations. Thus, the correlations are based on 72 participants who had measurable levels of E and P for their first test session.

There were no significant correlations between performance on either motor task and either E or P concentrations. The only significant correlation between the cognitive tasks and either E or P concentrations was a small negative correlation between performance on Mental Rotations and E concentration, $r(71) = -.21, p < .05$. A previous study had reported a curvilinear relation between E concentration and performance on tasks of spatial abilities (Hampson, 1990a). However, for our participants, a similar stepwise multiple regression failed to yield a significant curvilinear relation between E concentrations and performance on the Mental Rotations task, $t(71) = 0.72$, ns. Instead, in our participants, lower E concentrations were associated with better performance on the Mental Rotations task.

Results Based on Self-Report

Eighteen women who had reported that they had been in the appropriate phase during testing were excluded based on their hormone levels. These women ranged in age from 19 to 27 years, with a mean of 20.0 years, and were significantly younger than the mean age of 22.3 years for the participants who were included, $t(1, 50) = 3.16$, $p < .01$. In younger women, the incidence of ovulation is lower (Metcalfe & MacKenzie, 1980). Thus, the failure to find hormonal levels corresponding to their menstrual phase in these 18 women may reflect the fact that some of them may not have ovulated in that cycle. We nevertheless examined the data for the entire group of 51 participants who reported that they had been in the appropriate phase (either midluteal or menstrual) for both test sessions. The same statistics were performed on this group of 51 women as had been performed on the initial sample of 33. The pattern of results was essentially similar, but levels of significance were generally reduced.

For the targeting data, there was no significant effect of phase, $F(1, 50) = 1.18$, ns, and there was a significant effect of hand, $F(1, 50) = 58.52$, $p < .0001$. There was also a significant interaction between phase and hand, $F(1, 50) = 17.86$, $p < .0001$.

For the Manual Sequence Box task, there were no significant differences during the either the acquisition or performance phases. However, the pattern of results for the performance phase was similar to our results with the 33 participants, with a trend for better performance in the midluteal phase. There were no significant differences between the phases for the cognitive tasks, but again, a similar trend was noted for Mental Rotations as before.

Thus, the use of hormonal assays as the basis for selecting participants allowed us to observe effects that otherwise may have been missed.

DISCUSSION

Although the performance of intrapersonal (Manual Sequence Box) and extrapersonal (Targeting) motor tasks were both related to the phase of menstrual cycle, they showed a different pattern of results. Performance on the Box task was enhanced during the midluteal phase, consistent with previous research (Hampson, 1990a, 1990b; Hampson & Kimura, 1988), but the overall performance on the Targeting task did not differ between the midluteal and menstrual phase. Targeting did, however, demonstrate an influence of hormonal phase on relative hand accuracy, which did not appear on the Box task. Thus, performance on intrapersonal motor tasks and extrapersonal motor tasks were differentially affected by hormonal variations across the menstrual cycle, confirming that they represent different functions.

Although both tasks require motor programming, they differ in rather fundamental ways. The sequence of movements required to perform intrapersonal motor tasks, such as the Box task, involve minimal spatial analysis or visual control, particularly once they have been executed several times (Kimura, 1977, 1993). Thus, once initial contact has been made with the Box, the movements could be performed with minimal visual guidance, and with only the body framework as a referent. Where excursions from one part of the task to another are much larger (Peters & Servos, 1989), this might not be the case. In contrast, the movements required to perform an extrapersonal motor task such as Targeting, rely heavily on external visual information and spatial analysis to achieve accurate performance on each trial (Kimura, 1993). Performance on the Box task is known to require the participation of left-hemisphere praxis systems (Kimura, 1977), whereas the performance on the Targeting task may demand more integration of motor and visual systems. Thus, although both tasks ultimately engage the corticospinal system, the antecedent sources of control differ.

Nevertheless, the results for both the Box task and the Targeting task are consistent with left-hemisphere activation during high levels of E. Enhancement of left-hemisphere activity might be expected to affect the intrapersonal movements of either hand fairly equally, as the left-hemisphere praxis system exerts bilateral control over the hands (Kimura, 1993). Thus, the finding of faster overall performance, but no phase by hand interaction, for the Box task during the midluteal phase is consistent with an enhancement of the left-hemisphere praxis system during this phase.

The extrapersonal motor task is presumed to depend less exclusively on left-hemisphere praxis systems than do intrapersonal tasks, because we know that accurate location of external loci is more dependent on the right hemisphere (Kimura, 1969; Saucier & Kimura, 1996).

The results of this study have parallels in other research on the effects of estrogen variation. The right-hand facilitation on Targeting during the high-E menstrual phase is consistent with the relative enhancement of the right-ear effect on dichotic listening (Hampson, 1990a). The overall efficiency on the Box task, coupled with no such effect on Targeting is consistent with a study comparing women in high- and low-E phases of oral contraceptive use (Szekely, Hampson, Carey, & Goodale, this issue). As they predicted, women were faster at the Box task during the high-E phase, but their accuracy on pointing to or between visual targets was not consistently related to contraceptive phase.

On the cognitive tests, as expected, there was no effect of the phase of menstrual cycle on the performance of the Advanced Vocabulary task, a task included to measure general intelligence levels. There was no effect of the phase of the menstrual cycle on performance on the Math Aptitude task, in contrast to reports that spatial ability is affected by hormonal variation during the menstrual cycle. This result is consistent with a previous report (Gouchie & Kimura, 1991) that failed to find a relation between testosterone levels and performance on the Math Aptitude test for women, although present in men. Thus, in women, performance on the Math Aptitude task may be less linked to hormonal levels than are tests of spatial abilities.

There was a weak trend for performance on the Mental Rotations task to be better in the menstrual phase. As well, the only significant correlation between E concentration and performance on cognitive tasks occurred with the Mental Rotations task, although it was not a curvilinear function. Taken together, these results suggest that performance on the Mental Rotations task is related to E concentrations. Peters et al.'s (1990) negative data are difficult to interpret because menstrual phase was neither very precisely determined, nor were hormone levels assayed. Thus, performance on a male-advantaged spatial task, but not a mathematical reasoning task, appears to be related to circulating E concentrations. Not all male-advantaged tasks are necessarily sensitive to fluctuations in hormone levels.

Although there is a spatial component to Targeting, performance on the Targeting task was not related to performance on Mental Rotations in our participants. This result was consistent with the findings of Watson and Kimura (1991), who also failed to find a relation between targeting and performance on several spatial tasks. Together, these two studies suggest that the spatial component of the Targeting task, emphasizing location of an external target, is distinguishable from that of paper-and-pencil spatial tasks that measure spatial visualization and orientation.

In summary, it appears that the performance of intrapersonal and extrapersonal motor tasks are differently affected by the hormonal fluctuations during the menstrual cycle, although both are consistent with an enhancement of left-hemisphere activity during the high-E midluteal phase. These results also suggest that the two tasks are served by different brain systems, with the intrapersonal Box task more reliant on the left-hemisphere praxis system than is the Targeting task.

ACKNOWLEDGMENTS

Deborah M. Saucier is now at the Department of Psychology, University of Regina, Regina, Saskatchewan, Canada.

This research was funded by a grant from the Medical Research Council of Canada to Doreen Kimura.

REFERENCES

Benbow, C. P. (1988). Sex differences in mathematical reasoning ability in intellectually talented preadolescents: Their nature, effects, and possible causes. *Behavioral and Brain Sciences, 11*, 169–232.

Ekstrom, R. B., French, J. W., Harman, H. H., & Dermen, D. (1976). *Kit of factor referenced cognitive tests.* Princeton, NJ: Educational Testing Service.

Gesell, A. (1940). *The first five years of life: A guide to the study of the preschool child.* New York: Harper & Brothers.

Gouchie, C., & Kimura, D. (1991). The relationship between testosterone levels and cognitive ability patterns. *Psychoneuroendocrinology, 16*, 323–334.

Hall, J. A. Y., & Kimura, D. (1995). Sexual orientation and performance on sexually dimorphic motor tasks. *Archives of Sexual Behavior, 24*, 395–407.

Halpern, D. F. (1992). *Sex differences in cognitive abilities* (2nd ed.). Hillsdale, NJ: Lawrence Erlbaum Associates, Inc.

Hampson, E. (1990a). Estrogen-related variations in human spatial and articulatory-motor skills. *Psychoneuroendocrinology, 15*, 97–111.

Hampson, E. (1990b). Variations in sex-related cognitive abilities across the menstrual cycle. *Brain and Cognition, 14*, 26–43.

Hampson, E., & Kimura, D. (1988). Reciprocal effects of hormonal fluctuations on human motor and perceptual-spatial skills. *Behavioural Neuroscience, 102,* 456–459.
Harshman, R. A. (1988). Can dichotic listening measure "degree of lateralization?" In K. Hugdahl (Ed.), *Handbook of dichotic listening: Theory, methods, and research* (pp. 215–282). New York: Wiley.
Hyde, J. S., Fennema, E., & Lamon, S. J. (1990). Gender differences in mathematics performance: A meta-analysis. *Psychological Bulletin, 107,* 139–155.
Jardine, R., & Martin, N. G. (1983). Spatial ability and throwing accuracy. *Behavior Genetics, 13,* 331–340.
Kimura, D. (1969). Spatial localization in left and right visual fields. *Canadian Journal of Psychology, 23,* 445–458.
Kimura, D. (1973). Manual activity during speaking: Left handers. *Neuropsychologia, 11,* 51–55.
Kimura, D. (1977). Acquisition of a motor skill after left-hemisphere damage. *Brain, 100,* 527–542.
Kimura, D. (1993). *Neuromotor mechanisms in human communication.* New York: Oxford University Press.
Kimura, D. (1996). Sex, sexual orientation and sex hormones influence human cognitive function. *Current Opinion in Neurobiology, 6,* 259–263.
Linn, M. C., & Petersen, A. C. (1985). Emergence and characterization of sex differences in spatial ability: A meta-analysis. *Child Development, 56,* 1479–1498.
Lunn, D. (1987). *Foot asymmetry and cognitive ability in young children.* Unpublished masters thesis, University of Western Ontario, London, Canada.
Mead, L. A., & Hampson, E. (1996). Asymmetric effects of ovarian hormones on hemispheric activity: Evidence from dichotic and tachistoscopic tests. *Neuropsychology, 10,* 578–587.
Metcalfe, M. G., & MacKenzie, J. A. (1980). Incidence of ovulation in young women. *Journal of Biological Science, 12,* 345–352.
Nicholson, K. G., & Kimura, D. (1996). Sex differences for speech and manual skill. *Perceptual and Motor Skills, 82,* 3–13.
Peters, M. (1990). Subclassification of non-pathological left-handers poses problems for theories of handedness. *Neuropsychologia, 28,* 279–289.
Peters, M., Laeng, B., Latham, K., Jackson, M., Zaiyouna, R., & Richardson, C. (1995). A redrawn Vandenberg and Kuse mental rotations test: Different versions and factors that affect performance. *Brain and Cognition, 28,* 39–58.
Peters, M., & Servos, P. (1989). Performance of subgroups of left-handers and right-handers. *Canadian Journal of Psychology, 43,* 341–358.
Saucier, D. M., & Kimura, D. (1996). Dermatoglyphic asymmetry is related to perceptual asymmetry and to interhemispheric transmission. *Laterality, 1,* 185–198.
Silverman, I., & Phillips, K. (1993). Effects of estrogen changes during the menstrual cycle on spatial performance. *Ethology and Sociobiology, 14,* 257–270.
Szekely, C., Hampson, E., Carey, D. P., & Goodale, M. A. (1998/this issue). Oral contraceptive use affects manual praxis but not simple visually guided movements. *Developmental Neuropsychology, 14,* 399–420.
Tiffin, T. (1968). *Purdue Pegboard Examiner Manual.* Chicago: Science Research Associates.
Vandenberg, S. G., & Kuse, A. R. (1978). Mental rotations, a group test of three-dimensional spatial visualization. *Perceptual and Motor Skills, 47,* 599–601.
Vernon, P. E. (1971). *The structure of human abilities.* London: Methuen.
Watson, N. V., & Kimura, D. (1989). Right-hand superiority for throwing but not for intercepting. *Neuropsychologia, 27,* 1399–1414.
Watson, N. V., & Kimura, D. (1991). Nontrivial sex differences in throwing and intercepting: Relation to psychometrically-defined spatial functions. *Personality and Individual Differences, 12,* 375–385.
Wechsler, D. (1958). *The measurement and appraisal of adult intelligence.* Baltimore: Williams & Wilkins.

Oral Contraceptive Use Affects Manual Praxis but Not Simple Visually Guided Movements

Christine Szekely
Department of Psychology
University of Western Ontario
London, Canada

Elizabeth Hampson
Department of Psychology and Neuroscience Program
University of Western Ontario
London, Canada

David P. Carey
Department of Psychology
University of Aberdeen, Kings College
Old Aberdeen, Scotland

Melvyn A. Goodale
Department of Psychology and Neuroscience Program
University of Western Ontario

A detailed analysis of both motor sequencing and visually guided movements was carried out in a group of neurologically normal women who were receiving exogenous estrogen in the form of oral contraceptives. Women were tested under both low and high estrogen conditions, in order to examine any hormone-related facilitation in the speed or accuracy of movement. Kinematic parameters examined on the visually guided motor tasks included movement onset time, duration of the reach, peak

---

Requests for reprints should be sent to Elizabeth Hampson, Department of Psychology, The University of Western Ontario, London, Ontario, Canada N6A 5C2. E-mail: ehampson@uwovax.uwo.ca

velocity, deceleration time, and endpoint accuracy (resultant error). The results showed that variations in motor performance were associated with fluctuations in estrogen level, but that this hormone sensitivity was task selective. Improved performance on a test of speeded motor sequencing, the Manual Sequence Box, was found under higher estrogen conditions, but this effect did not occur consistently in tests of rapid prehensile movements. Results are interpreted in terms of differential reliance of these tasks on left-hemisphere praxic systems.

Evidence is accumulating to support the notion that gonadal hormones can affect certain nonreproductive behaviors in both humans and nonhuman animals (for reviews, see Beatty, 1992; Hampson & Kimura, 1992; Collaer & Hines, 1995). In the rat, behavioral and neurochemical studies suggest that ovarian hormones, specifically estrogens, may have a facilitatory influence on motor behaviors, including open field activity, wheel running, and sensorimotor tasks (Becker, Snyder, Miller, Westgate, & Jenuwine, 1986; Burke & Broadhurst, 1966; Colvin & Sawyer, 1969; Smith, Waterhouse, & Woodward, 1987; Vick & Banks, 1969).

Comparable studies across the human menstrual cycle suggest that estrogens may affect some overt motor behaviors (for reviews, see Hampson & Kimura, 1992; Sommer, 1992). The results of studies on general ambulation, reaction time, and athletic performance have been inconsistent due to methodological differences across studies as well as variability in the types of movements assessed. For example, some studies have shown improved performance under high estrogen conditions (Becker, Creutzfeldt, Schwibbe, & Wuttke, 1982; Hunter, Schraer, Landers, Buskirk, & Harris, 1979; Wearing, Yuhosz, Campbell, & Love, 1972; Zimmerman & Parlee, 1973;), some have failed to find any menstrual cycle-related changes (Jensen, 1982; Pierson & Lockhart, 1963; Stocker, 1973), and still others have reported ambiguous findings (Morris & Udry, 1970; Stenn & Klinge, 1972). More consistent results have been found in studies using a test of motor sequencing, the Manual Sequence Box (Kimura, 1977), in that speed and accuracy are reliably facilitated when circulating levels of estrogen are high. This result has been replicated in various groups, including women with normal menstrual cycles (Hampson, 1990c; Hampson & Kimura, 1988; Saucier & Kimura, this issue), postmenopausal women receiving estrogen-replacement therapy (Kimura & Hampson, 1993), and women taking oral contraceptives (OCs; Hampson 1990b; Szekely, 1992). Women taking OCs are one of the most convenient populations for investigating the potential effects of estrogens on motor skills because the hormonal milieu is tightly controlled. Serum levels of ethinyl estradiol rise after ingestion of OCs and are low when pill ingestion ceases (Dibbelt et al., 1989; Longcope & Williams, 1977). Furthermore, ethinyl estradiol is able to enter the central nervous system and bind to central estrogen receptors (Briggs & Briggs, 1983; Fishman & Norton, 1977; Stumpf & Sar, 1977; Vreeburg, Schretlen, & Baum, 1974).

Given that evidence is accumulating in support of the notion that endogenous and exogenous estrogens have activational effects on motor performance in humans and other animals, it would be useful to study these effects in greater detail. The measures of motor coordination used in past studies on humans are fairly crude in that the exact nature of changes across the menstrual cycle can usually not be attributed to a particular movement variable such as speed versus error (e.g., Hampson, 1990a, 1990b; Hampson & Kimura, 1988). Therefore, it is necessary to analyze the movements made during tasks of speed and coordination at a more basic level to determine which components of movement are hormone sensitive. This study examined the possible effects of changes in estrogen concentrations on movements that represent some of the fundamental components of the motor tasks used in previous studies. In particular, these movements share many features with the subcomponents of the Manual Sequence Box, which has demonstrated hormone sensitivity in a number of recent studies. Sex differences are often found on tasks that require the sequencing of multiple movements (Denckla, 1974; Kimura, 1986; Nicholson & Kimura, 1996), but have only rarely been reported on visually guided motor tasks of the sort to be used here (e.g., Jakobson, 1987).

In this study, it was hypothesized that women taking OCs would exhibit faster or more accurate motor performance while taking the medication (higher estrogen condition) than during the menstrual phase of the contraceptive cycle (lower estrogen condition) when pill ingestion ceases.

METHOD

Participants

Forty-six female volunteers were obtained through advertisements displayed around the University of Western Ontario campus. Participants ranged in age from 19 to 27 years old ($M = 21.5$ years). Handedness was confirmed with a behavioral handedness questionnaire (Hampson & Kimura, 1984) and only right-handed participants were included in the study. All participants had normal or corrected-to-normal vision, and had been taking OCs for an average of 29 months (range = 4–130 months). Only women using standard low-dose combination-type pills were included. Table 1 shows the brand names of the OCs used by women in the sample and the number of women taking each type of pill. All individuals were reimbursed for their participation.

General Procedure

All volunteers completed a confidential screening questionnaire over the telephone and eligible participants were then scheduled for a test session. Each participant was tested twice approximately 2 weeks apart; one half of the participants were

TABLE 1
Hormone Content of Oral Contraceptives Used by Women in the Sample

Brand	Hormone Content	Number of Participants
Monophasic		
Brevicon .5/35	EE 35ug NOR .5 mg	1
Cyclen	EE 35ug NOR .25 mg	6
Demulen 30	EE 30ug ED 2 mg	5
Loestrin 1.5/30	EE 30ug NOR 1.5 mg	2
Minovral	EE 30ug LEV 150 ug	3
Ortho .5/35	EE 35ug NOR .5 mg	2
Ortho 1/35	EE 35ug NOR 1 mg	3
Triphasic		
Ortho 7/7/7	EE 35ug NOR .5/.75/1 mg	12
Synphasic	EE 35ug NOR .5/1/.5 mg	4
Triphasil	EE 35ug LEV 50/75/125 ug	8
Total		46

Note. EE = ethinyl estradiol; NOR = norethindrone acetate; ED = ethynodiol diacetate; LEV = levonorgestrel.

tested first during the menstrual phase of the cycle. Women in this phase were not tested until the 5th, 6th, or 7th day after they had taken their last pill to avoid confounding variables such as physical or affective discomfort and to ensure that the contraceptive steroids had been maximally metabolized (Longcope & Williams, 1977; Marriott & Faragher, 1986). A second group of women was scheduled for the first testing after they had taken at least 11 pills of a new package and after at least two pills with the highest estrogen and progestin content had been taken. Verification of prescription information and of the number of pills remaining at the time of testing was provided by each participant at the test session. Of the original 46 women, 41 were available for testing at a second session at which the opposite phase was assessed.

Tests

Each test session was approximately 1 hr in length. Tests were given to all participants in the following order: bisection, pointing, Profile of Mood States (POMS; McNair, Lorr, & Droppleman, 1971), Mental Rotations (Vandenberg & Kuse, 1978), demographic questionnaire, reaching and grasping task, and the Manual Sequence Box (Kimura, 1977). All tests are described in detail later. The pointing and grasping tasks used in this study were developed by Goodale and colleagues for studies of visually guided movement and have been validated extensively (Goodale, Milner, Jakobson, & Carey, 1990; Jakobson & Goodale, 1991). Of the 41 women tested twice, 29 received the full test battery and an additional 12 participants received the POMS, Mental Rotations, demographic questionnaire, and Manual Sequence Box only.

Pointing and Bisection Tasks

Apparatus. Participants were seated in front of a black table surface and were required to point to an illuminated target (pointing task) or to the estimated midpoint between two illuminated targets (bisection task; see Figure 1). Infrared light-emitting diodes (IREDs) were attached to the tip and the base of the index finger. During each reach, the two-dimensional positions of the IREDs were monitored by two high-resolution infrared-sensitive cameras fixed above the testing apparatus in front and to the left of the participant. The coordinates of each IRED provided by each camera were digitized at a rate of 100 Hz and were fed into the data collection system of a WATSMART computer (Waterloo Spatial Motion Analysis and Recording Technique, Northern Digital Inc., Waterloo, Canada) that was calibrated daily. The spatial resolution of the WATSMART system is accurate to within < 1 to 2 mm (Servos, Goodale, & Jakobson, 1992).

At the beginning of each trial, the tip of the participant's right index finger rested on a start button that was located 7 cm from the table edge and 32 cm in front of the center of a horizontal target array. All trials were performed with the participant's head in a chin rest. The array consisted of light-emitting diodes (LEDs) embedded into a styrofoam surface covered by black speaker cloth. The row of LEDs was 2 cm above the surface of the table and the lights were only visible when illuminated. A fixation light was mounted 7 cm above the center of the horizontal LED array. Although five LEDs served as targets, data were collected on only three of these: one located at the center, one at 12 cm to the right of center, and one at 12 cm to the left of center. The distance to the center target was 32 cm but to the most peripheral targets was 34 cm, an increase of 5.8%; therefore the data were normalized before statistical analysis.

Procedure. Each session began with five practice reaches in the bisection task. The participants were asked to look at the fixation LED for the entire time it was illuminated (850 msec). The disappearance of the fixation light coincided with illumination of two target LEDs. Participants were asked to point with the right index finger as quickly and accurately as possible to the perceived midpoint between the two illuminated LEDs. The reach ended when the participant's finger came in contact with the LED display. The two LEDs illuminated for any particular bisection trial were positioned 12 cm apart and the actual midpoints were the same positions as the five targets used in the pointing task. The LEDs were extinguished after 400 ms. Each of the five targets was tested six times in a predetermined random

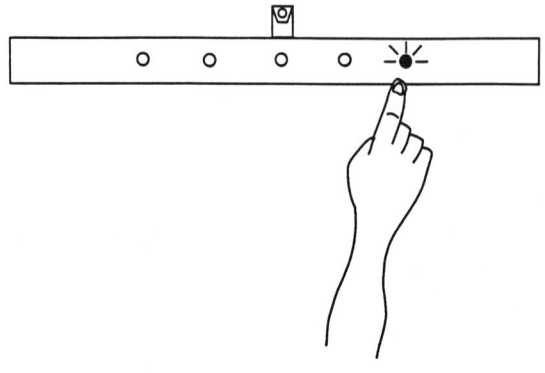

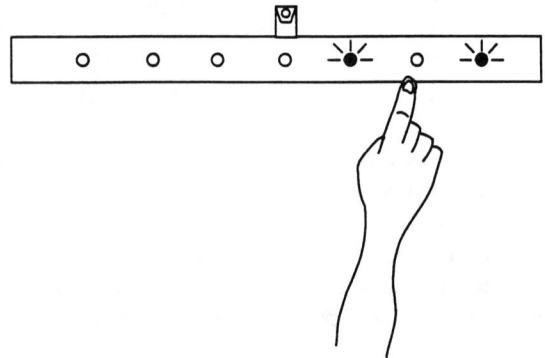

FIGURE 1   Schematic representation of pointing and bisection tasks. Filled circles represent illuminated light-emitting diodes (LEDs). Open circles represent other LED locations not visible until illuminated. Top: In the pointing task, participants were required to reach to a single LED location. Bottom: In the bisection task, they were required to reach to the midpoints between two illuminated LEDs. The actual midpoints between the LEDs corresponded to the five target locations in the pointing task.

sequence governed by an Apple IIe computer located in an adjacent room, to give a total of 30 reaches.

Following the bisection task, participants completed the pointing task. In this condition, the disappearance of the fixation light coincided with illumination of one of the target lights. The participant was instructed to point with the right index finger to the target light as quickly and accurately as possible. The target LED remained on for the entire duration of the reach (1,500 msec). Once again, five different target positions were used and each LED was illuminated six times in a predetermined random sequence to give a total of 30 reaches.

Dependent measures. The coordinates of the IREDs during each trial were reconstructed by the WATSMART software in three dimensions and filtered offline with a 7-Hz cutoff using a second order Butterworth filter. A number of kinematic parameters were extracted from the three-dimensional data in order to give a detailed description of each reach. *Movement onset time* or reaction time (in milliseconds) was determined as the point at which the mean velocity of the index finger over three consecutive frames was equal to or exceeded 5 cm/sec. The *duration* of the reach in pointing was calculated by subtracting the movement onset time from the time in the terminal portion of the reach when the finger was moving at less than 5 cm/sec for at least five frames. The *peak velocity* (centimeters per second) of the reach was also extracted using the position of the tip of the index finger. The *time spent decelerating* (milliseconds) was considered the time from the peak velocity to the end of the entire reach. *Resultant error* (millimeters) was calculated as the straight line distance between the fingertip IRED at the termination of the reach and the actual target position.

Reaching and Grasping Task

Apparatus. Each participant began the task sitting in a dark room facing a black table surface. Three red magnetized blocks (2 × 5 cm, 3 × 7.5 cm, and 5 × 12.5 cm) all 2 cm in height were used as target objects. These objects appeared in front of the participant along the midline axis one at a time in one of three positions: They were placed over a magnetic switch that was located at 20 cm, 30 cm, or 40 cm from the start position. For additional details, see Jakobson and Goodale (1991).

Three IREDs were attached to the participant's right hand: one on the lower left corner of the index fingernail, one on the lower right corner of the thumbnail, and one on the inside of the right wrist across from the styloid process of the ulna. The locations of these IREDs were monitored by the WATSMART recording system as described earlier.

Procedure. Participants began each trial with the right thumb and index finger in a pinch formation depressing a start key that was located at midline 15 cm from the edge of the table. The testing began with five practice trials. The participant was seated and was instructed to keep her eyes closed between trials and to open them only at the experimenter's command. When the participant opened her eyes the room was initially dark, but after a variable time period (a few seconds) a small lamp above the tabletop was illuminated. Participants were instructed to pick up the object as quickly and accurately as possible as soon as it became visible. Between each reach the experimenter placed one of the three different-sized blocks at one of the three different distances from the participant according to a presequenced random order, resulting in a total of 36 trials. Data collection began immediately when the light came on and ceased when the magnetic contact between the block and the table was broken. The overhead light remained illuminated for the entire duration of the reach.

Dependent measures. As with the pointing data, a number of kinematic parameters were extracted from the three-dimensional reaching and grasping data. *Movement onset time* was determined as the point at which the mean velocity of the wrist over three consecutive frames was equal to or exceeded 5 cm/sec. The *duration* of movement (milliseconds) was calculated by subtracting the movement onset time from the time when the magnetic contact between block and table was broken, signaling the end of the reach. The *peak velocity* (centimeters per second) and *time spent decelerating* (milliseconds) were also extracted using the wrist IRED.

Other Tasks

In order to demonstrate comparability of this sample with previous research, two tasks were given that have been used in other menstrual cycle studies—the Mental Rotations test and the Manual Sequence Box.

In the Mental Rotations test (Vandenberg & Kuse, 1978), the participants were asked to look at line drawings of abstract three-dimensional block constructions. For each item, the participant must choose the two objects from a set of four that are rotated versions of a target object. Alternate halves of the test were given on the two testing occasions with order counterbalanced across participants. Four minutes were allowed to complete 12 items. The traditional scoring method was used (Vandenberg & Kuse, 1978).

The Manual Sequence Box (Kimura, 1977) was used to assess manual praxis. The participants were required to learn a sequence of hand movements with the right hand, consisting of pushing a button, pulling out a handle, and pressing down on a bar. Following a series of learning trials, participants were required to perform this sequence of movements as quickly as possible until they achieved a criterion of 10 consecutive sequences without error (Hampson, 1990a). The overall score on this task was the cumulative time required to reach criterion after the learning trials had been successfully completed. Speed of the last 10 trials only gave an error-free score. To evaluate the total number of errors, participants' performance was videotaped with two videocameras and the two images were combined on videotape using a screen splitter so that performance from both the front and side views could later be verified. An intraclass correlation of $r = .89$ indicated high interrater reliability for error judgment across two independent observers. The traditional Manual Sequence Box apparatus was also adapted for this study so that any manipulation of the box automatically triggered a millisecond timer, enabling performance on the task to be precisely timed and recorded by computer.

The POMS (McNair et al., 1971) was administered to assess self-reported mood in order to determine if the menstrual cycle had effects on emotional state that might indirectly influence performance on the experimental motor tasks.

RESULTS

Variations in performance across the two phases of the contraceptive cycle were analyzed using analyses of variance (ANOVAs) incorporating phase of cycle (contraceptive, menstrual) as a within-subjects factor and test order (contraceptive first, menstrual first) as a grouping factor. Analysis of the reaching and pointing tasks included additional factors, as described later. To assess whether hormone influences were present, two major effects were examined for each variable. The main effect of Phase of Cycle was examined because it illustrates any overall change in performance between the two estrogen conditions. In addition, the Phase × Test Order interaction was examined because this could indicate either a simple practice effect or *differential* change across test sessions in the two order-of-testing groups attributable to hormonal influences acting additively with practice. To more clearly isolate the hormonal component and evaluate it for significance, it was necessary to calculate a change value for each participant by subtracting the score on the first session from the score on the second session for a particular dependent variable. A planned t test comparison was then performed on the change values with test order as the between-subject factor. Other main effects and interactions are described only insofar as they influence the interpretation of the Phase or Phase × Test Order effects.

Manual Sequence Box

Total time to criterion, time for the last 10 sequences, and total number of errors on the speeded trials of the Manual Sequence Box were analyzed using separate 2 × 2 ANOVAs. Only the time scores recorded by the millisecond timer were analyzed because these scores were found to be highly correlated with the times obtained using the traditional stopwatch method, $r(37) = .92, p < .001$. Figure 2 shows the average time needed to reach criterion and the mean number of errors made on the Manual Sequence Box as a function of contraceptive status.

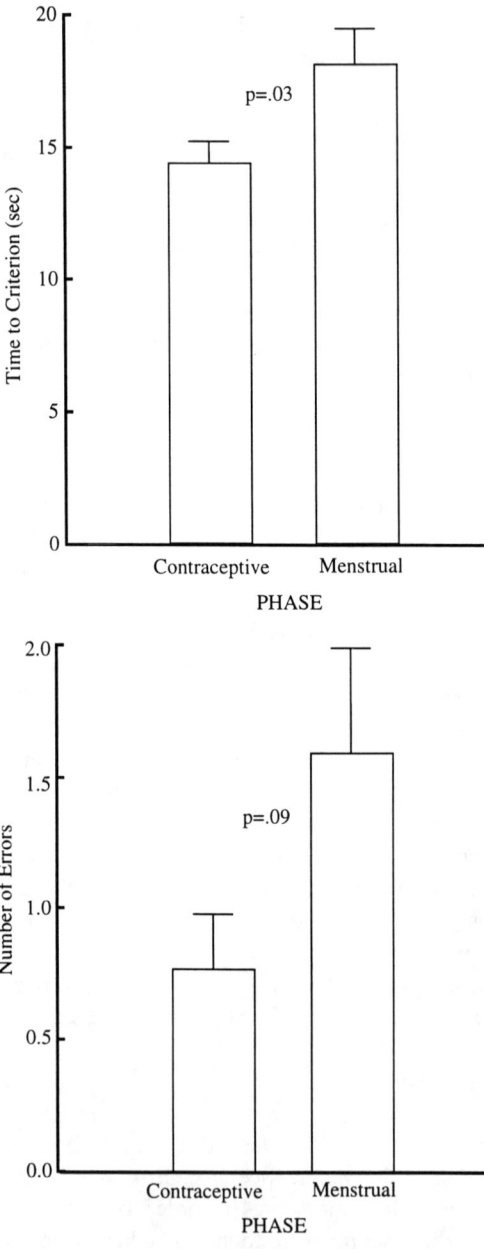

FIGURE 2 Mean time to reach criterion (Top) and the mean number of errors committed (Bottom) on the Manual Sequence Box as a function of oral contraceptive status.

As expected, for total time to criterion there was a main effect of phase of cycle. Women showed reduced time to reach criterion on the speeded trials of the Manual Sequence Box during the contraceptive portion of the cycle as compared to the menstrual phase, $F(1, 35) = 4.89$, $p < .05$. The Test Order × Phase interaction was not significant. This reduced time to criterion could mean either fewer errors or faster speed or both at the contraceptive phase. As Figure 2 illustrates, there was in fact a trend for the total number of errors to show a main effect of phase of cycle, $F(1, 35) = 3.03$, $p = .09$. Fewer errors were made at the contraceptive phase than at the menstrual phase. To determine whether speed was also faster at the contraceptive phase, the time to complete the last 10 (errorless) sequences was analyzed. There was no significant difference in speed between the two estrogen conditions (contraceptive = 12.04 sec, menstrual = 12.01 sec). In this study, therefore, the shorter total time to reach criterion on the Manual Sequence Box at the contraceptive phase was due to fewer errors rather than faster execution of movements per se.

Grasping, Bisection, and Pointing

The most novel aspect of this study was the inclusion of exploratory visual-motor tasks. In general, participants showed the expected effects of target distance, size, and eccentricity on the kinematics of their reaches. An effect of estrogen state, however, was only weakly and inconsistently found. Means and standard deviations for peak velocity, duration of the reach, deceleration time, and movement onset time for the three visual-motor tasks, as a function of test session and contraceptive status, are shown in Table 2.

Grasping

For grasping, a mean was calculated from the four reaches to each size and distance condition in each estrogen phase for each dependent measure. The means for each participant were then entered into a 2 × 3 × 3 × 2 ANOVA for each dependent measure, with phase of cycle (menstrual, contraceptive), object size (small, medium, large), and object distance (20 cm, 30 cm, 40 cm) as within-subjects factors and test order (contraceptive–menstrual [CM], menstrual–contraceptive [MC]) as a grouping factor.

The expected effects of object size and object distance were found, replicating the results of previous studies that have used this task (Jakobson & Goodale, 1991; Servos et al., 1992). Specifically, the duration of the reach increased as the distance of the target object increased, $F(2, 35) = 309.38$, $p < .001$.[1] Participants attained higher peak velocities as the target object was positioned farther away, $F(2, 30) =$

---

[1] Degrees of freedom were corrected using the Huynh–Feldt adjustment, where appropriate, to correct for violations of the circularity or homogeneity of variance assumption.

TABLE 2
Peak Velocity, Duration, Deceleration Time, and Movement Onset Time as a Function of Test Session and Contraceptive Status

	Session 1				Session 2			
	Contraceptive		Menstrual		Contraceptive		Menstrual	
	M	SD	M	SD	M	SD	M	SD
Mean peak velocity (cm/sec)								
Grasping	119.25	21.71	112.80	19.00	117.36	20.33	117.60	21.67
Bisection	117.00	12.27	121.60	23.53	127.29	25.06	120.89	17.05
Pointing	123.06	11.94	124.95	20.99	122.93	26.65	127.14	15.76
Duration of reach (msec)								
Grasping	582.33	146.39	601.81	90.46	570.15	72.88	573.72	162.89
Bisection	470.05	77.39	461.93	81.27	431.23	72.19	454.61	81.64
Pointing	447.03	49.75	468.63	101.86	474.43	117.19	450.16	62.71
Deceleration time (msec)								
Grasping	325.00	113.70	344.74	73.18	317.64	60.48	319.41	131.26
Bisection	285.89	75.12	281.85	66.05	260.47	44.47	287.39	60.71
Pointing	281.86	56.21	300.59	81.75	301.69	71.06	299.92	59.20
Movement onset time (msec)								
Grasping	375.75	63.89	370.20	29.78	355.94	50.97	368.95	73.61
Bisection	264.83	68.58	258.38	54.07	224.40	55.88	227.75	50.03
Pointing	208.47	49.52	211.83	31.55	203.05	44.18	196.06	32.37

507.16, $p < .001$. Duration and velocity also increased as the size of the target object increased; for duration, $F(2, 38) = 64.51$, $p < .001$; for velocity, $F(2, 44) = 16.59$, $p < .001$. This suggests that our participants were not atypical in terms of their basic reaching patterns.

Analysis of the grasping data revealed no significant effect of phase on movement onset time. In general, if movement amplitude is held constant, a decrease in the duration of a reach is accompanied by an increase in peak velocity and a decrease in the deceleration time. As such, it was not unexpected that these movement parameters would show correlated hormonal effects in this study. Although the duration of the entire reach appeared slightly shorter and the peak velocities slightly faster when women were tested while taking OCs as compared to the menstrual phase of the cycle, these effects did not reach conventional levels of significance. The main effect of phase on time spent decelerating was also nonsignificant.

A significant interaction between phase and test order was found on both duration, $F(1, 22) = 5.87$, $p < .025$, and deceleration time, $F(1, 22) = 4.22$, $p < .05$. For duration, a follow-up t test confirmed a trend for differential change across test sessions in the two order of testing groups, $t(22) = 1.39$, $p = .09$, one-tailed.

Women who were tested at the menstrual phase in the first session and the contraceptive phase in the second session tended to show a disproportionate reduction in movement duration on the second session (mean change = -31.66 msec) compared with women who were tested at the menstrual phase on the second session (mean change = -8.61 msec). A similar trend was evident for deceleration time, $t(22) = 1.35, p = .096$, one-tailed, with women on OCs in the second session tending to show greater improvement in deceleration time (mean change = -27.10 msec) than women who were at the menstrual phase in the second session (mean change = -5.59 msec). For peak velocity, the differential change across test sessions was significant, $t(22) = 1.67, p < .05$, one-tailed, with women on OCs in the second session showing greater improvement in peak velocity (mean change = 45.57 mm/sec) than women at the menstrual phase (mean change = -16.47 mm/sec), consistent with their presumed higher estrogen state on the second test session.

Pointing and Bisection

For bisection and pointing, a mean was calculated across the six reaches to each target location for each participant in each estrogen condition. The means for each participant were then entered into a separate 2 × 3 × 2 ANOVA for each dependent variable. Phase of cycle (contraceptive, menstrual) and target location (left, center, right) were within-subjects factors and test order (CM, MC) was a grouping factor.

In these tasks, the location of the target influenced the duration of movement in that reaches took increasingly longer from right to left targets; for pointing, $F(2, 48) = 80.63, p < .001$; for bisection, $F(2, 48) = 53.57, p < .001$. Similarly, peak velocity increased according to target location, with higher velocities being obtained for targets situated farther to the right; for pointing, $F(2, 33) = 242.38, p < .001$; for bisection, $F(2, 34) = 139.97, p < .001$. These findings are consistent with prior studies employing the bisection and pointing tasks with regard to reaching with the right hand (Carey, 1994), again suggesting that our participants are a representative sample.

No significant main effects of phase were found on any of the four kinematic variables examined, for either the pointing or bisection task. In the bisection task, there were interactions between phase and test order for movement onset time, peak velocity, and duration of the reach, but these reflected only simple practice effects in which onset time, $F(1, 24) = 14.28, p < .001$, and duration, $F(1, 24) = 3.56, p = .07$, were shorter in the second test session and peak velocity tended to be faster, $F(1, 24) = 3.34, p = .08$. For deceleration time, there appeared to be a differential pattern of change across the test sessions on the bisection task, with women on OCs on the second session showing a larger reduction in deceleration time (mean change

= −21.38 msec) than women at the menstrual phase (mean change = 1.50 msec), but this pattern was nonsignificant. In short, there was little evidence of a hormone-related effect on any of the kinematic speed variables for bisection, and not even a statistical trend for pointing.

An important and unique feature of the bisection and pointing tasks was that they allowed the endpoint accuracy of each reach to be assessed precisely by computing resultant error. A subtle increase in error at the contraceptive phase was not unexpected, given findings in other studies of decreased spatial skills during higher estrogen states (Hampson, 1990a; Hampson & Kimura, 1988; Silverman & Phillips, 1993). Any increase in error was expected to be more evident on the bisection task, as it arguably involves greater spatial demands than pointing (Goodale et al., 1990). Figure 3 shows the mean resultant error for the bisection and pointing tasks at the two test sessions as a function of OC status. There was no main effect of phase on resultant error in either pointing or bisection. The Phase × Test Order interaction was evaluated using a planned t test, which revealed a trend for differential change across test sessions in bisection, $t(19) = 1.55$, $p = .069$, one-tailed, but not in pointing. Despite previous practice on the bisection task, an increase in resultant error was seen in women who were on OCs in the second session (mean change = 2.60 mm of error per reach), whereas a negligible improvement in endpoint accuracy was seen in women at the menstrual phase (mean change = −0.11 mm of error per reach). Overall, on the second session, women on OCs displayed significantly higher resultant error scores than women in the menstrual group, $t(20) = 2.20$, $p < .025$.

Other Tasks

Mental Rotations Test

Scores on the Mental Rotations test were analyzed using a 2 × 2 (Phase of Cycle × Test Order) ANOVA. There was a tendency in the first session data for women at the menstrual phase to have higher Mental Rotations scores than women at the OC phase, $t(44) = 1.22$, $p = .11$, but the main effect of phase in the overall within-subjects analysis was not significant.

POMS

On the POMS questionnaire, there were no significant phase-related differences in the Tension, Anger, or Fatigue subscales. However, there was a trend for a decrease in Depression, $F(1, 39) = 3.80$, $p = .059$, and Confusion $F(1, 39) = 3.40$, $p = .073$, and an increase in Vigor, $F(1, 39) = 3.91$, $p = .055$, when women were taking OCs. Entering each of these variables as covariates in analyses of covariance

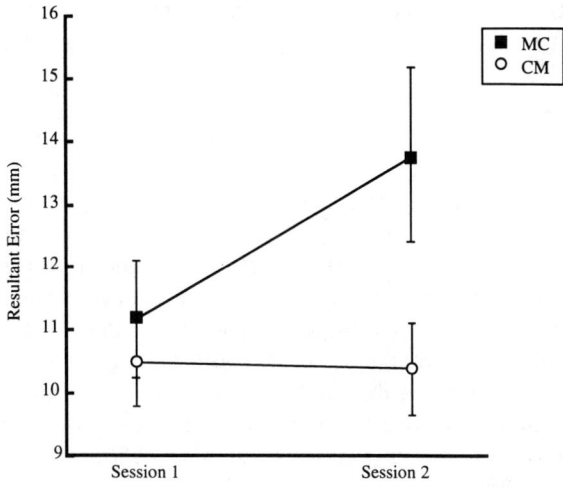

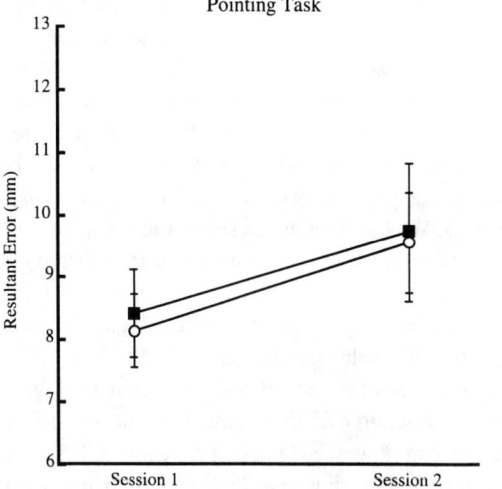

FIGURE 3 Mean resultant error on the two test sessions as a function of oral contraceptive status, for the bisection (Top) and pointing (Bottom) tasks. MC denotes participants tested at the menstrual phase first; CM denotes participants tested at the contraceptive phase first.

to control for changes in mood did not alter any of the patterns reported already for the visual-motor measures. Similarly, with regard to both the speed and error components of the Manual Sequence Box, none of the three covariates was significant (p values > .56), suggesting that changes in mood did not account for the motor changes seen across the contraceptive cycle.

DISCUSSION

The data from this study suggest that variations in motor performance do occur in OC users in accordance with changes in estrogen levels and, furthermore, that this hormone sensitivity may be task specific. The higher estrogen condition was associated with better performance on the Manual Sequence Box, a test of speeded motor programming, relative to performance at menses. This same facilitatory effect of estrogen occurred only weakly and inconsistently in tests of prehensile and aiming movements. Although there was a slight reduction in negative affect and an increase in positive affect at the higher estrogen phase, consistent with the results of some other studies (Marriott & Faragher, 1986), these did not account for the changes in motor performance.

One unexpected finding was the lack of hormone-related change in performance on the Mental Rotations test. Past studies have shown enhanced performance on a variety of spatial measures during the menstrual phase of the cycle when estrogen is at low levels as compared to time periods when estrogen levels are greatly increased (Hampson, 1990a; Hampson & Kimura, 1988; Silverman & Phillips, 1993). However, because the pattern of results was in the predicted direction in this study, it is possible that the inclusion of a larger battery of spatial tests, similar to those used in previous studies (Hampson, 1990a, 1990c), would have increased the reliability of the measure of spatial performance and thus increased the likelihood of finding significant differences. We note that in this study, only half the usual number of items was given at each session on the Mental Rotations test, which may have attenuated its reliability. Alternatively, the spatial effect may show more variability among OC users, perhaps varying with the estrogen and progestin content or schedule of the pills, or timing of testing in the OC cycle (see Hampson, 1990b).

The finding in this study of enhanced performance in the high estrogen condition on the computer modification of the Manual Sequence Box is consistent with previous literature (for review, see Hampson & Kimura, 1992). In fact, every study employing this motor sequencing task has shown an improvement in ability at higher estrogen levels. Furthermore, this effect has been achieved in a variety of populations, including spontaneously cycling women (Hampson, 1990a, 1990c; Hampson & Kimura, 1988; Saucier & Kimura, this issue), women receiving exogenous natural estrogen (Kimura & Hampson, 1993) or synthetic estrogen (Hampson, 1990b; Szekely, 1992), and women with athletic amenorrhea (Stokes

& Kimura, 1992). A novel finding of this study was that this effect may depend more on a reduction in errors at higher estrogen levels than on an increase in speed.

It is unlikely that these behavioral effects are primarily dependent on progestins, whose levels also change across the contraceptive cycle, for several reasons. First of all, improved performance on the Manual Sequence Box has been found at the preovulatory peak in estradiol in spontaneously cycling women, which is a phase of the menstrual cycle when progesterone levels are quite low (Hampson, 1990a). Facilitation of Manual Sequence Box performance has also been found in postmenopausal women on estrogen-alone replacement therapy (Kimura & Hampson, 1993). Interestingly, clinical cases of women with OC-induced chorea show that patients maintained on progesterone alone have no further choreic symptoms (Barber, Arnold, & Evans, 1976). Therefore, although we cannot completely rule out a contribution of progestins, it seems unlikely that these are a primary cause of the facilitation observed in Manual Sequence Box performance.

Animal studies have shown that estrogen can influence activity in extrahypothalamic brain regions involved in motor coordination such as the striatum and cerebellum (Becker & Beer, 1986; Becker & Cha, 1989; Smith, 1989). Estrogen improves sensorimotor coordination in the rat (Becker et al., 1986), but human studies using measures of motor skills such as reaction time, ambulation, arm movement, and line tracing have produced inconsistent findings (Becker et al., 1982; Hunter et al., 1979; Jensen, 1982; Morris & Udry, 1970; Pierson & Lockhart, 1963; Stenn & Klinge, 1972; Stocker, 1973; Wearing et al., 1972; Zimmerman & Parlee, 1973). Although the grasping, bisection, and pointing tasks were used in this study because they each involve movements that are inherent in the Manual Sequence Box, the results were equivocal and were not consistent among the three tasks. The reliable effect seen on the Manual Sequence Box coupled with the inconsistent results found when other motor skills were studied (including prehensile movements) may be related to the fact that the neural mechanisms underlying these tasks are different and that, consequently, the tasks vary in their hormone sensitivity.

Evidence from the neurological literature suggests that different types of movements rely on different underlying neural systems, at least to some degree. For example, people with manual apraxia show an inability to carry out learned movements with either hand, although strength and range of motion of the hands and arms are intact. This disorder almost exclusively follows damage to the left hemisphere, at least in right-handers (for review see Kimura, 1993). Kimura and colleagues noted that the reproduction of single hand postures is less affected than is a series of integrated movements of the hands and arms (Kimura, 1982; Kimura & Archibald, 1974). When apraxic patients were tested on the Manual Sequence Box, there was a high incidence of perseverative movements leading Kimura (1993) to suggest that the praxic system is primarily a movement selection system and that when several different movements must be carried out in rapid succession, especially high demands are placed on the system.

It could be argued that the motor demands of the reaching and pointing tasks do not, to the same extent as the Manual Sequence Box, place demands on the left-hemisphere praxic system. These tasks involve the selection and execution of only one type of movement, a movement that is then repeated over a series of trials. In contrast to the Manual Sequence Box, the reaching and pointing tasks do not require rapid changes in hand posture and continuous selection of distinctly different movements. Although evidence suggests that the organization of reaching and pointing movements may involve mechanisms within the left hemisphere as well (Fisk & Goodale, 1988; Goodale, 1988; Goodale et al., 1990), the degree of dependence of these prehensile movements on the praxic system may be considerably less than that of motor tasks that require the sequencing and integration of multiple movements.

Hampson and Kimura (1988, 1992) hypothesized that the left-hemisphere praxic system may be one of the specific brain areas sensitive to the effects of circulating estrogens in adults. This prediction was based, in part, on observations that verbal articulation and manual movements that are thought to be dependent on the left-hemisphere praxic system often show improvement at higher estrogen levels in women (Hampson 1990a, 1990b, 1990c; Hampson & Kimura, 1988; Stokes & Kimura, 1992). In favor of this hypothesis is the fact that this system shows a sex difference in cortical localization. Evidence from patients with localized brain damage has shown that, in women, specialized oral and manual praxic functions are dependent on the anterior left hemisphere, whereas in men, a more diffuse organization throughout the left hemisphere is seen (Hier, Yoon, Mohr, Price, & Wolf, 1994; Kimura, 1983). This sex difference in cortical organization favors the notion that this system may be hormone sensitive because, in other species, sex differences in brain organization arise under the influence of gonadal hormones (Breedlove, 1992). Sex differences also have been found in performance on the Manual Sequence Box and other tasks requiring sequencing of multiple movements (Denckla, 1974; Kimura, 1986; Nicholson & Kimura, 1996), whereas there is little evidence for sex differences in the proficiency of the visual-motor tasks used in this study (cf. Jakobson, 1987).

In further accounting for the lack of congruence between the Manual Sequence Box and the grasping, bisection, and pointing tasks, consideration must be given to the relative contribution of visuospatial information to the two types of tasks. Whereas the visual contribution to the Manual Sequence Box is almost certainly minimal once the task is acquired (Kimura, 1993), Goodale and colleagues have shown that changes in the spatial elements of reaching and pointing tasks may profoundly alter the movement kinematics of the reach. For example, peak velocity and duration of the reach have been shown to change as a function of object distance and, in some studies, object size (Jakobson & Goodale, 1991; Servos et al., 1992). Indeed, these findings were replicated in this study.

It is apparent that estrogen tends to influence visuospatial and motor tasks in opposite directions across the menstrual cycle; that is, as previously mentioned, several studies have revealed an increase in accuracy on visuospatial tasks and a decrease in speed or accuracy on motor tasks at menses. The fact that in the reaching and pointing tasks, the movement kinematics tend to be related to certain visuospatial parameters may mitigate against finding any significant changes in these motor skills across the menstrual cycle. Although performance on the Manual Sequence Box showed significant OC-related fluctuations in the predicted direction, the lack of significant changes in the kinematics associated with reaching and pointing could possibly be explained by the requirements of online estimation of object distance, object size, target location, or other visuospatial parameters of these tasks.

It should also be pointed out that the pointing and bisection tasks do allow for some separate assessment of the speed and accuracy components of limb placement, which could reflect the motor and visuospatial aspects of the tasks, respectively. One might have expected participants to have been faster at the OC phase when estrogen was relatively high while showing a simultaneous decrease in accuracy in relation to the target position. In this study, the resultant error showed a tendency for reduced accuracy in the high estrogen condition on the bisection task without a concomitant reduction in speed components of the reach. Indeed, the resultant error was significantly greater in the OC group than in the menstrual group on the second session. These results provide limited support for the notion that high levels of estrogen may decrease spatial accuracy because the visuospatial demands on the bisection task are arguably greater than on the pointing task even though the physical demands of the reach are very similar.

A final comment on these results concerns the central estrogen levels resulting from the low-dose OCs used in this study. Ethinyl estradiol levels could not be directly measured, and there is substantial individual variability in the metabolism of contraceptive steroids. Even so, pharmacokinetic studies support the assumption that the effective estrogen dose is higher during pill ingestion than during the menstrual washout phase of the contraceptive cycle, providing a variety of timing considerations are observed (Humpel et al., 1990; Longcope & Williams, 1977). It does not necessarily follow that effective estrogen levels are as high or higher in OC users than during the natural menstrual cycle.

This investigation was carried out in order to explore the effects of OC hormones on motor performance. Numerous measures were used, including tests of rapid prehensile movements and a motor sequencing task. A facilitatory effect of estrogen was found on the manual sequencing task but not on the reaching and pointing tasks, indicating that different motor measures may have varying hormone sensitivities. The Manual Sequence Box task differs from grasping, pointing, and bisection in at least two respects—the rapid selection and sequencing of discrete movements and the minimal use of ongoing visual guidance. The improved performance on the Manual Sequence Box supports the hypothesis that higher estrogen conditions facilitate functioning of specific left-hemisphere regions, including those subserving manual praxis.

ACKNOWLEDGMENTS

Christine Szekely is now at Sunnybrook Health Science Centre, Cognitive Neurology Unit, Toronto, Canada.

Elizabeth Hampson was supported by a New Faculty Research Fellowship from the Ontario Mental Health Foundation, Toronto, Canada. This work was done in partial fulfillment of the requirements of Christine Szekely's master's degree at the University of Western Ontario, London, Canada. We thank Lorna Jakobson for helpful discussions and Melonie Hopkins for scoring of videotapes.

REFERENCES

Barber, P. V., Arnold, A. G., & Evans, G. (1976). Recurrent hormone dependent chorea: Effects of oestrogens and progestogens. *Clinical Endocrinology, 5,* 291–293.

Beatty, W. W. (1992). Gonadal hormones and sex differences in nonreproductive behaviours. In A. A. Gerall, H. Moltz, & I. L. Ward (Eds.), *Handbook of behavioral neurobiology: Vol. 11. Sexual differentiation* (pp. 85–128). New York: Plenum.

Becker, D., Creutzfeldt, O. D., Schwibbe, M., & Wuttke, W. (1982). Changes in physiological, EEG, and psychological parameters in women during the spontaneous menstrual cycle and following oral contraceptives. *Psychoneuroendocrinology, 7,* 75–90.

Becker, J. B., & Beer, M. E. (1986). The influence of estrogen on nigrostriatal dopamine activity: Behavioral and neurochemical evidence for both pre- and postsynaptic components. *Behavioural Brain Research, 19,* 27–33.

Becker, J. B., & Cha, J. (1989). Estrous cycle-dependent variation in amphetamine-induced behaviours and striatal dopamine release assessed with microdialysis. *Behavioural Brain Research, 35,* 117–125.

Becker, J. B., Snyder, P. J., Miller, M. M., Westgate, S. A., & Jenuwine, M. J. (1986). The influence of estrous cycle and intrastriatal estradiol on sensorimotor performance in the female rat. *Pharmacology, Biochemistry, and Behaviour, 27,* 53–59.

Breedlove, S. M. (1992). Sexual dimorphism in the vertebrate nervous system. *The Journal of Neuroscience, 12,* 4133–4142.

Briggs, M., & Briggs, M. (1983). Oral contraceptives containing estrogen plus progestogen. In G. Benagiano & E. Diczfalusy (Eds.), *Endocrine mechanisms in fertility regulation* (pp. 17–48). New York: Raven.

Burke, A. W., & Broadhurst, P. L. (1966). Behavioural correlates of the oestrous cycle in the rat. *Nature, 209,* 223–224.

Carey, D. P. (1994). *Hand and hemispace differences in the visual control of aiming movements.* Unpublished doctoral dissertation, University of Western Ontario, London, Canada.

Collaer, M. L., & Hines, M. (1995). Human behavioral sex differences: A role for gonadal hormones during early development? *Psychological Bulletin, 118,* 55–107.

Colvin, G. B., & Sawyer, C. H. (1969). Induction of running activity by intracerebral implants of estrogen in ovariectomized rats. *Neuroendocrinology, 4,* 309–320.

Denckla, M. B. (1974). Development of motor co-ordination in normal children. *Developmental Medicine and Child Neurology, 16,* 729–741.

Dibbelt, L., Knuppen, R., Jutting, G., Heimann, S., Klipping, C. O., & Parikka-Olexik, H. (1989). Group comparison of serum ethinyl estradiol, SHBG and CBG levels in 83 women using two low-dose combination oral contraceptives for three months. *Contraception, 43*, 1–21.

Fishman, J., & Norton, B. (1977). Relative transport of estrogens into the central nervous system. In S. Garattini & H. W. Berendes (Eds.), *Pharmacology of steroid contraceptive drugs* (pp. 37–41). New York: Raven.

Fisk, J. D., & Goodale, M. A. (1988). The effects of unilateral brain damage on visually guided reaching: Hemispheric differences in the nature of the deficit. *Experimental Brain Research, 72*, 425–435.

Goodale, M. A. (1988). Hemispheric differences in motor control. *Behavioral Brain Research, 30*, 203–214.

Goodale, M. A., Milner, A. D., Jakobson, L. S., & Carey, D. P. (1990). Kinematic analysis of limb movements in neuropsychological research: Subtle deficits and recovery of function. *Canadian Journal of Psychology, 44*, 180–195.

Hampson, E. (1990a). Estrogen-related variations in human spatial and articulatory-motor skills. *Psychoneuroendocrinology, 15*, 97–111.

Hampson, E. (1990b). Influence of gonadal hormones on cognitive function in women. *Clinical Neuropharmacology, 13*(Suppl. 2), 522–523.

Hampson, E. (1990c). Variations in sex-related cognitive abilities across the menstrual cycle. *Brain and Cognition, 14*, 26–43.

Hampson, E., & Kimura, D. (1984). Hand movement asymmetries during verbal and nonverbal tasks. *Canadian Journal of Psychology, 38*, 102–125.

Hampson, E., & Kimura, D. (1988). Reciprocal effects of hormonal fluctuations on human motor and perceptual-spatial skills. *Behavioral Neuroscience, 102*, 456–459.

Hampson, E., & Kimura, D. (1992). Sex differences and hormonal influences on cognitive function in humans. In J. B. Becker, S. M. Breedlove, & D. Crews (Eds.), *Behavioral endocrinology* (pp. 357–398). Cambridge, MA: MIT Press.

Hier, D. B., Yoon, W. B., Mohr, J. P., Price, T. R., & Wolf, P. A. (1994). Gender and aphasia in the stroke data bank. *Brain and Language, 47*, 155–167.

Humpel, M., Tauber, U., Kuhnz, W., Pfeffer, M., Brill, K., Heithecker, R., Louton, T., & Steinberg, B. (1990). Comparison of serum ethinyl estradiol, sex-hormone-binding globulin, corticoid-binding globulin and cortisol levels in women using two low-dose combined oral contraceptives. *Hormone Research, 33*, 35–39.

Hunter, S., Schraer, R., Landers, D. M., Buskirk, E. R., & Harris, D. V. (1979). The effects of total oestrogen concentration and menstrual-cycle phase on reaction time performance. *Ergonomics, 22*, 263–268.

Jakobson, L. S. (1987). *Automatic recalibration following prismatic displacement.* Unpublished master's thesis, University of Western Ontario, London, Canada.

Jakobson, L. S., & Goodale, M. A. (1991). Factors affecting higher-order movement planning: A kinematic analysis of human prehension. *Experimental Brain Research, 86*, 199–208.

Jensen, B. K. (1982). Menstrual cycle effects on task performance examined in the context of stress research. *Acta Psychologica, 50*, 159–178.

Kimura, D. (1977). Acquisition of a motor skill after left-hemisphere damage. *Brain, 100*, 527–542.

Kimura, D. (1982). Left-hemisphere control of oral and brachial movements and their relation to communication. *Philosophical Transactions of the Royal Society of London, 298*, 135–149.

Kimura, D. (1983). Sex differences in cerebral organization for speech and praxic functions. *Canadian Journal of Psychology, 37*, 19–35.

Kimura, D. (1986). *Neuropsychology test procedures.* London, Canada: D. K. Consultants.

Kimura, D. (1993). *Neuromotor mechanisms of human communication.* Oxford, England: Oxford University Press.

Kimura, D., & Archibald, Y. (1974). Motor functions of the left hemisphere. *Brain, 97*, 337–350.

Kimura, D., & Hampson, E. (1993). Neural and hormonal mechanisms mediating sex differences in cognition. In P. A. Vernon (Ed.), *Biological approaches to the study of human intelligence* (pp. 375–397). Norwood, NJ: Ablex.

Longcope, C., & Williams, K. I. H. (1977). Ethynylestradiol and mestranol: Their pharmacodynamics and effects on natural estrogens. In S. Garattinni & H. W. Berendes (Eds.), *Pharmacology of steroid contraceptive drugs* (pp. 89–98). New York: Raven.

Marriott, A., & Faragher, E. B. (1986). An assessment of psychological state associated with the menstrual cycle in users of oral contraception. *Journal of Psychosomatic Research, 30,* 41–47.

McNair, D. M., Lorr, M., & Droppleman, L. F. (1971). *Profile of Mood States.* San Diego, CA: EdITS.

Morris, N. M., & Udry, J. R. (1970). Variations in pedometer activity during the menstrual cycle. *Obstetrics and Gynecology, 35,* 199–201.

Nicholson, K. G., & Kimura, D. K. (1996). Sex differences for speech and manual skill. *Perceptual and Motor Skills, 82,* 3–13.

Pierson, W. R., & Lockhart, A. (1963). Effect of menstruation on simple reaction time and movement time. *British Medical Journal, 1,* 796–797.

Saucier, D. M., & Kimura, D. (1998/this issue). Intrapersonal motor but not extrapersonal targeting skill is enhanced during the midluteal phase of the menstrual cycle. *Developmental Neuropsychology, 14,* 385–398.

Servos, P., Goodale, M. A., & Jakobson, L. S. (1992). The role of binocular vision in prehension: A kinematic analysis. *Vision Research, 32,* 1513–1521.

Silverman, I., & Phillips, K. (1993). Effects of estrogen changes during the menstrual cycle on spatial performance. *Ethology and Sociobiology, 14,* 257–270.

Smith, S. S. (1989). Estrogen administration increases neuronal responses to excitatory amino acids as a long-term effect. *Brain Research, 503,* 354–357.

Smith, S. S., Waterhouse, B. D., & Woodward, D. J. (1987). Sex steroid effects on extrahypothalamic CNS: I. Estrogen augments neuronal responsiveness to iontophoretically applied glutamate in the cerebellum. *Brain Research, 422,* 40–51.

Sommer, B. (1992). Cognitive performance and the menstrual cycle. In J. T. E. Richardson (Ed.), *Cognition and the menstrual cycle* (pp. 39–63). New York: Springer-Verlag.

Stenn, P. G., & Klinge, V. (1972). Relationship between the menstrual cycle and bodily activity in humans. *Hormones and Behavior, 3,* 297–305.

Stocker, J. M. (1973). Motor performance and state anxiety at selected stages of the menstrual cycle. *Dissertation Abstracts International, 34,* 3971A.

Stokes, K. A., & Kimura, D. (1992). *Menstrual cyclicity and cognitive ability patterns in athletes* (Department of Psychology Research Bulletin No. 705). London, Canada: University of Western Ontario.

Stumpf, W. E., & Sar, M. (1977). Sites of action of contraceptive drugs in the central nervous system. In S. Garattini & H. W. Berendes (Eds.), *Pharmacology of steroid contraceptive drugs* (pp. 43–52). New York: Raven.

Szekely, C. A. (1992). *Cognitive performance in oral contraceptive users.* Unpublished bachelor's thesis, University of Western Ontario, London, Canada.

Vandenberg, S. G., & Kuse, A. R. (1978). Mental rotations: A group test of three-dimensional spatial visualization. *Perceptual and Motor Skills, 47,* 599–604.

Vick, L. H., & Banks, E. M. (1969). The estrous cycle and related behavior in the Mongolian gerbil *meriones unguiculatus* milne-edwards. *Communications in Behavioral Biology, 3A,* 117–124.

Vreeburg, J. T. M., Schretlen, P. J. M., & Baum, M. J. (1974). Specific, high-affinity binding of 17ß-estradiol in cytosols from several brain regions and pituitary of intact and castrated adult male rats. *Endocrinology, 97,* 969–977.

Wearing, M. P., Yuhosz, M. D., Campbell, R., & Love, E. J. (1972). The effect of the menstrual cycle on tests of physical fitness. *Journal of Sports Medicine, 12,* 38–41.

Zimmerman, E., & Parlee, M. B. (1973). Behavioral changes associated with the menstrual cycle: An experimental investigation. *Journal of Applied Social Psychology, 3,* 335–344.

The Cognitive Neuropsychology of Sex Hormones in Men and Women

Jeri S. Janowsky, Bambi Chavez, and Brian D. Zamboni

Departments of Neurology and Behavioral Neuroscience
Oregon Health Sciences University, Portland

Eric Orwoll

Department of Medicine
Oregon Health Sciences University
and Veterans Affairs Medical Center, Portland

In this study, we examined sex differences in performance on a variety of cognitive tasks. Performance was correlated with estradiol and testosterone levels in both men and women in order to examine whether hormone levels are related to performance on tasks that do and do not show sex differences. Men showed an advantage in performance on tests of spatial cognition (block design and card rotation) as well as a dart throwing task that requires both motor skills and spatial cognition. Sex differences were not found for measures of verbal and nonverbal memory, verbal fluency, or fine motor performance. Hormone levels were related to performance on tasks that showed sex differences as well as those that did not. Estradiol, but not testosterone, was related to block design in women but not men. Women with higher estradiol levels showed better performance than women with lower estradiol levels. No relations between card rotation and hormone levels were found. Performance on the two spatial cognitive measures were related to each other in women, but not men, suggesting that men may use different processes than women to accomplish these tasks. Performance on the dart throwing task was not consistently related to the spatial cognitive measures in either men or women. Positive relations that will require confirmation were found between estradiol and spatial recall, and between testosterone and verbal recall, in men. In general, both men and women showed a negative relation between both estradiol and testosterone and dart throwing performance.

Requests for reprints should be sent to Jeri Janowsky, Department of Neurology, Oregon Health Sciences University, CR131 3181 S.W. Sam Jackson Park Road, Portland, Oregon 97201–3098. E-mail: janowskj@ohsu.edu

These results do not support the notion that sex differences will necessarily predict the direction of the relation (positive or negative) between estrogen or testosterone and behavior in adulthood.

Many previous studies have shown sex differences in performance on a variety of cognitive tasks. Other studies have shown relations between hormone levels and performance on cognitive tasks. Very few studies have examined both sex differences and the relation between sex hormones (estrogen and testosterone) and performance in the same individuals. Therefore, it is not known whether circulating hormone levels influence sex differences in performance and whether circulating sex hormones influence performance on tasks for which sex differences have not been previously described. The purpose of this study was to examine both sex differences and the relation between hormones and performance in men and women. We do not review all of the studies on sex differences or hormone effects here, but focus on those directly relevant to this study.

Men and women differ systematically on tests of spatial cognition (for a review, see Halpern, 1986; Hampson & Kimura, 1992; Kimura, 1996; Maccoby & Jacklin, 1974; McGlone, 1980; Voyer, Voyer, & Bryden, 1995). Relevant to this study are studies showing that, on average, men have an advantage on tasks of spatial cognition such as the Viewfinding Task (Watson & Kimura, 1991), localization (Gordon & Lee, 1986), orientation (Gordon & Lee, 1986), and mental rotation (Gouchie & Kimura 1991; Moffat & Hampson, 1996; Sanders, Soares, & D'Aquila, 1982; Tapley & Bryden, 1977). Men also show an advantage on tasks that require both motor skills and spatial cognition, such as catching an object (Watson & Kimura, 1991) or throwing darts (Watson & Kimura 1989, 1991).

On average, women have an advantage on tasks requiring perceptual speed and fine motor skills, such as identification of pictures (Watson & Kimura, 1991) or sequenced hand movements (Nicholson & Kimura, 1996). In general, women are reported to be more verbally fluent than men (Stumpf, 1995), although mixed results have been obtained. For instance, studies have shown a female advantage for quickly producing words from a particular semantic category (e.g., foods; Gordon & Lee, 1986) but no sex difference for rapidly producing words beginning with a particular letter (Gordon & Lee, 1986). Others have found no sex difference for either type of fluency measure (e.g., Moffat & Hampson, 1996; for a review, see Hampson & Kimura, 1992) or a task of rapid articulation (Gouchie & Kimura, 1991).

A female advantage on word list learning tasks (Geffen, Moar, O'Hanlon, Clark, & Geffen, 1990; Kramer, Delis, & Daniel, 1988; Trahan & Quintana, 1990) as well as a slower rate of forgetting of words in women (Hart & O'Shanick, 1993) have also been reported. To our knowledge, sex differences on other forms of verbal and nonverbal learning and memory tasks have not been reported. We investigate here sex differences and hormone effects on both verbal and nonverbal memory measures.

Sex differences in spatial cognition, verbal fluency, or memory are not found in all studies. Differences among studies may be due, in part, to weak sex differences (small effects) that require large numbers of participants for identification. In addition, the hormonal status of participants may modify the degree of sex differences found. Several studies show that cognitive performance is modifiable in adulthood by the hormonal status of participants (Chiarello, McMahon, & Schaefer, 1989; Gouchie & Kimura, 1991; Hampson, 1990; Hampson & Kimura, 1988; Kampen & Sherwin, 1994, 1996; Phillips & Sherwin, 1992; Sherwin & Tulandi, 1996; Shute, Pellegrino, Hubert, & Reynolds, 1983). For instance, women at the low-estrogen phase of their menstrual cycle show enhanced spatial cognition, with the opposite being true at the high-estrogen phase (Hampson, 1990). Women show enhanced motor skills during the high-estrogen phase as compared to the low-estrogen phase (Hampson & Kimura, 1988). Women on estrogen replacement therapy show enhanced verbal memory, but no change in spatial memory, as compared to women not on replacement (Kampen & Sherwin, 1994; Sherwin, 1988; Sherwin & Tulandi, 1996; for a review, see Sherwin, 1994). Estrogen levels were also significantly related to visual memory in men such that men with higher estrogen had better visual memory than men with lower levels (Kampen & Sherwin, 1996). Szekely, Hampson, Carey, and Goodale (this issue) show that oral contraceptives affect manual praxis, and we have shown that estradiol is related to performance on a manual sequence task in women but not men (Jennings, Janowsky, & Orwoll, 1998). Finally, older men show enhanced spatial cognition when supplemented with testosterone to levels similar to that of younger men (Janowsky, Oviatt, & Orwoll, 1994). None of the studies just cited compared the cognitive performance of participants to those of the opposite sex. Therefore, the degree to which circulating hormone levels affects sex differences in performance between men and women has not been directly examined. We address this in this study by examining sex differences in performance as well as the circulating hormone levels of both men and women.

Differences among studies with regard to hormone effects or sex differences may also be due to the specific measures used suggesting that particular cognitive processes are influenced by hormones or are sexually dimorphic, or both. Comparing a participant's performance across cognitive measures is a method used in neuropsychology, and more recently cognitive neuroscience, to isolate the brain regions critical for a particular cognitive task or process. Impairments on tasks by participants with circumscribed brain injury, but relative preservation of performance on other tasks, suggest regions that are critical for task performance. In this study, we also compare across measures to examine which measures do and do not show sex differences or are affected by circulating sex hormones (see Nicholson

& Kimura, 1996; Szekely et al., this issue; Watson & Kimura, 1991, for a similar method of analysis).

Differences in cognition and behavior between men and women have been attributed to ontogenetic sex differences in brain development (Nordeen & Yahr, 1982; Phoenix, Goy, Gerall, & Young, 1959; for a review, see Berenbaum, Korman, & Leveroni, 1995; Collaer & Hines, 1995). Studies using techniques such as dichotic listening (McGlone, 1980), the examination of sexual dimorphism in language disorders after unilateral cerebrovascular accidents (Kimura, 1983; McGlone, 1977), behavior genetics (Resnick, Gottesman, & McGue, 1993), surgery for intractable epilepsy (Trenerry, Jack, Cascino, Sharbrough, & Ivnik, 1995), brain metabolism (Andreason, Zametkin, Guo, Baldwin, & Cohen, 1996; Gur et al., 1995), blood flow as assessed with functional magnetic resonance imaging (fMRI; Shaywitz et al., 1995), or brain morphology (Aboitiz, Scheibel, & Zaidel, 1992; Cowell et al., 1994; Gur et al., 1995; Witelson, 1989) suggest that cognitive differences are due to neural organizational differences between men and women's brains. For example, the posterior part of the corpus callosum is larger in women (DeLacoste-Utamsing & Holloway, 1982; but see Bishop & Wahlsten, 1997) and this is also found in the very old (Salat, Ward, Kaye, & Janowsky, 1997). Women with left-hemisphere brain damage are less likely to show as severe impairments in language as men with similar damage (Kimura, 1983). Women show a more bilateral representation of language than men using fMRI (Shaywitz et al., 1995), and men show higher resting brain metabolism than women in temporal lobe regions (Gur et al., 1995). A sex difference in neural organization does not preclude modification of sex differences due to task difficulty (Collins & Kimura, 1996) or life experiences (Baenninger & Newcombe, 1989, 1995). For instance, sports experience or using a nonpreferred (inexperienced) hand on a motor task modifies the degree of sex difference but does not eradicate a sex difference in performance (Hall & Kimura, 1995).

It is likely that ontogenetically established sexual dimorphisms, as well as the hormonal state of the participant, influence cognition. Although circulating hormones may affect the same regions that are organized by hormones during brain development, numerous recent studies have identified mechanisms by which hormones can affect other nonsexually dimorphic regions as well. Circulating androgens and estrogens can modify neural activity in adulthood (McEwen, 1991). Androgens and estrogen can act on intracellular genomic receptors to influence gene expression resulting in changes in receptors, neuropeptide availability, and synaptogenesis (McEwen, Jones, & Pfaff, 1987; for a review, see Pfaff, 1980). This has been described for brain areas related to sexual behaviors and sex organ morphology such as the hypothalamus. Recently, however, effects of estrogen and testosterone have been found in neural systems that do not have steroid receptors and are not strictly involved in sexual behavior. For instance, estrogen and testosterone can work indirectly on brain activity by being converted to metabolites that affect neurotransmitter receptor function. One example is that estrogen affects the gamma aminobutyric acid receptor chloride channels in the hippocampus (Gee, 1988) and increases the density of one form of serotonin receptor (5-HT_{2A}) in frontal cortex of rats (Sumner & Fink, 1995). Estrogen modifies dendritic branching and synapse formation in the hippocampus during development and in adulthood (Woolley & McEwen, 1992, 1993). This occurs in a cyclical pattern in relation to the estrus cycle in studies using a rat animal model. Estradiol also modulates dopamine-mediated striatal sensorimotor function despite the fact that there are few or no estrogen receptors in the striatum (Becker & Beer, 1986; Becker, Snyder, Miller, Westgate, & Jenuwine, 1987). It was recently found that this occurs by estrogen's modification of calcium channels at the cell membrane (Melmerstein, Becker, & Surmeier, 1996). It is likely that other neurobiological mechanisms for sex hormone effects on brain activity will be described in the future. Therefore, sex hormones can act on many cortical brain regions, including those for which ontogenetic sexual dimorphisms in morphology or function have not been found.

The effects of circulating hormones on behavior have been called *activational effects* (Kimura & Hampson, 1994; Phoenix et al., 1959). Activation implies the initiation of a previously absent behavior. Although this is an apt description of the effects of sex hormones on the control of sexual behavior, this may not be the best descriptor for the neuromodulatory roles of sex hormones on neural activity and anatomy in the cortex just described. Instead, *modulation* may better describe the moment-to-moment, or day-to-day, effects of hormones on the brain and behavior. We hypothesize that sex hormones have effects both in cognitive domains (and their underlying neural bases) that show ontogenetic sex differences as well as those that do not. We hypothesize that neuromodulation may be sex specific. For instance, estrogen but not other sex hormones, affects membrane calcium currents in basal ganglia neurons, and the effects are greater for neurons from female rats than for those from male rats (Melmerstein et al., 1996). Therefore, we would expect the neuromodulatory effects of sex hormones to differentially affect behavior in men and women, and enhance or impair performance depending on the neural system affected (Leiberburg & McEwen, 1977). The study reported here investigates the relation between hormone levels and performance on tasks that have previously been shown to have sex differences as well as those that have not.

In this study, we compare sex differences and the relation between hormone levels and performance in multiple cognitive measures in the same participants. These data were collected to set the stage for studies of the effects of hormone loss and hormone supplementation in the aged as well as studies that seek to isolate the cognitive processes and neural basis of hormone action in adults.

METHOD

Participants

Eighteen men and 30 women participated in the study. They were part of a larger study concerning the effects of hormones on cognition in the aged. Participant demographics are shown in Table 1. Briefly, participants were 23 to 34 years of age and had 12 to 24 years of education. Men and women did not differ in age or education, $t(46) < 1.4, p > .10$. Men and women also did not differ in their performance on the Vocabulary subtest of the Wechsler Adult Intelligence Scale–Revised (WAIS–R; Wechsler, 1981) as an index of general cognitive functioning, $t(46) < 1.0, p > .10$. One man and 3 women reported they were left-handed (see Data Analysis section for special consideration of these participants). Participants were recruited via advertisements in a university newsletter. All participants received $10 per hour. Participants were aware that this was a study of the role that sex hormones play on cognition, although they were not aware of specific hypotheses regarding the effects of hormones on the cognitive measures studied.

Participants were screened for a variety of health and hormone factors. These 48 participants met screening and health criteria that matched them to participants in an older cohort for a parallel study of sex hormone supplementation effects in the aged. Health status was assessed through a short health questionnaire concerning hospitalizations and current medications. Participants were sought who did not smoke, drank fewer than three alcoholic beverages per day, were not taking medicines likely to affect cognition or sex hormones (e.g., oral contraceptives), and had no neurologic (e.g., epilepsy, significant head injury) or psychiatric history (currently, or in the last year on medication or hospitalized for psychiatric or

TABLE 1
Participant Characteristics

	Men[a]			Women[b]		
	M	SD	Range	M	SD	Range
Age	28.5	3.1	23–34	29.8	3.2	24–34
Education	16.1	1.6	14–19	16.4	2.6	12–24
WAIS–R Vocabulary[c]	12.3	1.2	9–14	12.1	1.7	8–16
Estradiol (pg/ml) Session 1	23.6	7.9	10.0–37.5	122.3	59.5	4.9–248.9
Estradiol (pg/ml) Session 2	26.7	10.8	9.5–50.5	104.5	66.0	4.9–105.5
Free testosterone (pg/ml) Session 1	26.5	7.1	15.7–43.4	1.40	0.79	0.65–3.40
Free testosterone (pg/ml) Session 2	24.2	7.9	12.5–34.2	1.54	0.84	0.65–3.60

Note. WAIS–R = Wechsler Adult Intelligence Scale–Revised.
[a]$n = 18$. [b]$n = 30$. [c]WAIS–R scaled score.

emotional problems). Those qualifying were then further screened with a detailed health questionnaire (Cornell Medical Index, 1974), blood screening (cholesterol, blood chemistry, estradiol, free testosterone; normal for sex and the 23–35-year-old age range; see Table 2), normal length of the menstrual cycle for women (> 25 and < 35 days), and the Geriatric Depression Scale (GDS; Yesavage, Brink, & Rose, 1983). The GDS was used because depression is common in the elderly and we were matching the young participants' data to subsequently obtained data from an older sample of participants who were also screened with the GDS for depression. One woman was excluded due to her GDS score (> 10) and her endorsement of emotional problems on the Cornell Medical Index. Women reporting irregular cycles, 1 woman who became pregnant, and 1 man with an abnormally low testosterone level were excluded. One woman did not complete the study due to illness. Four other participants meeting criteria chose not to participate in the study. Thus, a total of 48 participants' data are reported here.

Procedure

After completing the screening visit, individuals participated in two test sessions. The second test session was approximately 4 weeks after the first test session and was scheduled to try to be at approximately the same point in the menstrual cycle for the women as the first test session. Men and women had comparable intertest session intervals (an average of 28.7 days for men and 29.5 days for women). Data from the second test session are utilized here to examine the consistency of findings with repeated testing. The data were also obtained to match the study design of the parallel study of hormone supplementation effects in the aged.

Our goal was to test women at the midluteal phase of their menstrual cycle, approximately 4 to 10 days before their menstrual period, when estrogen is relatively high. We reasoned that this phase, when hormonally men and women differ the most, would be when the largest differences in cognition between men and women would likely be found. Women were contacted by telephone after the test sessions to confirm the date of menstruation and to estimate the length of the cycle (Hampson, 1990). The average length of women's cycles between the first and second test session was 30.6 days ($SD = 4.8$). One woman's menstruation was greatly delayed for unknown reasons. Due to a scheduling problem, another woman was tested in the second session after her cycle ended. One woman whose hormone levels were normal at screening were low at both test sessions. The data from these women are included here, as they did not change the findings reported. All test sessions were in the morning. During both test sessions, participants had their blood drawn to assess hormone levels and they completed a set of cognitive measures.

Serum hormone levels were analyzed by the Clinical Research Center Laboratory at Oregon Health Science University with radioimmunoassay as per standard procedures for the assay (Diagnostic Products). Duplicate samples were run for each participant for each test session along with duplicate control samples. Samples for each participant from the two test sessions were run in the same assay to prevent interassay variability that would affect data on hormone levels across sessions. On rare occasions when duplicate samples differed widely, the samples were run again. The hormone levels reported for each session are the average of the duplicate samples. Approximately 15 participants' samples were run in a single assay, so that approximately three assays were necessary to process all of the samples for this study. The interassay standard variability for the Clinical Research Center averaged 8.0 for estradiol and 11.0 for free testosterone. These are in close agreement with the variability reported by the manufacturer (8.1 and 12.8, respectively). We examined free testosterone as opposed to total testosterone because we were interested in whether the testosterone available, or circulating, had effects on cognition.

Cognitive Measures

The measures chosen for study come from four major cognitive domains: spatial cognition, memory, verbal fluency, and motor function. These were chosen because they have not been studied together in both men and women, and relations between these measures and both estrogen and testosterone levels have not been examined previously in both men and women.

Spatial cognition. The spatial cognitive measures examined in this study have been reported by others to favor men, although these measures have not been examined together in the same participants. In addition, performance on these tasks has not been related to hormone status in both men and women.

The Block Design subtest of the WAIS–R (Weschler, 1981) was administered and scored according to standard testing procedures. This is a complex visual-construction task, and damage to many different brain regions disrupt performance, suggesting multiple brain systems and cognitive processes are required. However, patients with damage to the parietal lobe, particularly in the right hemisphere, have disrupted performance on this task that cannot be attributed to motor or cognitive planning disorders (Warrington, James, & Maciejewski, 1986). Functional neuroimaging studies have shown increased glucose metabolism in posterior parietal regions during performance (Chase, Fedio, & Foster, 1984). A previous study of older men showed that testosterone treatment enhanced performance, and estradiol was negatively related to performance on this task (Janowsky et al., 1994).

The Card Rotation task was administered in the standard manner (Ekstrom, French, Harman, & Derman, 1976). On each problem set, participants assessed whether each of eight figures were the same as or different from a model figure. Some of the figures were mirror reversed ("different" judgment) and some were rotated ("same" judgment). Participants had to mentally rotate the figures to make their assessment. There were 160 problems on the test. Participants completed as many problems as possible in 3 min. Correct responses minus incorrect responses was the measure used for analysis. Like the Block Design test, this test assesses parietal lobe functioning (Farah, Hammon, Levine, & Calvanio, 1988; Lezak, 1983), but does not require a complex motor response and does not have the cognitive planning components that are critical for optimal performance on the Block Design task. Thus, comparisons of sex differences or hormone effects on this task versus Block Design may suggest which particular processes and neural systems have sex differences or are modulated by sex hormones in adulthood.

Fluency. Two verbal fluency tests were administered (Benton & Hamsher, 1976). Letter fluency was assessed by participants producing as many words as they could beginning with the letters *F, A,* or *S*. Proper nouns (e.g., *Bob* or *Boston*) and repeating a word with a different suffix (e.g., *eat* and *eating*) were not allowed. Category fluency was assessed by participants producing as many words as possible that belonged to a particular category (e.g., animals). Participants had 1 min to respond to each letter or category. Different letters (*F-A-S, P-R-W*) and categories (foods, animals) were used for each session to avoid test–retest learning effects. These stimulus sets have been used in many neuropsychological studies and are used here because of their comparable and high verbal association frequency (Borkowski, Benton, & Spreen, 1967; Lezak, 1995). Responses were audiotaped and subsequently scored. This task is sensitive to left prefrontal cortex damage (Janowsky, Shimamura, Kritchevsky, & Squire, 1989). Some but not all studies have found a female advantage on verbal fluency measures (for a review, see Hampson & Kimura, 1992).

Memory. The Toy Task was used to assess verbal and nonverbal memory (Cave & Squire, 1991; Smith & Milner, 1984). The testing procedures for this task are described in detail elsewhere (see Janowsky, Carper, & Kaye, 1996). Briefly, participants viewed 16 three-dimensional toy objects arranged on a 60-cm^2 piece of paper. They were asked to point to each object, name the object, and price each object as if it were real. They were also told to try to remember the objects and their locations for a subsequent memory test later in the session. All participants viewed the same objects in the same spatial array. A different but comparable set of objects was used in the second session.

Recall of the names of the toy objects ("Name the toy objects I showed you a while ago") was obtained after a 40-to 50-min retention interval. Participants then completed a verbal recognition test in which they chose the name of the actual toy object they had seen from a set of eight possible object names printed on a card. The distractors were all objects that could be found as small toys, and each set of distractors contained an item of the same category as the target item (e.g., if the target was a toy car, then the distractor list would have the word *truck*).

Spatial recall was assessed immediately after the verbal recognition test by having participants replace the objects on a blank 60-cm^2 sheet of paper. Participants were given the objects and instructed to replace them in their original location. They were allowed to work at their own pace and could replace them in any order. They were also allowed to rearrange or adjust toys after all were replaced. Spatial recall was calculated by measuring the absolute distance (in centimeters) between the center of each replaced object and the location of the object in its original location.

Spatial recognition was tested by having participants choose the correct location of each object from eight photos showing each object in different locations on the paper. The percentage of correctly recognized object locations was the measure of interest.

The verbal recall, spatial recall, and spatial recognition measures are sufficiently sensitive that we did not anticipate either ceiling or floor levels of performance levels that would preclude findings of sex differences or hormone effects.

Performance on this memory task has been directly related to the medial temporal lobe memory system. Patients with damage to the left medial temporal lobe have difficulty recalling the names of the objects, whereas patients with damage to the right temporal lobe have difficulty recalling both the names and the locations of the objects (Smith & Milner, 1981). Patients with amnesia due to diencephalic damage (Korsakoffs patients), or those with bilateral damage to the temporal lobe, have comparable difficulty on both the verbal and nonverbal aspects of the task (Cave & Squire, 1991). Damage to the frontal lobes does not impair performance on the mnemonic aspects of the task but does impair the accuracy of the pricing of the objects. Thus, neural specificity of hormone effects or sex differences can be derived from this measure, in which verbal and nonverbal memory measures are derived from the same stimuli.

Motor function. The Grooved Pegboard Test (Klove, 1963) was administered to assess fine motor dexterity and speed using the standard testing procedures. The dominant and nondominant hands were tested. Participants placed small key-shaped pegs in a pegboard with the holes arranged in different directions. The time required to place all pegs was recorded for each hand. Fine motor dexterity is mediated by the motor cortex and is critical for performance on this task (Haaland & Delaney, 1981).

Women show an advantage over men on some tasks of distal motor control (finger and hand movements) and performance in women is reported to improve at high-estrogen points in the cycle. It has recently been proposed that the sex difference and hormonal control of sequential movement may be due to motor programming of movement (Jennings et al., 1998) or the accuracy of movement (Szekeley et al., 1998) and not absolute speed.

Dart throwing was used to assess target-directed visual-motor skills (Watson & Kimura, 1991). Participants threw 20 darts with each hand, beginning with the dominant hand. The target consisted of a circle 47.5 cm in diameter drawn on a 60-cm^2 piece of newsprint. A new target was used for each hand. Participants stood 10 ft from the target, and the center of the target was 5 ft high. The median distance for each participant from the center of the target to the points of impact was the measure of interest. This task was chosen because it assesses action on visual and spatial information. Men, on average, have shown an advantage over women on this task even when participants were asked to throw the darts in an unfamiliar way (Watson & Kimura, 1991). The Grooved Pegboard and dart throwing tasks investigated here have not previously been related to both estrogen and testosterone in both men and women.

Data Analysis

Differences in performance between men and women were assessed with a repeated measures analysis of variance, with session as the repeated measure for each hormone and cognitive task. The relations between hormones and cognitive performance in men and women were assessed with Pearson correlations. Correlations were also performed between particular cognitive measures as one means of assessing whether the processes involved in performance were similar across those measures (for a similar analysis method, see Watson & Kimura, 1991). Significance levels ($p < .05$) were calculated with two-tailed tests, and values between .05 and .10 are described as marginal. For marginal p values, the actual value found was reported.

RESULTS

Sex Differences

Spatial cognition. Men performed better than women on Block Design and the Card Rotation task, $F(1, 46) > 4.14$, $p < .05$. Men and women improved in performance on both tasks across the two sessions, $F(1, 46) > 18.0, p < .01$, and the improvement was comparable in men and women as there were no Group × Session interactions, $F(1, 46) < .10, p > .10$.

Memory. Verbal recognition performance was at ceiling (perfect performance) for many participants, thus it was not useful in distinguishing sex differences or hormone effects and is not discussed further. Men and women performed similarly on verbal and spatial recall, and spatial recognition, $F(1, 46) < 1.70, p > .10$. Performance on verbal recall marginally improved across sessions, $F(1, 46) = 3.69, p = .06$. Performance on spatial recall and recognition improved across sessions, $F(1, 46) > 6.0, p < .05$. There were no significant Sex × Session interactions for verbal or spatial recall, or spatial recognition, $F(1, 46) < .60, p > .10$.

Fluency. Men and women performed similarly on both letter and category fluency, $F(1, 46) < 2.40, p > .10$. Performance improved across sessions on letter fluency, $F(1, 46) = 12.9, p < .01$, and there was no Sex × Session interaction, $F(1, 46) = .11, p > .10$. Category fluency performance did not improve across sessions, $F(1, 46) = .01, p > .10$, however a significant Sex × Session interaction was found, $F(1, 46) = 8.84, p < .01$. This was due to a marginal decline in fluency in men between Sessions 1 and 2, $t(17) = 2.11, p = .05$, whereas women's performance improved across sessions, $t(29) = 2.26, p < .05$.

Motor performance. Men and women performed similarly with either hand on the Grooved Pegboard Task, $F(1, 46) < 70, p > .10$. Performance improved across sessions for both hands, $F(1, 46) > 4.70, p < .05$, and there were no Sex × Session interactions for either hand, $F(1, 46) < 2.60, p > .10$.

Men performed better than women on the dart throwing task with either hand, $F(1, 46) > 13.0, p < .01$. Performance did not improve across sessions for either hand, $F(1, 46) < 1.0, p > 10$, and there were no Sex × Session interactions for either hand, $F(1, 46) < .50, p > .10$.

There were 4 participants (1 man and 3 women) who reported their left hand as their dominant hand. None of the results change when the data are analyzed without these participants.

Relations Between Hormone Levels and Performance

These analyses should be considered exploratory due to the number of correlations relative to the number of participants. We were interested in patterns of relations between hormones and performance on measures that did and did not show sex differences, not each correlation per se. Correlations between hormone levels and performance are summarized in Table 2. With this number of comparisons, one would expect approximately five comparisons to be significant by chance (Type I error). We found 10 significant correlations between hormone levels and performance; therefore, we used two criteria to determine which to emphasize and which should be pursued with further studies. We discuss here those significant relations that were found in both test sessions and those that show sufficient power to suggest they are reliable. With a sample size of 30 women, a correlation of $r > .44$ has a good level of power at .70. With a sample size of 18 men, a correlation of $r > .55$

TABLE 2
Correlations Between Sex Hormones and Cognition

	Session 1				Session 2			
	Estradiol		Free Testosterone		Estradiol[a]		Free Testosterone	
	Men	Women	Men	Women	Men	Women	Men	Women
Spatial Cognition								
Block Design	.17	.40**	−.31	−.14	.05	.34*	−.16	−.06
Card Rotation	.04	.11	−.14	−.05	.25	.22	.006	.10
Fluency								
Letter Fluency	−.09	.05	−.04	.14	−.11	.09	.04	−.12
Category Fluency	−.40*	.02	−.33	.14	−.31	.14	−.22	.14
Memory								
Verbal Recall	.10	.06	.34	.17	.34	−.13	.51**	−.02
Spatial Recall	.25	.04	−.07	−.001	.52**	−.20	.46**	−.26
Spatial Recognition	−.10	−.17	−.09	−.12	−.003	.17	.22	−.02
Motor Performance								
Grooved Pegboard								
Dominant Hand	−.08	.16	.33	.03	−.18	.05	.09	−.23
Nondominant Hand	−.38	.28	.19	−.002	−.16	.18	−.04	−.28
Dart Throwing								
Dominant Hand	−.13	−.21	−.15	−.05	−.16	−.14	−.57***	.35**
Nondominant Hand	−.02	−.23	−.35	−.06	−.16	−.36*	−.50**	−.47***

[a]Correlations are based on 17 men and 29 women.
*$p \leq .10$. **$p \leq .05$. ***$p \leq .01$, two-tailed tests.

is necessary for the same level of power. Lack of relations between hormones and cognitive performance may be due to a restricted range of hormone levels in this healthy group of younger participants, small effects, insufficient participants (false negative or Type II error), or, in fact because task performance may not be related to circulating hormone levels. The power of .70 minimizes Type I error at the expense of Type II errors. This is a common trade-off in psychological studies (see review in Keppel, 1991).

Estradiol was positively related to Block Design performance in both sessions in women but not men. No significant relations were found between hormones and Card Rotation performance.

No significant relations were found between hormones and letter fluency. Men consistently showed relatively large, negative relations between category fluency and both estrogen and testosterone ($rs > .22$). These will require further study for confirmation as the relations did not reach significance in both sessions and did not have sufficient power to be considered reliable. No significant relations between hormone levels and category fluency for women were found.

Spatial recall was positively related to estradiol and testosterone in men. A weak positive relation was found between verbal recall and testosterone in men. Both of these relations will require further study for confirmation as the correlations were not significant in both sessions. No significant relations were found between hormone levels in women and any of the memory measures.

No consistent, significant relations between hormone levels and Grooved Pegboard performance was found. In general, dart throwing performance was negatively related to both hormones for both sexes except that the dominant hand in women was positively related to performance. This will require further study as the relations between hormone and performance did not reach significance in both sessions.

In order to begin to specify which cognitive processes are sexually dimorphic, previous studies have compared performance among measures. For instance, Watson and Kimura (1991) showed that although both dart throwing and mental rotation were advantaged in men, dart throwing was not correlated with mental rotation performance. This suggested that the male advantage in the two tasks was due to at least two distinct independent processes, not a single cause (Watson & Kimura, 1991). Although both Block Design and Card Rotation show a male advantage, performance on these tasks was not correlated with each other or with dart throwing in men in either session ($rs < .37$, $ps > .10$). Block Design and Card Rotation were correlated with each other in women in both sessions ($rs > .45$, $ps < .05$) but in general were not correlated with dart throwing, with the exception that in Session 2, Card Rotation performance was correlated with dart throwing performance with the nondominant hand ($r = .39$, $p < .05$).

DISCUSSION

We found a male advantage on two tests of spatial cognition: the Block Design and Card Rotation tasks. A male advantage was also found on the dart throwing task. A male advantage has also been found by others on these or similar tasks (e.g., Collins & Kimura, 1996; Gordon & Lee, 1986; Gouchie & Kimura, 1991; Watson & Kimura, 1991; for a review, see Hampson & Kimura, 1992; Maccoby & Jacklin, 1974). Sex differences in performance were not found for tests of memory, fluency, or rapid fine motor function.

The lack of sex effects on fluency and the Grooved Pegboard task is somewhat surprising given other reports of a female advantage on these measures. Our participants were tested twice and sex differences did not approach significance in either test session on these measures, although we did find sex differences on the spatial cognitive tasks in the same participants. We suspect that sex differences in fluency and fine motor performance may be small and thus require larger sample sizes. It is also possible that aspects of the tasks or study design, such as testing the women at the high-estrogen and high-progesterone phase of the cycle, modified women's performance and, thus, performance differences between men and women.

The correlational data between performance and hormone levels should be viewed as preliminary due to the numbers of comparisons made. Still, there were some interesting contrasts in the data. We found that estradiol was positively related to Block Design performance in women, and no relation was found between hormone levels and Card Rotation performance. This is surprising considering that both these measures showed a male advantage, and in women, performance on these two tasks was correlated. On the other hand, these two tasks are quite different in the cognitive processes required. It may be that estrogen is affecting aspects of Block Design other than mental rotation. One might have expected that the poorer performance of women than men on spatial cognitive tasks would be associated with a negative relation between estrogen and spatial cognition. Similarly, one might have expected that dart throwing performance would show a positive relation with testosterone in men, but a negative relation was found. Together, these data suggest that men and women may use different underlying processes to solve spatial cognitive tasks. In addition, the processes that cause the male advantage on the tasks are independent of the hormonal relation with performance in adulthood. Thus, it is possible that a sex difference in performance can be caused by hormonally induced ontogenetic neural sexual dimorphisms (Berenbaum et al., 1995) or life experience (Baenninger & Newcombe, 1995), but that hormones in adulthood have independent effects on sexually dimorphic brain regions as well as other nondimorphic regions that impact cognition.

The lack of hormonal effects on memory performance in women is puzzling in light of several studies showing enhancement of memory, particularly verbal memory in women on medical, surgical, or age-related estrogen replacement (Phillips & Sherwin, 1992; Sherwin, 1988; Sherwin & Tulandi, 1996). It is unlikely that our results are due to the sensitivity of the verbal or spatial recall measures, as participants were not at either ceiling or floor levels of performance. The stimuli (the recall of names of toys) in this study were different from those of Sherwin and Tulandi (1996), who used a paragraph recall task. Preliminary data from our laboratory suggest that the effects seen here in younger women are not due to task differences between the studies. We have found that estrogen replacement does enhance verbal memory on the task used here (unpublished data). One possibility is that estradiol effects on verbal memory are not linear. Rather, there may be a threshold level below which estrogen is critical for verbal memory. A second possibility is that progesterone modifies estrogen's effects on memory. We studied young women at a point in their cycle when both estradiol and progesterone were relatively high. In animal models, estradiol induces synaptogenesis in hippocampus but progesterone reverses this increase in synapse number in the same region (Woolley & McEwen, 1993). Therefore, we may not find verbal memory effects because the high progesterone would cancel the enhancing effects of estradiol on hippocampal memory function. Our tentative findings of a correlation between spatial memory and estradiol in men is similar to that found recently by Kampen and Sherwin (1996), although our data suggest that both estrogen and testosterone may play a role in memory in men.

It is not clear if the effects we and others report are sex specific or if they may be due, in part, to the large differences in estrogen and testosterone in men versus women. However, our goal was to ask whether normal circulating hormone levels are related to cognitive performance. The selectivity of the findings to particular sexes and tasks likely reflects the ways everyday hormone levels are related to cognition in healthy adults. Others have reported curvilinear relations between sex hormones and cognition when men's and women's data are combined (Moffat & Hampson, 1996) or when comparing participants with high versus low hormone levels (Gouchie & Kimura, 1991; McKeever & Deyo, 1990). Studies of participants with a broader range of performance on these tasks and a broader range of hormone levels will help address whether some of the effects we see are due to curvilinear relations between hormones and performance on some tasks. Estrogen and testosterone can function competitively or synergistically to influence neural activity. Therefore, multiple regression analysis with both estrogen and testosterone and the examination of estrogen to testosterone ratios may further elucidate hormone effects in men and women.

In summary, we suggest these initial data from normal participants suggest that sex hormones may play a modulatory role on many aspects of cognition in adulthood. We expect that the neural basis of these effects is not the same as those that cause ontogenetic sex differences during brain development but are due to effects on numerous cortical regions. As we learn more about the neural basis of other cognitive tasks, we will be able to further investigate the brain basis of hormonal effects on cognition. Finally, functional neuroimaging studies in the future, in which brain activation is examined under different hormonal and behavioral conditions, will provide direct evidence for the neural basis of hormone effects on cognition.

ACKNOWLEDGMENTS

This study was supported in part by NIA AG12611 and a pilot grant from the Oregon Alzheimer's Disease Research Center NIH 5P30 AG08017. The Oregon Health Sciences University Clinical Research Center was supported in part by Grant NIH M01RR0034. We gratefully acknowledge the assistance of Leeza Maron, Kellie Spooner, Kirsten Silvey, and biostatistician Gary Sexton.

REFERENCES

Aboitiz, F., Scheibel, A. B., & Zaidel, E. (1992). Morphometry of the sylvian fissure and the corpus callosum, with emphasis on sex differences. *Brain, 115,* 1521–1541.

Andreason, P. J., Zametkin, A. J., Guo, G. C., Baldwin, P., & Cohen, R. M. (1996). Gender-related differences in regional cerebral glucose metabolism in normal volunteers. *Psychiatric Research, 51,* 175–183.

Baenninger, M., & Newcombe, N. (1989). The role of experience in spatial test performance: A meta-analysis. *Sex Roles, 20,* 327–344.

Baenninger, M., & Newcombe, N. (1995). Environmental input to the development of sex-related differences in spatial and mathematical ability. Psychological and psychobiological perspectives on sex differences in cognition: I. Theory and research [Special issue]. *Learning and Individual Differences, 7,* 363–379.

Becker, J. B., & Beer, M. E. (1986). The influence of estrogen on nigrostriatal dopamine activity: Behavioral and neurochemical evidence for both pre- and postsynaptic components. *Behavioral Brain Research, 19,* 27–33.

Becker, J. B., Snyder, P. J., Miller, M. M., Westgate, S. A., & Jenuwine, M. J. (1987). The influence of estrous cycle and intrastriatal estradiol on sensorimotor performance in the female rat. *Pharmacology, Biochemistry, and Behavior, 27,* 53–59.

Benton, A. L., & Hamsher, K. D. (1976). *Multilingual Aphasia Examination.* Iowa City: University of Iowa Press.

Berenbaum, S. A., Korman, K., & Leveroni, C. (1995). Early hormones and sex differences in cognitive abilities. Psychological and psychobiological perspectives on sex differences in cognition: I. Theory and research [Special issue]. *Learning & Individual Differences, 7,* 303–321.

Bishop, K. M., & Wahlsten, D. (1997). Sex differences in the human corpus callosum: Myth or reality? *Neuroscience and Biobehavioral Reviews, 21,* 581–601.

Borkowski, J. G., Benton, A. L., & Spreen, O. (1967). Word fluency and brain damage. *Neuropsychologia, 5,* 135–140.

Cave, C. B., & Squire, L. R. (1991). Equivalent impairment of spatial and nonspatial memory following damage to the human hippocampus. *Hippocampus, 1,* 329–340.

Chase, T. N., Fedio, P., & Foster, N. L. (1984). Wechsler Adult Intelligence Scale performance cortical localization by fluorodex\oxyglucose F18-positron emission tomography. *Archives of Neurology, 41,* 1244–1247.

Chiarello, C., McMahon, M. A., & Schaefer, K. (1989). Visual cerebral lateralization over phases of the menstrual cycle: A preliminary investigation. *Brain Cognition, 11,* 18–36.

Collaer, M. L., & Hines, M. (1995). Human behavioral sex differences: A role for gonadal hormones during early development? *Psychological Bulletin, 118,* 55–107.

Collins, D. W., & Kimura, D. (1996). *A large sex difference on a two-dimensional mental rotation task* (Research Bulletin No. 739). London, Canada: University of Western Ontario, Department of Psychology.

Cornell Medical Index. (1974). Ithaca, NY: Cornell University Medical Center.

Cowell, P. E., Turetsky, B. I., Gur, R. C., Grossman, R. I., Shtasel, D. L., & Gur, R. E. (1994). Sex differences in aging of the human frontal and temporal lobes. *Journal of Neuroscience, 14,* 4748–4755.

DeLacoste-Utamsing, C., & Holloway, R. L. (1982). Sexual dimorphism in the human corpus callosum. *Science, 216,* 1431–1432.

Ekstrom, R. B., French, J. W., Harman, H. H., & Derman, D. (1976). *Kit of factor-referenced cognitive tests.* Princeton, NJ: Educational Testing Service.

Farah, M. J., Hammon, K. M., Levine, D. N., & Calvanio, R. (1988). Visual and spatial mental imagery: Dissociable systems of representation. *Cognitive Psychology, 20,* 439–462.

Gee, K. (1988). Steroid modulation of the GABA/benzodiazepine receptor-linked chloride ionophore. *Molecular Neurobiology, 2,* 291–317.

Geffen, G., Moar, K. J., O'Hanlon, A. P., Clark, C. R., & Geffen, L. B. (1990). Performance measures of 16–86 year old males and females on the auditory verbal learning test. *Clinical Neuropsychologist, 4,* 45–63.

Gordon, H. W., & Lee, P. A. (1986). A relationship between gonadotropins and visuospatial function. *Neuropsychologia, 24,* 563–576.

Gouchie, C., & Kimura, D. (1991). The relationship between testosterone levels and cognitive ability patterns. *Psychoneuroendocrinology, 16,* 323–334.

Gur, R. C., Mozley, L. H., Mozley, P. D., Resnick, S. M., Karp, J. S., Alavi, A., Arnold, S. E., & Gur, R. E. (1995). Sex differences in regional cerebral glucose metabolism during a resting state. *Science, 267,* 528–531.

Haaland, K. Y., & Delaney, H. D. (1981). Motor deficits after left or right hemisphere damage due to stroke or tumor. *Neuropsychologia, 19,* 17–27.

Hall, J. A. Y., & Kimura, D. (1995). Sexual orientation and performance on sexually dimorphic motor tasks. *Archives of Sexual Behavior, 24,* 395–407.

Halpern, D. F. (1986). *Sex differences in cognitive abilities.* Hillsdale, NJ: Lawrence Erlbaum Associates, Inc.

Hampson, E. (1990). Estrogen-related variations in human spatial and articulatory-motor skills. *Psychoneuroendocrinology, 15,* 97–111.

Hampson, E., & Kimura, D. (1988). Reciprocal effects of hormonal fluctuations on human motor and perceptual-spatial skills. *Behavioral Neurosciences, 102,* 456–459.

Hampson, E., & Kimura, D. (1992). Sex differences and hormonal influences on cognitive function in humans. In J. B. Becker, S. M. Breedlove, & D. Crews (Eds.), *Behavioral endocrinology* (pp. 357–398). Cambridge, MA: MIT Press.

Hart, R. P., & O'Shanick, G. J. (1993). Forgetting rates for verbal, pictorial, and figural stimuli. *Journal of Clinical and Experimental Neuropsychology, 15,* 245–265.

Janowsky, J. S., Carper, R. A., & Kaye, J. A. (1996). Asymmetrical memory decline in normal aging and dementia. *Neuropsychologia, 34,* 527–535.

Janowsky, J. S., Oviatt, S. K., & Orwoll, E. S. (1994). Testosterone influences spatial cognition in older men. *Behavioral Neuroscience, 108,* 325–332.

Janowsky, J. S., Shimamura, A. P., Kritchevsky, M., & Squire, L. R. (1989). Cognitive impairment following frontal lobe damage and its relevance to human amnesia. *Behavioral Neuroscience, 103,* 548–560.

Jennings, P., Janowsky, J. S., & Orwoll, E. (1998). Estrogen and sequential movement. *Behavioral Neuroscience, 112,* 154–159.

Kampen, D. L., & Sherwin, B. B. (1994). Estrogen use and verbal memory in healthy postmenopausal women. *Obstetrics & Gynecology, 83,* 979–983.

Kampen, D. L., & Sherwin, B. B. (1996). Estradiol is related to visual memory in healthy young men. *Behavioral Neuroscience, 110,* 613–617.

Keppel, G. (1991). *Design and analysis: A researcher's handbook.* Englewood Cliffs, NJ: Prentice Hall.

Kimura, D. (1983). Sex differences in the cerebral organization for speech and praxic functions. *Canadian Journal of Psychology, 37,* 19–35.

Kimura, D. (1996). Sex, sexual orientation and sex hormones influence human cognitive function. *Current Opinion in Neurobiology, 6,* 259–263.

Kimura, D., & Hampson, E. (1994). Cognitive pattern in men and women is influenced by fluctuations in sex hormones. *Current Directions in Psychological Science, 3,* 57–61.

Klove, H. (1963). Clinical neuropsychology. In F. M. Forster (Ed.), *The medical clinics of North America* (pp. 1647–1658). New York: Saunders.

Kramer, J. H., Delis, D. C., & Daniel, M. (1988). Sex differences in verbal learning. *Journal of Clinical Psychology, 44,* 907–915.

Leiberburg, I., & McEwen, B. S. (1977). Brain cell nuclear retention of testosterone metabolites, 5a-dihydrotestosterone and estradiol-17b, in adult rats. *Endocrinology, 100,* 588–597.

Lezak, M. D. (1983). *Neuropsychological assessment.* New York: Oxford University Press.

Lezak, M. D. (1995). *Neuropsychological assessment* (3rd ed.). New York: Oxford University Press.

Maccoby, E. E., & Jacklin, C. N. (1974). *The psychology of sex differences.* Stanford, CA: Stanford University Press.

McEwen, B. S. (1991). Steroids affect neuronal activity by acting on the membrane and the genome. *Trends in Pharmacological Science, 12,* 141–147.

McEwen, B. S., Jones, K., & Pfaff, D. (1987). Hormonal control of sexual behavior in the female rat: Molecular, cellular and neurochemical studies. *Biology of Reproduction, 36,* 37–45.

McGlone, J. (1977). Sex differences in the cerebral organization of verbal function to patients with unilateral brain lesions. *Brain, 100,* 775–793.

McGlone, J. (1980). Sex differences in human brain asymmetry: A critical survey. *The Behavioral and Brain Sciences, 3,* 215–262.

McKeever, W. F., & Deyo, R. A. (1990). Testosterone, dihydrotestosterone, and spatial task performances of males. *Bulletin of the Psychonomic Society, 28,* 305–308.

Melmerstein, P. G., Becker, J. B., & Surmeier, J. D. (1996). Estradiol reduces calcium currents in rat neostriatal neurons via a membrane receptor. *Journal of Neuroscience, 16,* 595–604.

Moffat, S. D., & Hampson, E. (1996). A curvilinear relationship between testosterone and spatial cognition in humans: Possible influence of hand preference. *Psychoneuroendocrinology, 21,* 323–337.

Nicholson, K. G., & Kimura, D. (1996). Sex differences for speech and manual skill. *Perceptual and Motor Skills, 82,* 3–13.

Nordeen, E. J., & Yahr, P. (1982). Hemispheric asymmetries in the behavioral and hormonal effects of sexually differentiating mammalian brain. *Science, 218,* 391–394.

Pfaff, D. W. (1980). *Estrogens and brain function.* New York: Springer-Verlag.

Phillips, S. M., & Sherwin, B. B. (1992). Effects of estrogen on memory function in surgically menopausal women. *Psychoneuroendocrinology, 17,* 485–495.

Phoenix, C. H., Goy, R. W., Gerall, A. A., & Young, W. C. (1959). Organizing action of prenatally administered testosterone propionate on the tissues mediating mating behavior in the female guinea pig. *Endocrinology, 65,* 369–382.

Resnick, S. M., Gottesman, I. I., & McGue, M. (1993). Sensation seeking in opposite-sex twins: An effect of prenatal hormones? *Behavior Genetics, 23,* 323–329.

Salat, D., Ward, A., Kaye, J. A., & Janowsky, J. S. (1997). Sex differences in the corpus callosum with aging. *Neurobiology of Aging, 18,* 191–197.

Sanders, B., Soares, M. P., & D'Aquila, J. M. (1982). The sex difference on one test of spatial visualization: A nontrivial difference. *Child Development, 53,* 1106–1110.

Shaywitz, B. A., Shaywitz, S. E., Pugh, K. R., Constable, R. T., Skudlarski, P., Fulbright, R. K., Bronen, R. A., Fletcher, J. M., Shankweiler, D. P., Katz, L., & Gore, J. C. (1995). Sex differences in the functional organization of the brain for language. *Nature, 373,* 607–609.

Sherwin, B. B. (1988). Estrogen and/or androgen replacement therapy and cognitive functioning in surgically menopausal women. *Psychoneuroendocrinology, 13,* 345–357.

Sherwin, B. B. (1994). Sex hormones and psychological functioning in postmenopausal women. *Experimental Gerontology, 29,* 423–430.

Sherwin, B. B., & Tulandi, T. (1996). "Add-back" estrogen reverses cognitive deficits induced by a gonadotropin-releasing hormone agonist in women with leiomyomata uteri. *Journal of Clinical Endocrinology & Metabolism, 81,* 2545–2549.

Shute, V. J., Pellegrino, J. W., Hubert, L., & Reynolds, R. W. (1983). The relationship between androgen levels and human spatial abilities. *Bulletin of the Psychonomic Society, 21,* 465–468.

Smith, M. L., & Milner, B. (1981). The role of right hippocampus in the recall of spatial location. *Neuropsychologia, 19,* 781–793.

Smith, M. L., & Milner, B. (1984). Differential effects of frontal lobe lesions on cognitive estimation and spatial memory. *Neuropsychologia, 22,* 697–705.

Stumpf, H. (1995). Gender differences in performance on tests of cognitive abilities: Experimental design issues and empirical results. Psychological and psychobiological perspectives on sex differences in cognition: I. Theory and research [Special issue]. *Learning & Individual Differences, 7,* 275–287.

Sumner, B. E. H., & Fink, G. (1995). Estrogen increases the density of 5-hydroxytryptamine$_{2A}$ receptors in cerebral cortex and nucleus accumbens in the female rat. *Journal of Steroid Biochemistry and Molecular Biology, 54,* 15–20.

Szekely, C., Hampson, E., Carey, D. P., & Goodale, M. A. (1998/this issue). Oral contraceptive use affects manual praxis but not simple visually guided movements. *Developmental Neuropsychology, 14,* 399–420.

Tapley, S. M., & Bryden, M. P. (1977). An investigation of sex differences in spatial ability: Mental rotation of three-dimensional objects. *Canadian Journal of Psychology, 31,* 122–130.

Trahan, D. E., & Quintana, J. W. (1990). Analysis of gender effects upon verbal and visual memory performance in adults. *Archives of Clinical Neuropsychology, 5,* 325–334.

Trenerry, M. R., Jack, C. R., Cascino, G. D., Sharbrough, F. W., & Ivnik, R. J. (1995). Gender differences in post-temporal lobectomy verbal memory and relationships between MRI hippocampal volumes and preoperative verbal memory. *Epilepsy Research, 20,* 26–76.

Voyer, D., Voyer, S., & Bryden, M. P. (1995). Magnitude of sex differences in spatial abilities: A meta-analysis and consideration of critical variables. *Psychological Bulletin, 117,* 250–270.

Warrington, E. K., James, M., & Maciejewski, C. (1986). The WAIS as a lateralizing and localizing diagnostic instrument. *Neuropsychologia, 24,* 223–239.

Watson, N. V., & Kimura, D. (1989). Right-hand superiority for throwing but not for intercepting. *Neuropsychologia, 27,* 1399–1414.

Watson, N. V., & Kimura, D. (1991). Nontrivial sex differences in throwing and intercepting: Relation to psychometrically-defined spatial functions. *Personality and Individual Differences, 12,* 375–385.

Wechsler, D. A. (1981). *The Wechsler Adult Intelligence Scale–Revised.* San Antonio, TX: Psychological Corporation.

Witelson, S. F. (1989). Hand and sex differences in the isthmus and genu of the human corpus callosum. *Brain, 112,* 799–835.

Woolley, C. S., & McEwen, B. S. (1992). Estradiol mediates fluctuations in hippocampal synapse density during the estrous cycle in the adult rat. *Journal of Neuroscience, 12,* 2549–2554.

Woolley, C. S., & McEwen, B. S. (1993). Roles of estradiol and progesterone in regulation of hippocampal dendritic spine density during the estrous cycle in the rat. *Journal of Comparative Neurology, 336,* 293–306.

Yesavage, J. A., Brink, T. L., & Rose, T. L. (1983). Development and validation of a geriatric depression screening scale: A preliminary report. *Journal of Psychiatric Research, 17,* 37–49.

Acknowledgment

Grateful acknowledgment is made to the following individuals who served as reviewers of one or more articles in this special issue.

Jill Becker
Ray Blanchard
M. Barbara Bulman-Fleming
Lisabeth F. DiLalla
Judith Semon Dubas
Harold W. Gordon
Gina Grimshaw
Elizabeth Hampson
Lorna Jakobson
Jocelyn Keillor
Catherine Leveroni

Neil J. MacLusky
Larissa A. Mead
Michael Peters
Tony M. Plant
Susan Resnick
Judith L. Ross
Irwin Silverman
Jane Stewart
Neal Viemeister
Fred vom Saal
Sandra Witelson

Psychobiology

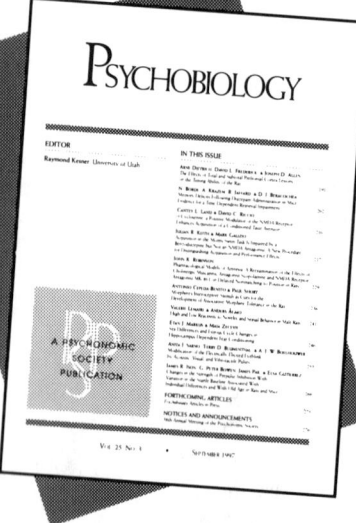

EDITOR
Raymond Kesner,
University of Utah

Psychobiology examines the biological substrates of behavior and cognitive function, encompassing all of the allied fields of the neurosciences that relate directly, or potentially, to these areas. Experimental, review, and theoretical papers from many disciplines — psychology, biology, pharmacology, anatomy, physiology, electrophysiology, clinical neurophysiology, neuroendocrinology, and autonomic functions — are included.

SPECIAL ISSUES, 1998

In 1998, Psychobiology will publish two special issues:

The Role of the Parietal Cortex in Mediating Cognitive Function

Review articles and empirical contributions relating the latest findings and
 theoretical ideas concerning cognitive functions (e.g., attention, egocentric and allocentric spatial representations) associated with parietal cortex in rats and monkeys.

The Cognitive Neuroscience of Object Representation & Recognition

Focus on the neural mechanisms underlying object processing from
 an interdisciplinary perspective. The authors show how converging
 methodologies, including functional neuroimaging, single-unit recordings, computational models, and neuropsychological case studies
 advance our understanding of recognition mechanisms.

Published quarterly, beginning in March. Institutions, $94; Individuals, $45; Students, $23.
Students: enclose proof of student status. Add $7 postage outside U.S. Canadian orders add 7% GST;
15% HST on orders from Newfoundland, Labrador, Nova Scotia, and New Brunswick.

Psychonomic Society Publications • 1710 Fortview Road, Austin, TX 78704
Phone: (512) 462-2442 • Fax: (512) 462-1101
http://www.sig.net/~psysoc/home.htm

Subscription Order Form

Please ☐ enter ☐ renew my subscription to

DEVELOPMENTAL NEUROPSYCHOLOGY
Volume 14, 1998, Quarterly

Subscription prices per volume:

Individual: ☐ $55.00 (US/Canada) ☐ $85.00 (All Other Countries)
Institution: ☐ $330.00 (US/Canada) ☐ $360.00 (All Other Countries)

Subscriptions are entered on a calendar-year basis only and must be prepaid in US currency -- check, money order, or credit card. **Offer expires 12/31/98. NOTE: Institutions must pay institutional rates. Individual subscription orders paid by institutional checks will be returned.**

☐ **Payment Enclosed**
   Total Amount Enclosed $_____

☐ **Charge My Credit Card**
   ☐ VISA   ☐ MasterCard   ☐ AMEX   ☐ Discover

   Exp. Date_____

   Card Number _____

   Signature _____
   (Credit card orders cannot be processed without your signature.)

Please print clearly to ensure proper delivery.

Name _____

Address _____

_____

City _____ State _____ Zip+4 _____
Prices are subject to change without notice.

Lawrence Erlbaum Associates, Inc.
Journal Subscription Department
10 Industrial Avenue, Mahwah, NJ 07430
(201) 236-9500   FAX (201) 236-0072

RECOVERY AFTER TRAUMATIC BRAIN INJURY

edited by
Barbara P. Uzzell
Memorial Neurological Association
Henry H. Stonnington
Memorial Rehabilitation Center
A VOLUME IN THE INSTITUTE FOR RESEARCH IN BEHAVIORAL NEUROSCIENCE SERIES

Emotions, behaviors, thoughts, creations, planning, daily physical activities, and routines are programmed within our brains. To acquire these capacities, the brain takes time to fully develop — a process that may take the first 20 years of life. Disruptions of the brain involving neurons, axons, dendrites, synapses, neurotransmitters or brain infrastructure produce profound changes in development and functions of the one organ that makes us unique. To understand the functions and development of the brain is difficult enough, but to reverse the consequences of trauma and repair the damage is even more challenging. To meet this challenge and increase understanding, a host of disciplines working and communicating together are required.

The International Association for the Study of Traumatic Brain Injury tried to correct this limitation during its meetings of international clinicians, researchers, and scientists from many fields. It was felt that many of the outstanding thoughts and ideas from the most recent meeting and from others working in the field of traumatic brain injury (TBI) should be shared in written communication. Hence, this book was conceived not as proceedings of the conference, but as a collection of knowledge for those working in the acute and chronic recovery aspects of head injury.

This book reflects the importance of the team treating patients with TBI in that the chapter authors come from a diverse array of disciplines — basic science, neurosurgery, neurology, radiology, psychology, neuropsychology, and legal, consumer, and speech/language science. Their contributions provide the most current research and the latest ways of managing a variety of aspects of TBI.

Contents: B.P. Uzzell, H.H. Stonnington, Introduction. Part I: *Diagnoses and Management.* J.D. Lewine, W.W. Orrison, J.T. Davis, B. Hart, J. Spar, P.W. Kodituwakku, D. Hill, S. Chang, V.A. Waldorf, P. Shaw, C. Edgar, J.H. Stone, Neuromagnetic Evaluation of Brain Dysfunction in Postconcussive Syndromes Associated with Mild Head Trauma. J.T.L. Wilson, D.M. Hadley, L.C. Scott, A. Harper, Neuropsychological Significance of Contusional Lesions Identified by MRI. J.L. Dowling, R.G. Dacey, Jr., Factors Affecting Brain Injury in Subarachnoid Hemorrhage. Y. Katayama, A. Yoshino, T. Kawamata, T. Tsubokawa, Role of Excitatory Amino Acids in Neuronal and Glial Responses to Trauma Brain Injury. W.D. Dietrich, Light and Electron Microscopic Studies of Fluid Percussion Brain Injury in Rats: Posttraumatic Considerations. T. Tsubokawa, Chronic Brain Simulation as a Restorative Treatment for Brain Damage. W.E. Lux, Pharmacological Strategies in the Management of Cognition and Behavior Following Traumatic Brain Injury. Part II: *Clinical States.* B. Johnstone, T.S. Callahan, Neuropsychological Evaluation of Traumatic Brain Injury in the United StatesL A Critical Analysis. J.D. Corrigan, Assessment of Agitation During the Acute Phase of Recovery. J.D. Corrigan, The Incidence and Impact of Substance Abuse Following Traumatic Brain Injury. Z. Kalisky, B.P. Uzzell, Florid Confabulation Following Brain Injury. B.E. Murdoch, Physiological Rehabilitation of Disordered Speech Following Closed Head Injury. N.D. Zasler, Vegetative State: Challenges, Controversies, and Caveats. A Physiatric Perspective. Part III: *Timing and Outcomes.* B. Kolb, Brain Plasticity and Behavior During Development. J.L. Ponsford, J.H. Olver, C. Curran, Outcome Following Traumatic Brain Injury: An Australian Study. A-L. Christensen, C. Caetano, G. Rasmussen, Psychosocial Outcome After an Intensive, Neuropsychologically Oriented Day Program: Contributing Program Variables. M.J. Fuhrer, J.S. Richards, Medical Rehabilitation Outcomes for Persons with Traumatic Brain Injury: Some Recommended Directions for Research. P. Wehman, Traumatic Brain Injury: Work Outcome and Supported Employment. Part IV: *Family and Community.* J.E. Farmer, R. Stucky-Ropp, Family Transactions and Traumatic Brain Injury. F. Krause, The Development of Grassroots Support for Research and Services in Brain Injury. D.N. Cope, A Databased Managed Care System of Catastrophic Neurologic Injury Rehabilitation. J.S. Taylor, Neurolaw: Medicolegal Aspects of Traumatic Brain Injury. B.P. Uzzell, H.H. Stonnington, Speculations for the Future.
0-8058-1823-5 [cloth] / 1996 / 360pp. / $69.95
0-8058-1824-3 [paper] / 1996 / 360pp. / $34.50
Prices subject to change without notice.

Lawrence Erlbaum Associates, Inc.
10 Industrial Avenue, Mahwah, NJ 07430
201/236-9500   FAX 201/236-0072

Call toll-free to order: 1-800-9-BOOKS-9...9am to 5pm EST only.
e-mail to: orders@erlbaum.com
visit LEA's web site at http://www.erlbaum.com

THE MYTHOMANIAS
The Nature of Deception and Self-Deception

edited by
Michael S. Myslobodsky
Tel-Aviv University

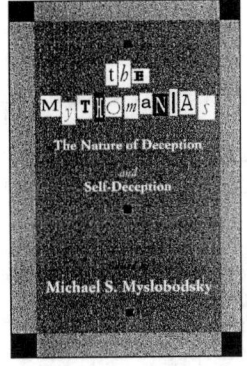

Recently, there has been a renewal of interest in the broad and loosely bounded range of phenomena called deception and self-deception. This volume answers this interest of philosophers, social and clinical psychologists, and more recently, neuroscientists and cognitive scientists. Expert contributors provide timely, reliable, and insightful coverage of the normal range of errors in perception, memory, and behavior. They place these phenomena on a continuum with various syndromes and neuropsychiatric diseases where falsehood in perception, self-perception, cognition, and behaviors are a peculiar sign. Leading authorities examine the various forms of "mythomania," deception, and self-deception ranging from the mundane to the bizarre such as imposture, confabulations, minimization of symptomatology, denial, and anosognosia. Although the many diverse phenomena discussed here share a family resemblance, they are unlikely to have a common neurological machinery. In order to reach an explanation for these phenomena, a reliable pattern of lawful behavior must be delineated. It would then be possible to develop reasonable explanations based upon the underlying neurobiological processes that give rise to deficiencies designated as the mythomanias. The chapters herein begin to provide an outline of such a development. Taken as a whole, the collection is consistent with the emerging gospel indicating that neither the machinery of "nature" nor the forces of "nurture" taken alone are capable of explaining what makes cognition and behaviors aberrant.

Contents: I. Maltzman, Foreword. **M.S. Myslobodsky,** Living Behind a Facade: Notes on the Agenda. **J. Agassi,** Self-Deception: A View From the Rationalist Perspective. **A.G. Greenwald,** Self-Knowledge and Self-Deception: Further Consideration. **D. Zakay, J. Bentwich,** The Tricks and Traps of Perceptual Illusions. **Y. Trope, B. Gervey, N. Liberman,** Wishful Thinking From a Pragmatic Hypothesis-Testing Perspective. **M.K. Johnson,** Identifying the Origin of Mental Experience. **M. Ross, T.K. MacDonald,** How Can We Be Sure? Using Truth Criteria to Validate Memories. **A. Rechtshaffen,** The Single-Mindedness and Isolation of Dreams. **H. Ben-Zur, S. Breznitz,** Denial, Anxiety, and Information Processing. **L.A. Wells,** Imposture Syndromes: A Clinical View. **I. Nachson,** Neuropsychology of Self-Deception: The Case of Prosopagnosia. **L. Hicks, M.S. Myslobodsky,** Mnemopoesis: Memories That Wish Themselves to Be Recalled? **M. Devor,** Phantom Limb Phenomena and Their Neural Mechanism. **M.S. Myslobodsky,** Awareness Salvaged by Cunning: Rehabilitation by Deception in Audiovisual Neglect.
0-8058-1919-3 [cloth] / 1997 / 424pp. / $79.95
Special Prepaid Offer! $39.95
No further discounts apply.

Lawrence Erlbaum Associates, Inc.
10 Industrial Avenue, Mahwah, NJ 07430
201/236-9500   FAX 201/236-0072

Prices subject to change without notice.

Call toll-free to order: **1-800-9-BOOKS-9**...9am to 5pm EST only.
e-mail to: orders@erlbaum.com
visit LEA's web site at http://www.erlbaum.com

CLINICAL NEUROPSYCHOLOGY
Theoretical Foundations for Practitioners
edited by
Mark Edward Maruish, *Health Outcomes Institute*
James A. Moses, *VA Medical Center*

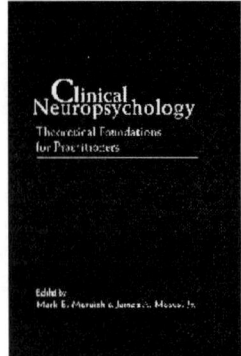

For nearly two decades, the level of interest, study, and practice devoted to clinical neuropsychology has enjoyed a rate of growth that may be unprecedented in the behavioral science field. The number of doctoral-level training programs with clinical neuropsychology tracks increased dramatically. This has been accompanied by an increase in the number of predoctoral clinical psychology internships with neuropsychology rotations, and in the number of predoctoral internships and postdoctoral fellowships focused solely on clinical neuropsychological training. Membership in professional organizations such as the American Psychological Association's Division of Clinical Neuropsychology, the National Academy of Neuropsychology, and the International Neuropsychological Society has also grown steadily. In addition, the number of journals that has been proliferated from the growing interest in and need for information in the area further reflect how far the field has progressed. However, it probably is the American Board of Professional Psychology's acknowledgement of clinical neuropsychology as a specialty that most strongly identifies the field as being a discipline in its own right rather than being a subspecialty of clinical psychology.

With the emergence of the field as one of the fastest growing specialties in psychology comes the need for current and future practitioners to stay abreast of the most recent research. The professional journals mentioned above more than adequately meet this need. At the same time, there is also a need to stay up to date on the current thinking on topics and issues that are important to the practice of the profession. For this reason, the editors set out to produce this volume. Drawing upon the expertise of some of the leaders in the field, their intent was to provide the practitioner with a source for discussions of topics that are important to their ongoing development as clinical neuropsychologists but which generally are not addressed in the literature to any great degree.

Contents: M.J. Meier, The Establishment of Clinical Neuropsychology as a Psychological Specialty. J.E. Shuren, Interdisciplinary Relationships: Behavioral Neurology. F.J. Friedrich, S.D. Rader, Component Process Analysis in Experimental and Clinical Neuropsychology. D.A. Pritchard, Forensic Neuropsychology. L.I. Cripe, Personality Assessment of Brain-Impaired Patients. G.G. Kay, V.N. Starbuck, Computerized Neuropsychological Assessment. E.D. Bigler, S.S. Porter, C.M. Lowry, Neuroimaging: Interface With Clinical Neuropsychology. P. Klonoff, D.G. Lamb, D.A. Chiapelli, S. Kime, J. Shepherd, M. Cunningham Cognitive Retraining in a Milieu-Oriented Outpatient Rehabilitation Program. B.K. Schefft, J.F. Malec, B.K. Lehr, F.H. Kanfer, The Role of Self-Regulation Therapy With the Brain-Injured Patient. G. Goldstein, The Etiology of Mental Illness. J.G. Csernanky, K.J. Black, W.O. Faustman, The Interface Between Standard Psychiatric and Neuropsychological Diagnosis. C.R. Reynolds, E.M. James, Development of Neuropsychological Measures. K.R. Krull, R.L. Adams, Problems in Neuropsychological Research Methodology.
0-8058-1343-8 [cloth] / 1996 / 448pp. / $79.95
Special Prepaid Offer! $39.95
No further discounts apply.

Prices subject to
change without notice.

Lawrence Erlbaum Associates, Inc.
10 Industrial Avenue, Mahwah, NJ 07430
201/236-9500   FAX 201/236-0072

Call toll-free to order: 1-800-9-BOOKS-9...9am to 5pm EST only.
e-mail to: orders@erlbaum.com
visit LEA's web site at http://www.erlbaum.com